Manfred Porkert

The Essentials of Chinese Diagnostics

ACTA MEDICINAE SINENSIS
CHINESE MEDICINE PUBLICATIONS LTD.
ZÜRICH, SWITZERLAND

©1983 Manfred Porkert

THE ESSENTIALS OF CHINESE DIAGNOSTICS. Copyright © 1983 by Manfred Porkert. All Rights Reserved. Printed in the United States of America. No part of this book may be used or reproduced in any manner whatsoever electronic or mechanical or other without prior written persmission. Also no part of this book may be stored in a retrieval system or transmitted in any form or by any means without prior written consent and permission. Permission may be obtained from Manfred Porkert, Chinese Medical Publications, Ltd. or the U.S.A. Distributor.

First Published in German in 1976 as:
Lehrbuch der chinesischen Diagnostik

Translated and fully revised
First Published in English in 1983 as:
The Essentials of Chinese Diagnostics
©1983 Manfred Porkert
All Rights Reserved

By the same author:

THE THEORETICAL FOUNDATIONS OF CHINESE MEDICINE: Systems of Correspondence
East Asian Science Series, Vol. 3, 368 pages.
Published by MIT Press, 1974

PUBLISHED BY:

ACTA MEDICINAE SINENSIS
CHINESE MEDICINE PUBLICATIONS LTD
Beethovenstrasse 11,
8008 Zürich, Switzerland

DISTRIBUTED IN NORTH AMERICA BY:

The Centre for Traditional Acupuncture, Inc.
American City Building, (Suite 108)
Columbia, Maryland, 21044

DISTRIBUTED IN GREAT BRITAIN BY:

Acupuncture Supplies
Mile House, Luddington Road,
Stratford-on-Avon, Warwickshire, CV37 9SE, England

For distribution outside North American and Great Britain please contact the publisher.

ISBN 0-912379-00-6 Paper

Library of Congress Catalog Card Number: 83-70735

CONTENTS

Preface ix

Introduction 1
   Why Use Chinese Diagnostics? 1
   The Polarity of Western and Chinese Science 1
   Causal Analysis and Its Limitations 2
   Inductive Synthesis and Its Limitations 4
   The Consequence of Western Medicine's Limitation to Causal Analysis 5
   Why Chinese Medicine is Capable of the Specific Determination of
   Functional Disorders - The Importance of Inductive Synthesis . . 7
   Chinese Diagnostics as a Prerequisite to Rational Acupuncture . . 10
   The "Simplicity" of Chinese Diagnostics 11
   Objective Diagnostic Statements 12
   The Rational Quality of Chinese Diagnosis 13
   The Patient's Personality Under Diagnosis 14

PART ONE - THE THEORY OF CHINESE DIAGNOSTICS

Chapter One: General Standards and Correspondences 17
   General Conventional Standards 17
      Yin (Struction, Structivity) and Yang (Action, Activity) . . . 18
      The Five Evolutive Phases (The Five E.P.s - wuxing 22
   Orbisiconography 26

Chapter Two: Basic Concepts of Differential Diagnosis 31
   The Eight Guiding Criteria (bagang) 32
      Yin and Yang 33
      Deficiency of yin merum, Deficiency of yang merum 35
      Total Loss of Yin, Total Loss of Yang 36
      Species and Intima 39
      Species and Intima Symptoms 39
      The Combination of Species- and Intima-Symptoms with Algor and Calor,
      Inanitas and Repletio 41
      Symptoms of Part Species, Part Intima 42
      Combination and Interference of Species- and Intima-Symptoms . 42
      Algor and Calor ("Cold" and "Heat") 44
      The Combined Occurrence of Algor- and Calor-Symptoms 45
      Algor falsus, calor falsus 46
      Inanitas and Repletio 49
      The Symptoms of inanitas and repletio 50

The Combined Manifestation of <u>inanitas</u>- and <u>repletio</u>-Symptoms	52
False <u>inanitas</u> and False Repletion	53
The Agents of Disease (<u>bingyin</u>)	56
The Six Climatic Excesses (<u>liuyin</u>) and Their Symptoms	58
<u>Ventus</u> ("Wind")	58
<u>Algor</u> ("Cold")	58
<u>Aestus</u> ("Oppressive Heat of Summer")	59
<u>Humor</u> ("Humidity")	60
<u>Ariditas</u> ("Extreme Dryness")	60
<u>Ardor</u> ("Glare")	61
The Seven Emotions (<u>qiqing</u>) and Their Symptoms	61
Pleasure (<u>voluptas</u>)	61
Wrath (<u>ira</u>)	61
Anxiety (<u>sollicitudo</u>)	62
Reflection (<u>cogitatio</u>)	62
Sorrow (<u>maeror</u>)	62
Fear (<u>timor</u>)	62
Fright (<u>pavor</u>)	63
Neutral Agents and Their Symptoms	63
Unwholesome Diet	63
Excessive Bodily Stress	63
Sexual Excesses	63
Addenda	64
Epidemic Infections	64
Diseases Developing After a Time of Latency	64
Chapter Three: Pathology	65
The Pathology of the Orbs (<u>morbi varii, zabing</u>)	66
Diseases of the <u>orbes hepaticus et felleus</u>	66
Diseases of the <u>orbes cardialis et intestini tenuis</u>	73
Diseases of the <u>orbes lienalis et stomachi</u>	80
Diseases of the <u>orbes pulmonalis et intestini crassi</u>	87
Diseases of the <u>orbes renalis et vesicalis</u>	94
The Pathology of the Conduits (<u>algor laedens</u>, "Harmful Cold"-Diseases	**100**
<u>Yang maior</u> (<u>taiyang</u>) Diseases	103
<u>Splendor yang</u> (<u>yangming</u>) Diseases	105
<u>Yang minor</u> (<u>shaoyang</u>) Diseases	106
<u>Yin maior</u> (<u>taiyin</u>) Diseases	108
<u>Yin flectens</u> (<u>jueyin</u>, "Yielding Yin") Diseases	109
<u>Yin minor</u> (<u>shaoyin</u>) Diseases	110
The Pathology of the Forms of Energy (<u>morbi temperati, wenbing</u>)	113
Defensive Energy (<u>wei</u>, <u>qi defensivum</u>)	114
<u>Qi</u>, Individually Specific, Active Energy	114
Constructive Energy (<u>ying</u>, <u>qi constructivum</u>)	115

Xue, Individually Specific, Structive Energy 115
The Tricalorium ("Three Heated Spaces", sanjiao) 116

PART TWO - THE PRACTICE OF CHINESE DIAGNOSTICS

. . . . 121

Chapter One: The Diagnosis by Inspection (inspectio, wangzhen) . . . 123
  Inspection in General 123
    Inspection of the Configurative Force (wangshen) 123
    Inspection of Colour (wangse) 124
    Inspection of the Bodily Shape (wangxing) 126
    Inspection of Motions and Movements (wangdong) 127
    Inspection of the Tongue ("Tongue Diagnosis, shezhen, wangshe) . 129
      Inspection of the Body of the Tongue 135
      Inspection of the Coating of the Tongue 142
      Summary of Critical Symptoms 153
    Inspection of Different Parts of the Body 155
      Inspection of the Head 155
      Inspection of the Face and Complexion 156
      Inspection of the Eye 162
      Inspection of the Nose 165
      Inspection of the Ear 166
      Inspection of the Mouth and of the Lips 167
      Inspection of Teeth and Gums 167
      Inspection of the Inner Throat 168
      Inspection of the Members 169
      Inspection of the Index in Pediatric Diagnosis 169
      Inspection of the Skin 171
      Inspection of Excretions 171
      Inspection of Urine 172

Chapter Two: The Diagnosis by Auscultation and Olfaction (wēnzhen) . 173
  Auditive Diagnosis of Voice and Speech 173
    The Voice 173
    The Flow of Speech 173
    Respiration 174
    Ths Sound of Coughing 175
    The Sounds of Retching, Vomiting, Hiccup, Eructation . . . 176
  Diagnosis by Olfaction 178

Chapter Three: Interrogation Diagnosis (wēnzhen) 179
  Sensation of Temperature 179
  Perspiration 181

Pain	182
Defecation and Micturition	185
Appetite and the Intake of Food	186
Hearing	188
Eyes and Vision	189
Sleep and the Desire to Sleep	190
Menstruation	190
Chapter Four: Palpation Diagnosis (qiezhen, anzhen)	193
Palpation of the Pulses (qiemo, "Pulse Diagnosis")	193
Prerequisites for Mastering Pulse Diagnosis	193
Historical and Theoretical Background of Pulse Diagnosis	197
Technique I: Practical Requirements and Precautions	199
Fundamentals	199
Timing of Pulse Diagnosis	200
Accidental Influences to Be Reckoned With or Avoided	201
Topology and Significance of the General Body Pulses	202
Topology and Correlation of the Pulses in the ostium pollicare	205
General Remarks, History, Terminology	205
Regions of the Body and Radial Pulses	206
Orbs and Radial Pulses	208
Specific Iconography of the Radial Pulses: Iconograms (moxiang)	209
General Characteristics of the Pulses	209
Iconography of the Pulses: The Conventional Iconograms	210
Remarks on Reduced Iconographies of the Pulse	224
Comparison of Iconograms of the Pulse	225
Qualitative and Systematic Categories of the Pulse	228
Pulses of the Orbs	229
Pulses Defined by Their Form	229
The Modal Pulses	230
The Qualification of the Pulses by Yin and Yang	231
The Pulses Grouped Under Descriptive Characteristics	231
Technique II:	233
Position & Support of the Patient's Arm	233
Application of the Fingers	233
Applying and Slackening Pressure: Tilting and Sliding	235
Determining and Assessing the Frequency of the Pulse	238
Time Taken for Pulse Diagnosis	238
Quick, Summary and Emergency Diagnoses	239
Palpation of the Pulses of Infants and Adolescents	239
Sensations When Applying One or More Fingers; Halos	240
Recording Pulse Data	242
Evaluation of Pulse Data	243
The Normal Pulse	243
Varietes of the Normal Pulse	244

Classification of Symptoms; Priorities	248
The Significance of the Pulses of the Orbs	248
The Significance of the Site of the Pulse	249
The Significance of the Levels of the Pulse (Depth)	250
Summary of Practical Implications	251
Simple and Complex Iconograms of the Pulse	251
Critical Symptoms of the Pulse	252
Palpation in General	254
Palpation of the Inner Side of the Forearm (palpatio cutis pedalis)	254
Palpation of the Skin	254
Palpation of Ulcers at the Surface of the Body	255
Palpation in Pedriatrics	256
Palpation of the Foramina (Acupuncture Points)	256
Bibliography	259

INDEXES:

English General Index	263
Index of Symptoms	275
Index of Latin Terms	285
Index of Transcribed Chinese Terms and Names	291

PREFACE

PREFACE
to the Revised English Version

What follows is the thoroughly revised and extensively amended English version of my <u>Lehrbuch der chinesischen Diagnostik</u>, first published in Heidelberg in 1976. Just as that book was the first practicable treatment of the topic of Chinese diagnostics in any Western language, so the present version continues to offer the most comprehensive presentation of the subject even by textbooks in Chinese. And the chapter on pulse diagnostics, as regards completeness, systematic detail and didactic transparence, is unparalleled even by the best accounts in Chinese or Japanese. Of course, all the material presented here is taken directly from Chinese classical and secondary sources, from my practical training in East Asia, and from my experience in applying and teaching Chinese diagnostics there and in Europe.

This book is addressed essentially to Western general practitioners and medical research workers who have become aware of certain limitations of Western medicine inherent in its methodology and who, consequently, are convinced that a system of medical science comparable in rational maturity to that of modern Western medicine yet complementary to it, as far as methodology is concerned, is the only solution to their (our) dilemma.

Traditional Chinese medicine, to the extent that it is perceived and applied as stringent methodology, is the only system extant that fulfills the following conditions: It has, since its inception during the 3rd century B.C., consistently applied only one mode of cognizance: inductive synthesis - thus achieving extraordinary precision and reliability where the definition of and action on functions, on vital processes and on psychic phenomena are required. Of course, since inductive synthesis today represents the very opposite of what physicians are inculcated with during their training, <u>understanding</u> the rationale of Chinese medicine and effectively applying its mature insights usually entail a radical breach with patterns of thought and expression common to, not to say exclusively accepted by, their professional setting. It is this mental switch-over, this chasm to be bridged between two radically different modes of thought - inductive synthesis and causal analysis - which presents the only serious difficulty at the first attempt to penetrate the arguments of Chinese medicine.

This book, unlike most fashionable or conventional introductions to acupuncture, does not gloss over this difficulty. For in treating this subject we must inevitably deal with the very opposite of what we have been familiar with for centuries, the contact with notions, concepts, hence terminology very often radically different from what we are used to. (Anyone promising to circumvent or to mitigate this problem, in the end cheats himself and his readers).

As compensation this approach, which at first sight appears more difficult, holds the promise that mastery of this complementary perspective not only opens up new horizons to the mind; above all it enables the Western therapist to achieve cures which he hitherto could not even conceive of.

Because this book is written as a fairly self-contained practical introduction, it will leave not a few theoretical questions unanswered. Readers curious to advance further into the intricacies of Chinese medical theory should consult the bibliography at the end of this volume.

My express thanks go to Mr. Guy Hollyday, for his literary advice and corrections, and to Dianne Connelly and Robert M. Duggan, for their encouragement and assistance in connection with this English edition.

Stein, April 12th, 1981

INTRODUCTION

Why use Chinese Diagnostics?

Three arguments, with precedence over many others, make us realize why diagnostic procedures evolved and perfected within the framework of traditional Chinese medicine, can or even must be purposefully used in a medical system aiming at the rational treatment of all disease in a modern world, viz.

1. There exists a considerable number of functional disturbances without the corollary of precise, or absolutely without any, somatic symptoms - hence beyond the reach of any rational statement from Western medicine. In their case, only Chinese diagnosis can produce positive and specific diagnostic information indispensable for any rational therapy and certain prognosis.

2. The multifarious and subtle therapeutic methods and means of traditional Chinese medicine in pharmacotherapy, acupuncture, moxibustion, physiotherapy, can only be understood, applied in practice, criticized and elaborated on the basis of a Chinese diagnosis conforming to the specific methodology, used to develop these methods in the course of more than two millennia.

3. The comparative simplicity of Chinese diagnostics as well as its high stringency, wherever it applies, leads to greater transparence and hence to a very much lower error rate in the diagnostic findings - with all the felicitous consequences for physicians and patients and society.

These arguments by themselves are highly convincing. The fact that to many persons in the medical field they still appear as surprising perspectives is due to the complementarity, due to the methodological polarity of modern Western medicine and traditional Chinese medicine.

The Polarity of Western and Chinese Science

If we here use the term of "polarity", we do not do so in conforming to any momentary linguistic fashion, but rather because of its precise and narrow connotations: Polar statements are mutually exclusive, thus at the same time perfectly complementary of each other. Polarizing filters completely shut out light of one particular oscillation plane, letting that of all others pass to varying degrees of intensity. Any scientific method, and the terminology essential to it, may be compared to such a polarizing filter, in the sense that it conveys insights conforming to the method, with great fidelity, producing more or less extensive deformations of other data - and completely shutting out polar, i.e. perfectly complementary, statements. When we realize that up to now all publications in Western languages on such methods as acupuncture or qi-exercises have been produced by authors intrinsically familiar only with Western science, we begin to suspect the reasons why Western medicine, to this day, has barely caught a glimpse of some isolated findings of the systematic scientific legacy of Chinese medicine.

Why should there be a change in this attitude? Well, to the extent that we realize how exact science in the West in modern times succeeds in applying the criteria for heuristic methods of unprecedented precision and effectivenes, the more strikingly we become aware that such precision and effectiveness in Western medicine is in fact limited to a very small portion of medical endeavour: The majority of diagnostic and therapeutic action still remains on a proto-scientific level, hence is exercised on a proto-scientific level. Every practicing physician continuously is faced with this gradient in his everyday work, aware as he is that the degree of specificity of diagnosis and therapy on the one hand, and the precision of prognosis are directly indicative of the rational character, consequently of the scientific nature of statements made and used. In spite of this awareness, he usually lacks the leisure and the historical information to realize which epistemological factors have produced such uneven levels. This leads us back to the polarity and complementarity of Occidental and Chinese science.

Causal Analysis and its Limitations

It is common experience that not all phenomena, not all effects liable to be defined can be perfectly perceived from one particular perspective only. And of course such a statement applies not only to astronomers, compelled to erect their observatories in the Northern and Southern hemispheres as well as in particularly favourable sites, but practically to all other professions and sciences. And, indeed, it applies to any methodology and even to specific modes of cognizance. In order to positively grasp and perceive substratums, matter, bodies, somatic aspects, causal analysis is required; causal analysis implies the damping or even repression of actual, momentary, present impressions and the focussing of conscious perception on past effects, causes. Conversely, these statements imply that by causal analysis only substratums, matter, somatic effects, etc. come into view and can be positively defined. Just as from no vantage point, however judiciously chosen, the perspective of our vision - or of any instruments designed to boost that vision - can encompass all reality, no single and particular method or mode of cognizance corresponding to a particular cognitive horizon will let us take in perfectly all extant effects.

Consequently, there is a limit to the practicability of causal analysis from any human vantage point. This limit is in the decrease of what may be called the <u>homogeneity of substratums</u>. By such homogeneity we mean the comparative insignificance of individual differences between single data or effects and other similar data and effects. For example, the statements made in a textbook on an oxygen atom have not been derived from the observation of one particular oxygen atom, but rather from the observation of a large, statistically significant number of such atoms. The case of oxygen atoms is relevant because this method produces statements of a probability neigh to 1 (hence of a probability bordering on certainty) because, as we may put it, the homogeneity of such atoms is extremely high; hence their recognizable individual differences are extremely low.

Now such homogeneity appears to be greatest in the realm of elementary particles, from whence it decreases through atoms, molecules, cells, lower and higher organisms, human individuals, social, political and cultural communities, planetary systems, galaxies, etc. This decrease in homogeneity hence is tantamount to a decrease of the stringency, the probability, and hence of the positive quality of causal and analytical statements, of statements deduced by causal analysis.

The decrease in homogeneity is directly paralleled by a decrease in the significance of causal and analytical statements. Eventually, this significance attains a limit situated in the center of the field of biological phenomena, largely congruent with the field of human medicine. In other words, the probability of statements based upon causal analysis there approaches and eventually attains the average of all aleatory procedures. Or, worded still differently, the more complex and complicated biological structures or beings appear to be constituted (decreasing homogeneity of substratums), the less probability attaches to data gleaned from the observation of one single individual as regards the demeanour of all similar individuals; and the less stringency is there in the detailed prognosis of an individual case derived from the statistical evaluation of observations of a great number of similar cases. In brief, statements based upon causal analysis show a marked decline of their stringency in the field of human physiology, and they fade away into utter vagueness and uncertainty in the field of psychic or social phenomena.

Inductive[1] Synthesis and Its Limitations

The loss of significance of statments based upon causal analysis, as just described, however, does not imply the utter loss or impossibility of stringent and rational statements on the corresponding phenomena. For, after all, causal analysis <u>focussed on past events</u> is not the only mode of cognizance, not the only way of positively looking at reality; it is not the only perspective from which positive statements on reality can be made. In fact, in order to perceive and define functions, movement, dynamic effects, psychic or vital phenomena, inductive synthesis is required - in other words an approach viewing a given effect within its present setting of other likewise present phenomena. Or, reversing the statement: inductive synthesis, by focussing conscious perception on present, actual events, opens up the perspective on functions, movements, dynamic or psychic phenomena.

Such a view or perspective has its limitations also. In fact, the significance of statements based upon inductive synthesis from the viewpoint of any observer is limited by what is called the stability of function, in other words, the relative duration during which a given function is maintained without change of direction, without qualitative modification. Such stability of function, from the vantage point of any human observer, appears to be immensely great in the realm of galaxies, and it decreases continuously in the direction of planetary systems, cultural, political, social communities, human individuals, higher and lower organisms, cells, molecules, atoms, elementary particles. In other words, the stability of function develops in inverse proportion to the homogeneity of the corresponding substratums.

In practice, the theorem just summed up, expresses the complementarity of causal analysis and inductive synthesis: To the extent that the significance, the positive quality of statements derived by causal analysis decreases, the significance of statements based upon inductive synthesis increases - and vice versa. From this theorem it is but one step to the recognition of the fact that causal and analytical science and inductive and synthetic science or the positive statements based upon these can overlap only in a comparatively small central field of scientific endeavour

---

[1] The words "induction", "inductive", "inductivity", in philosphical, technical or methodological contexts, are used in fairly narrow but not congruent meanings. The meaning we lend these terms, since the 1963 publication of the German version of Marcel Granet's Pensée chinoise, within the context of Chinese epistemology, however, can be understood as the direct acceptance of the meaning which these terms connote in modern electrodynamics. Cf. also pp. 56 f., below.

INTRODUCTION

and that, for the rest, they permit of positive statements on widely divergent aspects and fields of reality.

The Consequences of Western Medicine's Limitation to Causal Analysis

The insights just expressed are of compelling evidence, and their recognition is long overdue. If the prominent champions of Western medicine and, hence, the majority of its representatives, have seemed reluctant to recognize them, this is not the consequence of posssessing original better insights but rather because of the perseverence of the blinding effect of an historical configuration.

Western medicine accomplished the transition from proto-science to the level of exact science fairly late in the second half of the 19th century - through the application of causal and analytical methods by men like Ehrlich, Koch, Pasteur, Virchow, etc. This switchover produced effects unprecedented in the history of mankind such as the control of infectious diseases, the increase in the statistical life expectancy, drastic lowering of the infant death rate etc. The overwhelming impact of these incisive changes has to this day kept Western medicine from realizing what methodological consequences accrued from certain discoveries which simultaneously were being accomplished then in the field of physics - the pace-maker of all modern exact science - in the work of men like Faraday and Maxwell: Their discoveries led physics out of the one-sided and partial determination by causal analysis in opening up the use of inductive and synthetic methods - thus paving the way for the "Revolution in Physics" which, since the beginning of the 20th century, engendered electrodynamics and nuclear physics, both disciplines relying essentially upon inductive synthesis. And even less was Western medicine prepared to recognize the importance of traditional Chinese medicine which, then, in the middle of the 19th century, had reached the lowest point in an historical crisis[2].

It is inevitable that by focussing our consciousness on the past, by exercising causal analysis and employing its terminology, we must of necessity obscure, cover up or even annihilate any datum or statement given in any Chinese source and based upon the direct perception of actual phenomena. In other words, by attempting to interpret the statements of Chinese texts by the use of the terminology evolved in our causal and analytical sciences, we are in fact destroying, obliterating or at least garbling all that

---

[2] Cf. Porkert, The Intellectual and Social Impulses Behind the Evolution of Traditional Chinese Medicine, Wenner-Gren Symposium No. 53 ("Toward the Comparative Study of Asian Medical Systems"), reprinted in Asian Medical Systems, Berkeley 1976, pp. 63 - 81.

information which we are so keen to get at, and so much in need of making accessible to our contemporary generations.

The inevitable consequence of this is that, if we want to investigate and to apply in practice the mature results of scientific medicine in China, we must 1. make sure that we maintain its own logical context and 2. see that we apply it in stringent conformity with its own rational arguments.

To make sensible use of Chinese diagnostics, consequently, when we meet with all the rules and theories developed below, our first question must not be: "What does this mean in terms of Western medicine?" For very often no close and precise correspondences exist in both systems, otherwise we would not be obliged to speak of complementarity. Instead, we must strive to grasp and experience these rules from the context of their own correspondence system and through clinical practice.

Take as an example disease symptoms accompanying what Western medicine calls Parkinsonism, epilepsy, mental disease. The striking behavioral changes characterizing such diseases or disturbances today may not be very different from what they were 2000 years ago. If we are to attempt their rational treatment, the outward signs and impressions gathered must, however, be elaborated and substantiated by diagnostic examinations, thus establishing unequivocal connections with other systematic medical insights. Now Western medicine correlates all these diseases to lesions of the nervous system and hence attempts to arrive at a diagnosis by somatic and, recently, also by functional examinations. But even if such diagnoses are given, they very rarely attain the specificity and univocality which are prerequisite to sure prognosis and effective and rapid treatment.

The scientific medicine of China, there constituted since the 3rd century B.C., interprets the diseases mentioned primarily as disturbances of the renal orb (orbis renalis, which, let us always remember[3], has very little in common with what Western physiology defines as "renal function". This diagnosis, as a rule, can be objectivated and substantiated by all available diagnostic procedures, such as inspection, auscultation/olfaction, interrogation and palpation, thus leading to precise prognoses and to highly specific therapeutic measures, including the application of acupuncture and moxibustion. This fairly common example shows why any attempt to reduce the statements of a medical system to those of another, as well as any hypotheses in the sense that Western physiology may not yet have explored the functions of the kidneys in certain respects or that, inversely, Chinese iconography of the renal orb might

---

[3] Cf. page 26 below, as well as the folding table following p. 30.

INTRODUCTION

contain "philosophical elements" requiring correction by research of modern Western science, are equally ineffective and misleading. The example also shows the real superiority of the Chinese – i.e. inductive and synthetic – view: Neurological theory is the very recent result of a very young science, closely dependent upon technical means and the still growing disciplines of neurological anatomy and histology. The postulate of a renal orb, already 2000 years ago, could be derived in its essential traits from very few present or anamnestic sensory data which, in turn, for fully two millennia, could be subjected to reviewing, checking and counterchecking within in the most populous civilization we know of.

Why Chinese Diagnostics Is Capable of the Specific Determination of Functional Disorders, or the Importance of Inductive Synthesis in Medical Practice

China's traditional medicine (for historical reasons we must not go into detail here) relies exclusively upon inductive synthesis. In its classical teachings, it perfectly complies with the general criteria of science in the modern sense, viz.

1. positive experience (to be checked and re-checked at will),
2. univocality of statements,[4] and
3. the stringent rational integration (systematization) of empirical data.

Chinese medicine hence must be distinguished qualitatively (i.e. as regards its perspective or methodological approach) from scientific medicine in the West, and as regards its methodological sophistication from all kinds of purely empirical medicines.

Let us first briefly dwell upon the difference between the statements of traditional Chinese medicine and those of causal and analytical Western medicine, whose physiology also deals with functions. It must be noted that Western physiology can define or postulate functions only with respect to, or by constant reference to, anatomical or histological data. It would be an affront to the logic and methodology of

---

[4] The univocality, hence exactitude and precision, of scientific statements is exclusively the result of these statements being consistently expressed with reference to so-called conventional standards. Thus, if a given science or scientific discipline relies upon measurements, these measurements must be expressed with consistent reference to conventions of quantity, conventional quantitative standards. (This is the case, as we all are aware, for causal and analytical science, using the quantitative standards of the metric system.) If a science deals with functions and, for distinguishing these, relies upon the definition of direction (directionality = quality), qualitative conventions, i.e. conventional standards of quality are required. (This is the case for all inductive and synthetic Chinese sciences, including Chinese medicine which, as we shall see, relies upon the qualitative conventions of yin, yang, the Five Evolutive Phases, the Eight Guiding Criteria etc.) Cf. also Porkert, The Theoretical Foundations of Chinese Medicine, Introduction, pp. 1 ff., as well further details given below on pp. 17 ff.

Western medicine to conceive of a function without knowledge of the existence of the corresponding substratums. By contrast, the teachings of orbisiconography ("the manifestations of functional orbs") takes its point of departure directly from the positive observations of momentary actual functions and <u>directly</u> integrates these into a rational system. By contrast, when it deals with statements about somatical data, these can be treated and formulated only with reference to such functional insights. This difference of perspective is the reason why positive findings obtained respectively by one or the other method are the less liable to direct mutual reduction or explanation, the greater the precision and positive character of these findings appears to be. At the same time, this difference of perspective and vantage point is the basis for specific superiorities of both methods in <u>different</u> fields, on different aspects.

As regards the functions, it should be perfectly clear that knowledge of these - vital phenomena, manifestations of life - can never be obtained directly from the dead substratums of anatomy and histology, and can only be indirectly deduced from analytical (= dissolving the momentary functional setup) experimental conditions. The direct and positive perception of function, life or movement is possible only through the continuous and comparative observation of healthy and ill human beings within their everyday settings.

A word must also be said about empirical methods and every kind of purely empirical medicine. Such procedures constituting a significant if not the better part of Western medicine establish a direct, but not a stringent, connection between any group of symptoms or syndromes and certain remedies and therapeutic measures. In other words, treatment is decided upon on the basis of the direct comparison between symptoms and the effects of certain medicines. In such cases, the application of treatment rests upon probability, as does prognosis: Only after application of the remedy can a prognosis be made as to the probable evolution of the symptoms (To increase probability, empirical medicine offers combinations of medicines for the treatment of certain symptomatic manifestations, "complex remedies", the application of which partially or completely dispenses the physician from producing an individually specific diagnosis).

As will become evident as the arguments of this book proceed, all symptoms registered in a patient must be univocally classed and defined by the use of general criteria and, after this, must be referred to the relevant general agents (<u>yin</u>) postulated as their ultimate conditioning factor. (Obviously, these agents are not

INTRODUCTION

postulated or found in the past, do not constitute causes but, instead, are seen as the factors <u>at present</u> inducing the disturbance or disease.) By a synthetic definition and qualification of all these factors, the physician arrives at therapeutic recommendations which, by definition, take care of all influences having a bearing on the present situation of the patient: constitutional weaknesses, momentary emotional imbalance, influences from the social setting or from climatic conditions etc. (Chinese medicine may and will revise such a highly specific diagnosis and adjust the therapeutic recommendations resulting from it within hours of its first proposal. A significant change of climate or the reaction of the patient stronger than expected rapidly warrants a new prescription.)

It was stated at the outset that at the present stage of medical science, Chinese diagnosis is unique in producing a <u>specific description of functional disorders</u> not accompanied by somatic changes or modifications. Although in the intervening paragraphs we had dropped some hints about the epistemological and methodological background of this statement, and although terms like "functional disturbance" or "functional disorder" are current vocabulary in the speech of Western doctors, and although many of these doctors reflect upon the reciprocal influences between soma and psyche, substratum and function, the comprehensive meaning of the statement can be realized only if we have an even more precise and clearcut notion of this mutual influence between function and substratum.

Movement, function, may be perceived directly and influenced positively only in the present. Such present effect (= function) is the product of past and future effects. Substratums, matter, are effects accumulated in the past, retreated, sunken back into the past. Viewed through the eyes of a physician, the somatic changes of the body are the result of past effects and constitute functions sunken back into the past. Likewise, pathological changes of the body, somatic disease, are the result of past functional disorders, of functional disorders sunken back into the past. Modern physiology, histology, neurology,etc. convey an approximate notion of the relative intensity and duration required to produce certain perceptible changes (traces) of functional disorders in the bodily substratum. But whereas a single thought, and even the multifarious sensory impressions, emotions and actions accomplished throughout one busy day may not produce any somatic traces which afterwards can be defined or isolated by causal analysis, such traces will appear when a disturbed psychological milieu, when a professional misuse of the body, wrong eating habits are maintained for months or years, or when an extreme environmental stimulus is maintained for weeks, days, or even only hours, when a strong poison or rough mechanical shock works upon the individual for minutes or only a fraction of a second. And it is only the latter - somatic changes - which come within the reach of Western causal and analytical diagnosis. Also, the precision of this diagnosis and the efficacy of the subsequent therapy will be the greater, the less malfunction has accumulated in the past, the more restrictedly, but also the more clearly the pathological influence has modified the somatic substratum. By contrast - as we already pointed out - such diagnosis will fade away into mere surmisal and vague alternatives as soon as the individual, the personality, the entire organism is affected as a consequence of constitutional weakness or of chronic but very subtle noxious influences and stimuli. It is here that Chinese medicine with its diagnoses (not very impressive in the somatic field) shows its strong points. Practically all factors, particularly those <u>not accompanied by somatic changes or modifications</u>, conditioning the momentary functional situation can, when Chinese diagnosis is properly exercised, be objectively defined and, more important still, specifically and individually specified - thus furnishing the prerequisite to any individual and highly effective therapy and significant prognosis.

The arguments developed thus far may be summed up as follows: Applying Chinese diagnosis opens up to scientific medicine possibilities hitherto closed to it, especially

> a. a genuine early diagnosis of functional disorders which, if left untreated, eventually will produce degenerative or malignant organic changes;
> b. the specific and comprehensive, all-inclusive determination of all factors having a bearing on complex pathological processes (at the roots of chronic or constitutional diseases);
> c. specific and comprehensive and direct appreciation of the immediate effects of any applied drug or therapeutic measure or agent (indispensable for the immediate follow-up of any therapeutic measure, as well as in the assaying of new drugs).

Chinese Diagnostics as a Prerequisite to Rational Acupuncture and Moxibustion

A thematic and logical connection must exist between diagnosis and effective therapy. Acu-moxi-therapy (i.e. acupuncture and moxibustion), to name but that method of Chinese medicine which, thus far, is best known in the West, is an integral part of Chinese medicine, and there has developed and reached relative maturity through an

INTRODUCTION

evolution of approximately 2200 years. Consequently, all measures and possibilities of acu-moxi-therapy are founded upon data arrived at by inductive synthesis, and on a very precise and subtle functional diagnosis. If acu-moxi-therapy, as today is the case worldwide, is divorced from its scientific context and "empirically" applied on the basis of causal and analytical diagnoses, such eclecticism must be qualified as irrational and uneconomical, a parody of scientific methodology - thus precluding many of the possibilities inherent in acu-moxi-therapy. And, of course, it prevents any consistent argument relative to the effectiveness of Chinese methods - which in turn would be prerequisite to full recognition of acupuncture as a scientific discipline. In other words, only the adequate use of Chinese diagnostics prevents this scission of logic and links any therapeutic method of Chinese medicine with its systematic foundations.

What has been said, of course also holds good for the therapeutic application of Chinese drugs, in China since early times the principal curative measure, and of considerably more subtle and wide applications than acupuncture.

The "Simplicity" of Chinese Diagnostics

Compared to many hypertrophic and oversophisticated diagnostic procedures of Western medicine, Chinese diagnostics is of <u>relative</u> simplicity. (However, its simplicity is not of the kind that its essentials can be grasped in a weekend course or be mastered within a few months in all its subtleties.) The relative simplicity of Chinese diagnostics is the consequence of an optimum congruence between method and purpose; it is not indicative of crudeness or primitivity. If Chinese diagnostics is perfectly served by sensory data, this is not because, as some authors rashly infer, in former times, no technical aids were available, but rather instead, because from the perspective of inductive synthesis, absolutely no relevant medical (we did not say "biological"!) changes are conceivable which lie beyond the reach of competent diagnosis of sensory data.

The distinction between health and disease primarily rests upon the subjective impression or feeling that one enjoys unrestricted presence of mind, energy, or that one's resources are limited, have been impaired. Still, a subjective impression or sentiment is no more than that, even when it prompts medical diagnosis. For diagnosis, properly speaking, presupposes systematic and consistent action and a scientific theory, in addition to a thorough training of the senses and the mind of the physician, just as we expect and require such training when reading and writing, distinguishing colours and sounds, or defining quantities and qualities. In other words, medical diagnosis relying exclusively upon the senses is intrinsically different from haphazard and accidental perception or self-observation. Such diagnosis produces specific findings far beyond the subjective threshold which make a patient decide that he is healthy or unwell.

The distinction may be illustrated by the fact that, for example, pulse diagnosis will produce individually significant findings on practically 100 percent of persons examined, yet that, at most 60 to 70 percent of these complain of any occasional or permanent disorders.

Functional disorders beyond the reach of Chinese diagnostics either constitute disturbances so insignificant that they will not induce even the most fleeting functional incapacity of the individual (and hence are medically irrelevant) or, on the contrary, already have materialized in somatic changes, for the diagnosis and treatment of which Western causal and analytical medicine takes precedence.

Objective Diagnostic Statements

The arguments just considered show the futility of claims and requirements repeated recently with increasing frequence with respect to Chinese diagnostics: It should be "rendered objective" by the use of technical implements. It is true that it was only after the invention of modern technical aids, that Western medicine could attain to some of its most essential statements. And yet even here we must beware of shallow generalizations such as: "the use of apparatus produces objectivity", or "technical refinement guarantees higher precision" in diagnosis. By using a fever thermometer, the resulting measurement is not directly being rendered objective[5]; it only gains in quantitative precision. And similar consequences obtain for many other technical aids of causal and analytical Western medicine: They render possible or increase the precision of quantitative statements. But, as we already pointed out, the definition of functions does not rest primarily upon quantitative, but rather upon qualitative

---

[5] If somebody feels that he cannot dispense with the term "objectivity", we must surely distinguish between potential and actual objectivity; in most medical publications, their identity is implicitly and inadvertently taken for granted - thus depriving corresponding arguments of most of their conviction. In using a fever thermometer, potential objectivity results when measures are taken to prevent arbitrary or inadvertent influences by the patient upon the measurement; actual objectivity is ensured when one (or several) competent persons ascertain fever, independent of the opinion of the patient - and possibly independent of the use of any fever thermometer.

INTRODUCTION

statements and data; and we never deal with absolute but always with data that are <u>relative</u> (here taken in the literal sense of denoting and expressing relations, relationships between simultaneous or synchronous events). For example, in formulating the diagnosis of the tongue, it will not do to simply describe the colour and thickness of the tongue's covering, the colour and form of the tongue's body; it will instead be necessary to define univocally the extension of the tongue's covering, its changes in relation to the different regions of the tongue, its apparent thickness, whether the covering is fast or can be rubbed off, whether it is sticky, slippery, wet, sleek or rough or dry, with or without protuberances, clefts, fissures, dental impressions etc. And similar distinctions must be made in pulse diagnosis. The absolute frequency of the pulse, very often the only sign dealt with in Western diagnosis, is by itself worthless for Chinese pulse diagnosis; even the relative pulse frequency (determined by comparison with the breathing rhythm) is only one among nearly a dozen other, equally significant and important criteria[6].

Today, surely it is technically feasible to register some of the signs just enumerated not simply through the sensory organs of the physician, but instead, by a sophisticated apparatus transmitting its data indirectly to the examiner. Proceeding thus is comparable to a healthy person who, in the morning, does not manipulate comb and tooth-brush with his right hand but instead operates a complicated robot: To achieve similar or diminished effectiveness, futile technology is expended. Worse still, such technical toys endanger that precious advantage consisting in the extraordinary dispatch and comprehensiveness with which even a fairly detailed and thorough examination according to the rules of Chinese diagnostics, can be carried out and taken in one sweep by the diagnosing physician: It is only extremely rare cases of intricate problems which will require up to two hours of diagnosis for a patient; the first examination of average cases will take 20 to 30 minutes; and routine diagnostic procedures on familiar patients may take minutes only.

The Rational Quality of Chinese Diagnosis

In any general diagnosis carried out in one sweep and established by one physician, the terseness and transparency of the data constitute factors which enhance the rational character, the logical consistency and univocality of the result. Hence, in this

---

[6] For details, cf. the chapter on Pulse Diagnostics infra pp. 193 ff.

respect also, the use of Chinese diagnostics adds an element making diagnosis more rational and more economical. If it is true that diagnostic methods of scientific Western medicine perfectly meet the tightest and most severe requirements wherever causal analysis is liable to produce optimum results, in the average medical practice, the historical curve showing the increase of effectivity, leveled off decades ago. The reason for this is that this kind of medicine vainly attempts to compensate the epistemological defects of methodology by increasingly complex and perfect technology - a vain and self-defeating enterprise. For, by splitting up diagnostic measures among several persons, by prolonging the process of diagnosis over hours or even days, occasions for error as well as the difficulties of correct evaluation or, more precisely, of correct and precise integration of the multiple diagnostic data increase in geometric proportions. This in turn not only occasions an increase in the per patient cost and time to obtain a diagnosis. The physician is thus constantly faced with the delusive alternatives either to use only a limited portion of the diagnostic instrumentarium put at his disposal by science, or to cause expense which burdens patients or insurance companies alike. We call these alternatives delusive because in the situation stated, whichever decision is taken, the consequences will be a disservice to all concerned: Superficial diagnoses may burden the conscience if not the reputation of the physician and may endanger the patient. A very complex diagnosis, on the other hand, raises the suspicion that the doctor is profiting beyond reason from the discomfiture of the patient, and of course, they also burden private as well as public budgets. Using Chinese diagnostics may show a way out of this dilemma, not by competing with Western diagnosis - precise somatic diagnosis today as in the future can only be arrived at by applying the rules of causal analysis - but instead by producing a rational diagnosis in that massive and still increasing group of cases without any clearcut or coherent statement at all, relating to the body.

The Patient's Personality under Diagnosis

For some time now, the impersonal if not indifferent attitude of modern physicians toward their patients and their patients' disturbances has been deplored. Such dissatisfaction is quite justified, but it is not justified to address it to the doctors exclusively. If man's view of the world through his organ of vision differs from that what the insect sees through its reticular eyes, such differences reflect neither personal nor collective merit, but simply the workings of nature. When doctors strive to apply causal analysis with care and consistency, after having been taught in the course of a

INTRODUCTION

prolonged learning phase, that its methods constitute the only scientific ones, such an attitude is neither their teachers' fault nor their own, but results from the logic of an historical situation. Part of this logic, however, is that, as indicated above[7], sufficient homogeneity of substratums constitutes an indispensable prerequisite for arriving at positive statements through causal analysis. Now the fact that causal and analytical science, of necessity operates upon the premise of "homogeneous substratums", in other words of the similarity, interchangeability of somatic, material data, for human medicine implies that only those aspects of an individual which it shares with all others are accessible to causal and analytical scientific appraisal and definition; it is only these general and common traits which can be positively defined and actively corrected by any such science. In other words, medical science consistently applying causal analysis, cannot conceive of a patient as a unique personality but, instead, by its intrinsic axiom, only as a random specimen of the human species. And, of course, neither moralizing exhortations nor the personal good will of the individual physicians can overcome this intrinsic logic, for the greater the consistency of a physician in his scientific statements, the less may he take into account the haphazard particularities of the individual case.

The diagnosis Chinese medicine strives for and produces is, by definition, <u>a synthesis of numerous individual factors</u>, assembled in each patient examined in a unique and characteristic manner. Moreover, the positive character of the statements of Chinese medicine rests upon the stability of function. In other words, only such functions will be attributed significance which, from a human perspective, offer sufficient stability to permit a precise and univocal definition. The upshot of this in practice is that, compared to the findings of causal and analytical Western medicine, considerably greater congruence between subjective and objective symptoms is arrived at. And these two factors, out of inner necessity and without outward compulsion or personal caprice, insure that each disease is seen and treated as an individual and unique event, as disorder in an individual personality. This is why we may expect that the more general application of Chinese diagnostics gradually will exercise a re-humanizing influence in general medical practice. And such re-humanizing will not be induced by the accidental and uncontrolled implementation of ethical commandments; rather does it constitute the inevitable consequence of the proper application of a scientific method.

---

[7] Cf. page 3 above.

PART ONE — THE THEORY OF CHINESE DIAGNOSTICS

The theoretical tools of Chinese diagnostics, of necessity, are largely congruent with those of most other disciplines of Chinese medicine. Insofar as, at this writing, no comprehensive knowledge of this system may be taken for granted, it may be helpful in summing up the essential conventions and theories.

Chapter One: General Standards and Correspondences

GENERAL CONVENTIONAL STANDARDS

Empirical data can be exchanged and conveyed with stringency and universal significance only if they are referred to conventional standards, in other words, if they are expressed with reference to normative conventions. Everybody is familiar with the fact that the exact disciplines of the West, focused upon matter, substratum, achieve the exact expression of their data by reference to the metric system. In Chinese science, the univocality in the expression of <u>functional</u> data is dependent upon the use of qualitative standards, since quality, direction, constitutes the only criterium by which simultaneous and similar functions can be distinguished or defined[8]. The qualitative standards common to all Chinese science are yin, yang and the Five Evolutive Phases (E.P.s, <u>wuxing</u>).

In some Western literature on our topic, these qualitative standards are interpreted as "symbols" or even as philosophical "principles" – an interpretation which collapses if one really

---

[8] By definition, no actual function, i.e. movement taking place presently, can be defined <u>quantitatively</u>. The duration of a movement (= function) can only be determined after it has come to an end, in other words, after it has sunken back into the past. - Cf. Porkert, <u>Klinische chinesische Pharmakologie</u>, pp. 3 - 14. - Movements, functions developing synchronously, that is to say within the same present, "at the same time", can positively be distinguished only by defining their individual direction, hence their quality.

looks closely at the scientific context. Perhaps we should add that in Chinese medicine – not different here from other sciences – the transition from symbols (more correctly "emblems") to simple qualitative standards is paralleled by the retreat from magic practices or religious ritual, as evidenced in the Chinese medical classics at the very latest since the 3rd century before our era.

YIN (STRUCTION, STRUCTIVITY) AND YANG (ACTION, ACTIVITY)

In Chinese medical texts, it is pertinent to understand yang as active aspect, activity, action, yin as structive aspect, structivity, struction, provided we keep in mind those distinctive and precise associations attributed them in this context[9].

Thus yang, activity, action, not only implies setting off, inducing, setting in motion, dynamizing, motion, dynamics, expansion and development but also something which transforms existing things, changes, modifies, disperses, dissolves or destroys them; it may appear as something dispersed or loose.

Care should be taken to properly understand the paradox, clearly realized in China, that action, on the one hand, is the source of all determinations (yang, activity, determines) but that, in itself, by itself, it escapes all definition or determination. If we are under the impression that we can perceive the effect or the extent of an action, or that we are even capable of controlling it, we have in fact registered or controlled only selected re-actions of the action in question. These re-actions have been registered structively through our human sensory organs or by the interposition of instruments. Action is the negation of existing things, of things positively extant; activity (yang) consequently is negative, negating effect, completely escaping all (direct) determination.

These seeming paradoxes today may be illustrated by referring to the physical phenomena of radiation. Radiation (= action) emanating from a body A (= position A) can be positively determined only then and to the extend that it strikes other bodies B, C, D, etc., and insofar as in these bodies specific qualities are being structed, that is rendered concrete, materialized. Comparing the concrete changes which a radiation emanating from A produces in the bodies B, C, and D, we are able to make a partial and random, but not any comprehensive and stringent statement about the radiation emanating from A. Strictly speaking, statements about the changes in B, C, and D are statements primarily and at first only about B, C, and D, in other

---

[9] Cf. Porkert, Theoretical Foundations... pp. 21 - 22.

GENERAL STANDARDS AND CORRESPONDENCES 19

words about the capacities of the bodies B, C, and D to produce the changes observed. Transferring these relationships to diagnostic practice: What we are positively capable of ascertaining is not the direct effects (= actions) of pathogenic or therapeutic agents; we can only register changes taking place in receptive organs or organisms and re-actively reflected upon the sensory receptors of a human observer. Consequently, an assay of drugs will never produce information about the total effects of a given drug nor even about its most powerful or long-lasting effects; the information will be solely about effects producing changes in certain organs and registered by human observers or instruments within the momentary context of his or their momentary attention or functional possibilities.

If we look for modern terms to define yang (action), words like extroversion, expansion, expansiveness, centrifugality, aggressiveness, appettitiveness, negative, negation come to our mind.

Yin can be rendered by structivity (struction, structive) - these terms derived from the Latin struere, "to erect", "to build" - hence, "to render concrete", "to present positively", "to materialize"[10]. Struction consequently implies a perfective, confirming, corresponding aspect; it is something which is quiescent or brings to rest, something static, something firming, confirming, consolidating, something freezing, stabilizing, dying off; something condensing, concentrating and hence, things compact, compaction; finally something which can be organized and hence appears as liable to determination.

Struction (yin) implies concretion, materialization, somatization in physiological as well as pathological respect. If we state that there is "deficiency of yin" or "inanitas yin", in other words deficient structivity, this statement implies a pathological deficiency of materializing energies in a given individual; inversely, "redundancy" of yin or repletio yin indicates a pathological excess of the same tendencies. (Cf. the next section but one, below.)

In the vocabulary of modern science, yin may be characterized by terms like contractive, introsusceptive, centripetal, responsive, conservative, positive. By focusing conscious perception on present phenomena and viewing reality through inductive synthesis, yin, struction, and yang, action, may serve as a basic polar qualification of all phenomena - and they are used in this way in all Chinese sciences. Indeed, after having become thoroughly familiar with the associations most directly linked with the

---

[10] Cf. op. cit. pp. 14 - 23.

qualitative standards, we will have no difficulty in qualifying correctly any dynamic or vital phenomena we meet with as a whole or in part. We then can dispense with those lists of "correspondences" given in popular and not so popular publications. If we here append two condensed lists, it is less for reference than for encouraging readers to exercise and check their ability of discrimination.

Thus the qualification of

YANG applies to	of YIN applies to
Heaven	Earth
Sun (taiyang, Major Yang)	Moon (taiyin, Major Yin)
Spring	Autumn
Summer	Winter
Maleness	Femaleness
Warmth	Cold, Coolness
Exterior	Interior
Brightness	Obscurity, Darkness
Power	Weakness, Smallness
Upper side	Lower side
Fire	Water
Movement	Quiescence
Day	Night
Left side	Right side[11].

And, within the restricted framework of medical disciplines,

YANG applies to	YIN applies to
Time between midnight and noon	Time between noon and midnight
Outer orbs (species)	Inner orbs (intima)[12]
Effects, functions on the surface	Effects, functions in depth

[11] In all cultures, the assignations of left and right are probably the result of early ritualizations of certain manual functions which, in historical times, have made their way into scientific disciplines in the guise of traditional conventions.

[12] On these terms see pp. 39ff. below.

GENERAL STANDARDS AND CORRESPONDENCES 21

Uplifting, raising to the surface	Sinking down, sinking in, making descend
Back side	Belly side[13]
Trunk above the diaphragm,	Trunk below the diaphragm
Aulic orbs (orbes aulici, fu)	Horreal orbs (orbes horreales, zang)
E.Ps Wood and Fire	E.Ps Metal and Water[14]
Configurative force (shen)	Structive potential (jing)[15]
Active individually specific energy (qi)	Structive individually specific energy (xue)
Defensive energy (wei)	Constructive energy (ying)
Active fluids (jin)	Structive fluids (ye)
Active aspect of the individually configurative force (hun)	Structive aspect of the individually configurative force (po)
Repletion (repletio, shi)	Depletion of energy (inanitas, xu)
Clear, refined energies	Murky, unrefined energies
Hardness	Softness
Sweet, pungent, bland sapors	Sour, bitter, salty sapors[16]
Odd numbers	Even numbers.

[13] The qualification of the surface of the human body by yin and yang is reminiscent of the polarization which modern embryology demonstrates for amphibia: the yang side (the back) extends from the perineum to the upper lip, the yin side (the belly) extends from the lower lip to the perineum. This parallel helps us understand why the front of the legs is also qualified as yang. For further references cf. also Porkert, Theoretical Foundations..., pp. 25 ff.

[14] See next Section.

[15] With the exception of shen and jing, all subsequent terms designate technical forms of energy, hence are distinguished and used only in applied medicine.
Shen is the force inducing (maintaining) all individual, personalized effects - including the development and maintenance of the human personality.
Jing, 'structive potential', is prerequisite to the empirical materializations of configurative force (shen).
All subsequent terms of energetics, useful to medical practice, viz. xue, 'individually specific structive energy', "blood", ying, 'constructive energy', but also the fluids, represent structive forms of energy. In certain contexts, these energies may in turn be polarized, e.g. into fluids attributed active functions (jin), and into fluids attributed structive functions (ye). For further details on energetics cf. Porkert, Theoretical Foundations..., pp. 166 - 169.

[16] The technical term sapor is an exact correspondence of the Chinese wei, designating - in Latin and Chinese - not only a flavour, but also food or medicine corresponding to that flavour or qualified by that flavour. For further information cf. Porkert, Klinische chinesische Pharmakologie, pp. 52 - 53.

THE FIVE EVOLUTIVE PHASES (THE FIVE E.P.s - wuxing)

Yin and yang constitute the basic qualitative standards of all Chinese science, including medicine. For the qualification of more intricate and elaborate cyclical patterns, another set of qualitative standards is used, elaborating on the former: the Five Evolutive Phases (wuxing). This set of conventional standards results from the combination of three polarizing criteria, viz.

activity: structivity,
potentiality: actuality,
distinctness: indistinction.

The combination of these polarities and the values of the resulting standards may best be grasped when arranged on the tips of a cross, a pattern also met with in Chinese texts (Fig. 1).

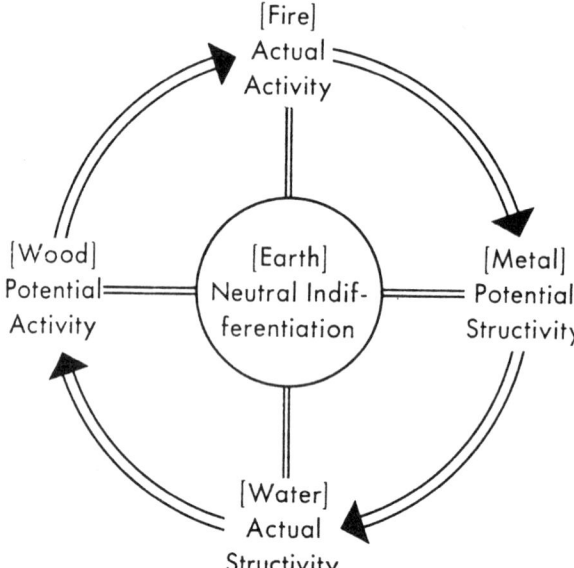

Fig. 1.

The four tips of the cross are marked with four distinct qualities termed "Wood", "Fire", "Metal" and "Water". The centre and intersection of the two axes, the origin of all distinct qualities, the spot in which qualities are mixed, transformed, exchange their attributes, the lieu of unity and indistinction, the pivot, the centre of gravity and zero, is termed "Earth".

GENERAL STANDARDS AND CORRESPONDENCES

One may easily imagine that these standards originally were derived from the experience of the movement of the seasons and hours, where "Wood" is correlated to morning, spring and the east, "Fire" correlated to noon, summer and the south, "Metal" to the evening, autumn and the west, "Water" to midnight, winter and the north. For the first two polarities can be derived without difficulty from such phenomena, viz. "Wood" and "Fire" (= morning + noon, spring + summer) may be designated as expansive or active (yang) phases; "Metal" and "Water" (= evening, midnight, autumn + winter) may be designated as contractive, conservative, structive (yin) phases. And these qualities are potentially present in "Wood" (morning, spring) and "Metal" (evening, autumn) and actually present in "Fire" (noon and summer) and "Water" (midnight and winter). Thus the qualitative standard of

Wood corresponds to a phase of potential activity,
Fire to a phase of actual activity,
Metal to a phase of potential structivity,
Water to a phase of actual structivity, and
Earth marks all phases of transition, inversion, transformation, equipoise, harmonization.

But let it be stressed once more, just as yin and yang, the five E.P.s constitute conventional standards of quality; they are means for univocally describing reality; <u>they do not, by themselves, constitute any description of reality</u>. They have no intrinsic value or function independent of the empirical data which can be expressed with reference to them. They do not represent any independent empirical or scientific discoveries or any philosophical postulates. Their sole purpose is to lend precision and univocality to statements and rules derived from the positive observation of dynamic phenomena. They make sense only if used as vehicles of such empirical data and of the systematic rules linking these.

Notable examples of rules expressed by means of the E.P.-conventions are the so-called phase sequences or simply sequences (<u>xu</u>), of which in medicine only three have significance, viz. the "production sequence" (sequence I), the "conquest or checking sequence" (sequence II) and the "violation sequence" (sequence III). All regular cosmic (hence also all biological) processes may be explained as the collusion, i.e. coöperation, of active impulse (= yang) and structive check (= yin). Active impulse acts in the direction of a mutual production sequence (<u>sequentia efficiens, xiangshengxu</u>) which, with reference to the E.P.s may be described thus: Wood -- Fire -- [Earth] --

Metal -- Water (Fig. 2).

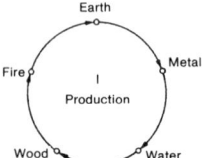

Fig. 2.

And the resistance of the substratum, in other words the structive check against this impulsion, has the direction of a checking or conquest sequence (sequentia vincens sive cohibens, xiangshèngxu, xiangkexu) which, with reference to the Five E.P.s may be described as Wood -- Earth -- Water -- Fire -- Metal. Mutual production as well as mutual checking and all processes corresponding to these in the microcosm may be understood as "physiological" effects which constitute the indispensable foundation of healthy function (Fig. 3).

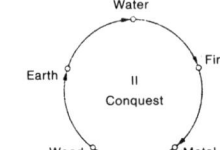

Fig. 3.

This physiological interaction, however, may be affected and disturbed by pathological agents. Such disturbances will at first manifest themselves as congestions of energy in some regions, energetic deficiencies in others; and they will eventually produce more or less extensive deformations, accroachments on the physiological relations between the phases. On such occasions, a pathological sequence, the so-called "violation sequence" (sequentia violationis, xiangwuxu) may occur. This constitutes a reversal of the sequence II, the so-called checking or conquest sequence, and expresses the fact that phases of insufficient energetic potential are overpowered by those which, under normal conditions, they would have to check: thus Wood overpowering Metal, Metal overpowering Fire, Fire overpowering Water, Water overpowering Earth, Earth overpowering Wood (Fig. 4).

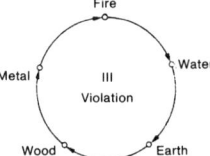

Fig. 4.

But it may also happen that certain phase qualities are represented by excessive energies (energetic redundancy). Consequently they will accroach phases which, physiologically, they should only check in accordance with sequence II, i. e. the conquest sequence.

The phase sequences just alluded to are the most succint systematic definitions for energetic relationships to be observed continuously. This explains their paramount significance when it comes to the diagnostic exploration or the therapeutic inferences to be drawn with reference to the functional orbs (orbes) - which we shall briefly deal with in the following paragraph.

26   THE ESSENTIALS OF CHINESE DIAGNOSTICS

ORBISICONOGRAPHY

Chinese medicine is oriented chiefly toward the description of positive function. Orbisiconography, "the theory of the manifestations of functional orbs" (zangxiang), is the system of postulates on which all practical disciplines of Chinese medicine are based. Orbisiconography thus is analogous to the combined theoretical disciplines of anatomy + physiology in Western medicine.

In judging the pronouncements of orbisiconography, we must avoid certain misunderstandings. In keeping with their inductive and synthetic view of phenomena, Chinese doctors and scientists always aimed at directly[17] establishing systematic links between biological functions. The results of such systematization is expressed in the word zang. Event today in the common usage of the butcher, housewife, and cook - just as in archaic, prescholarly times - the word signifies an organ, an intestine. Nevertheless, when espousing the view of Chinese physicians, we must not translate the Chinese term zang with the Western term "organ". Rather, we are compelled to render zang by "orb" (orbis), for, in orbisiconography (zangxiang)

1. only statements bearing upon functional relations may be verified positively and correlated rationally and with stringency;

2. by contrast, statements about the somatic substratums ("organs"), if they occur at all, are given with great vagueness, uncertainty, and appear restricted to exterior macroscopic details;

3. the illustrations of orbisiconography do not correspond to anatomical protocols or records, instead, they represent models of functional relationships; finally

4. in Chinese medicine there are zang ("orbs") for which there is no substratum (anatomical organ); inversely, in Western medicine there are organs or tissues for which Chinese medicine has no separate, distinct orb.[18]

Thus, despite their many similarities, it is incorrect and methodologically misleading to relate the zang ("orbs") of Chinese medicine to the organs of Western anatomy and

---

[17] In contradistinction to Western medicine, moulded by causal analysis, and in which, consequently, substratum-oriented anatomy constitutes the pacemaker of scientific progress. This is why Western physiology, although aiming at statements on function, may attempt these only by constant reference to anatomical data. Therefore all statements of Western physiology are only indirectly interrelated by their reference to basic anatomical data.

[18] Cf. e.g. below the information given on the o. renalis on pp. 94 ff.

GENERAL STANDARDS AND CORRESPONDENCES 27

physiology or, worse still, to identify the one with the other.[19] Here again we see why techniques derived from traditional Chinese medicine, such as acupuncture and moxibustion, can regain their reliability and breadth of application only if they are viewed in the context of their theoretical underpinnings. Only in this way can the logical connections between the theoretical insights on which the procedures are based and the technical details of these procedures be restored.

Orbisiconography describes three kinds of orbs, viz. 1. orbes horreales ("horreal orbs", zang), 2. orbes aulici ("aulic orbs", fu), 3. para-orbes ("para-orbs", qiheng zhi fu).

The horreal orbs, literally "storehouse orbs": the orbes hepaticus, cardialis, lienalis, pulmonalis, renalis, pericardialis, that is "liver", "heart", "spleen", "lung", "kidney", "percardium" orbs - are collectively qualified as structure orbs - a qualification expressing that within the total economy of the personality[20] they have constitutive, basic functions. In the classics[21] it is stated that they "store structure potential without leaking and are full (pleni, man), not replete (repleti, shi)". This simply means that the hypothetical substratum of these orbs is not subject to any physiological changes of form or consistency.

The aulic orbs (orbes aulici, fu), in English "transaction orbs", are the orbes felleus, intestini tenuis, stomachi, intestini crassi, vesicalis, tricalorii; that is, "gall-bladder", "small intestine" and "large intestine", "stomach", "urinary bladder" and "tricalorium" orbs. These are collectively qualified as active orbs, a qualification implying that they represent the personality in the face of external influences and forces. They mediate between the surface of the body (skin) and the inner structure, functional assemblies. The aulic orbs assimilate energies coming from without, including the energy ingested with food. Thus, as the classical quotation indicates, "They transport and assimilate but do not store; that is why they are [sometimes] replete (repleti), but never can be

---

[19] It should be perfectly clear tht the sorely awaited synthesis between modern Western and traditional Chinese medicine can, at this juncture, be undertaken only at and from the level of the positive experience of clinical medicine. Cf. Porkert, Der wissenschaftliche Ort der Akupunktur in Münchner Medizinische Wochenschrift, 14, 1976, pp. 421 - 424; also Porkert, The Quandary of Chinese Medicine, EASTERN HORIZON, Hongkong, December 1977.

[20] It should always be kept in mind that in traditional Chinese medicine, just as in all Chinese thought, the distinction between soma and psyche, body and mind, substratum and function, does not exist. This explains why the term 'personality', encompassing both body and mind, is the only acceptable translation for the corresponding Chinese term shen (first tone).

[21] Huangdi neijing Suwen, chapter 8; cf. Porkert, Theoretical Foundations..., p. 110.

full (pleni, man)[22]. In keeping with the roles postulated for the structive horreal orbs and the active aulic orbs, the former are called inner orbs (li, intima) and the latter outer orbs (biao, species).

Finally, there is the third category of the para-orbs (qiheng zhi fu), the paraorbes felleus, uteri, cerebri et meduallae. In this category are classed all empirical data that could not otherwise be integrated into the system.

To enable the reader to gain a quick grasp of all data of orbisiconography essential for diagnostics, the qualities, characteristics and relationships are assembled in a folding table. This table is based upon a simplified orbisiconographic paradigm comprising the following:

1. The qualification of the orb by an evolutive phase - corresponding to a comprehensive determination of the quality (= the directionality) of the energies operating in or through the orb.

2. Sapor, i.e. a taste quality which, when used in diagnostics, may point to a disturbance of the specific orb or, used in dietetics, may be taken into account for a specific therapy of the disturbance of the orb.

3. Smell - an olfactory affinity or quality gleaned from interrogation, and of possible relevance in assessing exhalations and other olfactory symptoms.

4. Vocal manifestation - which, if significant, may indicate a functional preponderance of the corresponding orb.

5. Colour - which, if of striking predominance in inspection, may point the disturbance of an orb.

6. Time and season - during which the orb shows a particular instability, and hence is particularly sensitive to disturbing as well as to therapeutic influences.

7. Complementary orb: designating the particular functional complement of an orb. Each horreal orb has as a complementary aulic orb, and vice versa. - Many diagnostic statements about the aulic orbs, i.e. the active outer orbs, rest solely upon this complementarity.

8. Checking orb: the orb exercising a physiological check upon the functions of another orb, to be ascertained according to the sequence II, the "conquest" or "checking sequence" of the E.P.s.

9. Sinartery - Each orb is represented at the surface of the body by a paired main

---

[22] Opus et loc. cit.

GENERAL STANDARDS AND CORRESPONDENCES

conduit (sinarteria cardinalis) qualified by the name of the orb. The foramina of this principal conduit ("acupuncture points") permit of diagnostic conclusions and therapeutic influences upon the functions of the orb)[23].

10. Specific unfoldment of the orbic function (chung, perfectio): Each orb "specifically unfolds" in certain parts of the body or its vital manifestations, and these phenomena and their modifications are of high diagnostic significance.

11. Outward manifestation (hua, flos): Each horreal orb is directly and each aulic orb indirectly represented in some part of the body easily accessible to diagnostic inspection.

12. Specific radial pulse: The more important horreal orbs are directly correlated to a particular site of the radial pulses[24]; and most aulic orbs are indirectly correlated to such a site[25].

13. Specific sensory organ (guan, organum) - correlated directly to most horreal orbs and indirectly to most aulic orbs.

14. Specific body opening (kai qiao) - This category only partially congruent with the preceding one is of similar diagnostic significance.

15. Emotion (zhi, qing): There is a specific correlation between each important orb and an emotion (emotio). The manifestation of such an emotion is dependent upon the energy level of the orb. The utter impossibility of provoking a given emotion or, on the contrary, the uncontrolled or too frequent manifestation of a particular emotion, either is a symptom of a lesion of that orb or will eventually produce such a lesion.

16. Specific function: This is a general category for the characteristic function distinguishing this particular orb from all others.

17. Dominant function: The functional qualitiy given here may be congruent with the preceding one or it may preponderantly refer to the phenomenal manifestation of the specific unfoldment (perfectio).

18. Constitutive function: Some orbs are assigned a comprehensive role in the maintenance of the temporal existence of the personality. This is expressed by the term: "the orb 'founds' (ben) the existence of the individual" in the manner defined.

---

[23] Each 'cardinal conduit', in turn, has collaterals called 'cardinal branch conduits', 'reticular conduits', 'reticular branch conduits', 'reticular conduits of the 3rd generation' and, finally, so-called 'skin zones' - regarding all of which cf. Porkert, Theoretical Foundations... pp. 203 ff.

[24] On this cf. pp. 205 ff. below.

[25] See the table on p. 208 below.

19. Storage function: Each horreal orb stores a particular form of physiological energy.

20. Multiple functions: Under this final item are listed additional functions assigned to some of the orbs to accommodate empirical data.

Inspection of the table appended will show that the paradigm just described is fairly complete only for the horreal orbs. The functions and qualities of the aulic orbs, according to Chinese theory, must be considered reflections, deflections or inflections of functions based upon the horreal orbs. The corresponding information must, consequently, be deduced indirectly from the iconograms of the corresponding "complementary orbs".

Chapter Two: Basic Concepts of Differential Diagnosis

Chinese medicine here dealt with is a scientific system[26]. Consequently, here as in modern Western medicine, therapeutic measures are never directly deduced from the symptoms observed and registered in diagnosis. Instead, between the former and the latter a complete system of rational considerations is interposed, with the purpose of reducing the multifarious phenomena of disease as well as the wealth of therapeutic possibilities to very precise and specific measures. This is achieved by introducing general and synthetic concepts and factors.

Such general factors in Chinese medicine are the so-called agents (yin[27]), in Western medicine the causes (causae). What is the difference between these two? An agent exists at the same time as, is co-existent with, the effect observed. It "induces" the effect, e.g. radiation of the sun and the increase or decrease of a migraine, the shivering under the influence of draft and so on. The cause, by contrast, precedes the phenomena observed, has "in the past" caused the present phenomena. If it is true that this distinction has only indirect[28], if any relevance for the practicing physicians, for compelling reasons it should not be passed over in silence.

Ascertaining general factors, hence differential diagnosis, in Chinese medicine is accomplished in two stages. During the first stage each symptom registered is qualified by a very important set of conventional standards called the "eight [diagnostic] guiding criteria" (ba gang). In this process it is univocally and precisely defined with respect to its energetic tendency, quality, directionality. In the second stage, a

---

[26] On this statement refer back to pp. 2 and 4 f. of our Introduction as well as to the Introduction of the Theoretical Foundations...

[27] This Chinese term yin is again a homonym (written with a different character!) of the term yin expressing structivity. Thus, in Chinese, to avoid confusion, very often the composite term of bingyin: 'agents of disease' is employed.

[28] It is true that this distinction does have considerable significance in physics where, due to confusions in terminology, since the 19th century mention is made of an "amendment" to the "law" of causality. In fact, causality does not represent a "law" but, instead, an axiom. An axiom cannot be "amended".
In the 19th century, classical causality: "Causes precede effects" - was thought to be amended by the clause: "Causes may exist synchronous with effects." This clause correctly would have to be: "Effects exist at the same time as agents inducing these effects". This formula represents another, a complementary axiom which, as everybody knows, is basic to electro-dynamics and nuclear physics.

synthesis of already precisely qualified data gleaned by all diagnostic methods[29], permits one to infer the pathological agent(s). A final step, the precise definition of the affected orb, and a recommendation of a specific therapy, as well as of a definition of certain prognoses, is the theme of pathology, which we shall briefly discuss in the next chapter.

THE EIGHT GUIDING CRITERIA *(ba gang)*

The eight guiding criteria of diagnosis are technical qualitative standards used to express the direction (= quality) in which a pathological function deviates from normal. These criteria are

yin and yang
species and intima
algor and calor
depletion (inanitas) and repletion (repletio).

Describing symptoms observed with reference to the guiding criteria not only brings clarity into an otherwise purely subjective description, it also is the first step toward a differentiation and generalization of symptoms. Among these criteria, yin and yang, structivity and activity, constitute a comprehensive set of standards, comprising in a way the three following pairs of qualitative conventions.

The degree of penetration of disease into a personality is expressed by the pair of species ("outer layer") and intima ("lining").

The general symptomatic quality of disease is defined by the values of algor ("cold") and calor ("heat").

Finally, depletion or exhaustion (inanitas), refers to a relative weakness of the orthopathy of an individual, in other words to a relative weakness of the faculty to maintain its normal functions, its homeostasis; by contrast, repletion, repletio, refers to the relative excessive strength of an individual heteropathy, i.e. a "biassing", detached function inducing or maintaining disease, malfunction.

The three last-named sets of criteria are hardly dependent upon each other. This is

---

[29] Note that the second part of this book is devoted to detailed descriptions of these diagnostic methods.

BASIC CONCEPTS OF DIFFERENTIAL DIAGNOSIS

why they may not only be met with independently when qualifying symptoms but more generally are used in all kinds of combinations. Thus we may speak (see below) of algor speciei, of calor speciei, of inanitas speciei, of repletio speciei, of inanitas intimae and so on. Indeed, it is the rule, not the exception that one and the same patient may show repletio speciei in one functional region and inanitas intimae in another. Such combinations give almost unlimited flexibility of precise qualification, further enhanced by reintroducing the basic qualities of yin and yang.

YIN AND YANG

Yin and yang, within the technical set of guiding criteria, play an eminent role because of their comprehensive significance. Thus, if we encounter a disease which has entered upon a critical stage and has produced striking symptoms requiring immediate help, we may at first limit ourselves to determining yin and yang. This is reflected in fundamental diagnostic statements like "the yang merum, the true yang is insufficient" or "the yin merum has been lost (the true yin has been lost)" - expressing fundamental diagnostic statements. For greater convenience let us also recall the qualification of the guiding criteria by yin and yang

Yin	Yang
intima	species
algor	calor
inanitas	repletio

Qualifying symptoms by yin and yang produces the following distinctions:

Diagnostic Method	Yin	Yang
INSPECTION	Physiognomy: sallow, pale, greenish white Demeanour: atonic, listless, tired appearance, looks, wasted, enfeebled, reclining patient, reluctant to move.	Physiognomy: intensely red or intermittently red Restless patient, dry or cracked lips

Diagnostic Method	Yin	Yang
	Body of the tongue pale, swollen, soft. Coating of the tongue moist, sleek slippery	Body of the tongue intensely red or scarlet. Coating of the tongue yellow to loamy colour, in extreme cases dry and cracked or even black with protuberances.
OLFACTION and AUSCULTATION	Low and weak voice, halting, faltering, reluctant speech, feeble or heavy breathing, shortness of breath	Loud, powerful, piercing voice; loquaciousness, noisy behaviour, loud breath, panting, rattling breath; raving speech, cries and swears.
INTERROGATION	Reduced appetite and thirst, refusal of food, sometimes demanding hot beverages. Urine clear and copious or reduced in quantity. Faeces smelling of fish or meat	Feeling of hotness, oppressive heat, asking for cool air, refusing food, finding even the smell of food repulsive; dry mouth, intense thirst. Urine reduced in quantity, of reddish colour. Faeces hard or difficult to expell, sometimes very malodorous.
PALPATION	Abdominal pains improved by pressure, cold body and extremities. Pulses: submerged, evanenscent, minute, grating, slowed down, infirm, always weak	Abdominal pains increased by pressure; hot or warm body and extremities. Pulses superficial, flooding, large, accelerated, slippery, replete, always strong.

Classical examples for combining yin and yang with other criteria: "If inanitas yang obtains, the patient will feel cold on the outside; if there is inanitas yin, the patient will feel heat within. If yang (active energies) is vigorously developed (vigens, sheng) the patient will feel heat without; if the structive energies (yin) are vigorously developed, he will feel cold within" (Huangdi neijing suwen, 62/547).

"If active energy (yangqi) is redundant, there will be heat without perspiration; if structive energy is redundant, the body will be cold with much perspiration" (Neijing suwen 17/178).

"Heat with shivering is the result of a faulty regulation of active energy; shivering without heat i.e. without fever, is the result of a faulty regulation of structive energy" (Shanghanlun, 1st section, p. 10).

Yin and yang, struction and action, are complementary concepts. Consequently, the

BASIC CONCEPTS OF DIFFERENTIAL DIAGNOSIS

rule is that if yang energy is redundant and excessively vigorous, yin energy appears to be enfeebled or deficient - and vice versa. In such relatively simple cases therapy aims at restoring a balance of energy. Thus, if in diagnosis the patient shows a flooding pulse (p. exundans), a red body of the tongue, a dry coating of the tongue, and if he complains about thirst, heat, etc., it is evident that yang is vigorous, yin, by contrast, dilabens, reduced, enfeebled. To correct this situation, the former must be pushed back, dampened, the latter increased, stabilized. If, on the contrary, diagnosis shows submerged or slowed-down pulses (pp. mersi sive tardi), a pale body of the tongue and a very moist coating of the tongue, if the patient complains of abdominal pains and diarrhea, we may conclude that the yin is vigens, vigorous, and yang dilabens, collapsing, that consequently active energy must be increased by applying warmth, and the structive energy must be collected, condensed.

Of course there are disturbances where we find exhaustion (inanitas) of structive energy without concomitant repletion of active energy - and vice versa. In such cases the necessary harmonization is achieved by concentrating therapy only on the one disturbed energetic aspect, e.g. inanitas yin or vigor yang.

Thus if in a patient we diagnose periodically recurring slight fever and a weak, minute and accelerated pulse (p. minutus et celer), a red, slightly moist body of the tongue without coating, red cheeks and intensely red lips, fever with restlessness, cough, and perspiration during sleep, we may conclude that the rise in temperature is due to the exhaustion of structive energy. If we bolster this structive energy by appropriate therapeutic measures, active energy producing the yang symptoms will automatically be contained and controlled.

Or it may occur that in a patient we observe a strong submerged pulse (p. mersus), a yellow, almost dry coating of the tongue with prickly protuberances, significant restlessness, panting, laboured breathing, constipation, raving speech, we may infer that active energy is redundant. By checking, reducing this redundancy, we will automatically contribute to the conservation of structive energy (yin).

Deficiency of yin merum, Deficiency of yang merum

The qi nativum, i.e. the store of energy received at birth and reflecting the constitution, is located in the orbis renalis ("kidney orb")[30]. Under certain

---

[30] Cf. the folding table inserted after page 30 as well as Theoretical Foundations... p. 144.

circumstances, any decrease or increase of the energy level in the o. renalis must be considered as a depletion or conservation of this constitutional reservoir. In classical Chinese texts, this leads to the idea that the energies of the o. renalis constitute "true" energy (zhen, merum) i.e. directly forming the basis of an individual. Consequently, deficiency of this energy has critical significance.

The expression "deficiency of yin merum" indicates a deficiency of the structive energies of the o. renalis. It is accompanied by symptoms such as intermittent manifestation of the "glare of exhaustion" (ardor inanitatis): pale complexion yet red cheeks, lips as if painted with cinnabar, dry mouth, deeply red yet dry tongue, dry throat, palpitations, dizziness, mouches volantes, tinnitus, pains and weakness of the loins, perspiration during sleep, nightmares, loss of semen during sleep, impeded micturition and defecation, hot palms and soles; the pulses, in particular the pedal pulses, are accelerated yet weak (pp. celeri et inanes).

Deficiency of yang merum indicates a deficiency of active energies of the o. renalis. This is accompanied by symptoms such as pale complexion, pale lips, pale body of the tongue, bland taste of food, reluctance to eat, heavy breathing, swollen abdomen, swollen legs, spontaneous perspiration, dizziness, cold skin[31], general diarrhea or morning diarrhea, atrophy of the genitals, impotence; weakness or paralysis of the feet; flooding and exhausted pulses (pp. exundantes et inanes), in particular at the pedal sites.

Total Loss of Yin (Structive Energy), Total Loss of Yang (Active Energy)

The total loss of one of the two forms of energy, if left untreated, rapidly ends in death. That is why the corresponding symptoms must be given proper attention. Corresponding diagnostic signs will often occur as sequels to high fever, heavy perspiration or generally after extreme loss of body fluids through perspiration, vomiting, diarrhea, hemorrhage.

The typical symptoms of the total loss of

---

[31] Literally: "cold flesh".

BASIC CONCEPTS OF DIFFERENTIAL DIAGNOSIS

STRUCTIVE ENERGY (yin)	ACTIVE ENERGY (yang)
Hot perspiration of salty taste, not sticky	Cold perspiration, tasteless, yet sticky
Extremities warm	Flexus, consequently cold extremities
Red and dry tongue	White and moist tongue
Pulses, especially at the pedal sites: exhausted and racing (pp. inanes et concitati), other pp. sometimes replete and flooding (repleti et exundantes)	Pulses especially at the pollex sites: exhausted and superficial and accelerated, minute and evanescent (pp. inanes, superficiales, celeri, minuti, evanescentes), also onion-stalk pulses (pp. cepacaulici)
Warm skin, heavy breathing	Cold skin, inaudible breathing
Thirst, desire for cold beverages	Lack of thirst, sometimes desire for warm beverages.
General situation aggravated by heat	General situation aggravated by cold.

To illustrate these considerations, we may adduce some quotations from Chinese clinical classics:

"If the pollex (also called pollicar) pulse is infirm (invalidus (the author thinks essentially of that of the left hand) - thus indicating inanitas of yang - one must not permit the patient to perspire. If one permitted him to perspire, he would completely loose all yang (active energy). If the pedal pulses are infirm (invalidi) - which lets us conclude that yin is exhausted (inanis) - we must likewise not permit the patient to perspire, for by perspiration total loss of yin may ensue."[32] For all body fluids, irrespective of their secondary qualifications, constitute structive forms of energy[33]. The extreme loss of fluid would entail the practically total loss of structivity - thus indirectly depriving active energy of its foundation.

"In the (Inner) Classic we have: 'If a patient has lost xue (the individually specific structure energy, partly manifesting itself as blood), he is without perspiration; if he has lost a great deal of sweat, he is without xue.' For xue is yin. By profuse perspiration one will eventually totally loose all yin. A method to control the loss of perspiration is the use of drugs which cool (refrigerate) the cardial orb, or which collect, concentrate the energy of the pulmonal orb - on the basis of the following considerations: The cardial orb regulates xue[34]; perspiration is the

---

[32] Section on sudatio (induced perspiration) in "Essential Insights into Medicine" (Yixue xinwu) by Cheng Zhongling.

[33] Cf. Porkert, Theoretical Foundations... pp. 190 and 195.

[34] Cf. op. cit. p. 126.

intermittently screted fluid corresponding to the cardial orb[35]. Therefore we must (at first) refrigerate <u>ardor o. cardialis</u> ("glare in the cardial orb")[36]. Perspiration diffuses outward through the skin and hair. The pulmonal orb regulates the functions of skin and hair[37]. Consequently, we must also contain, concentrate the energies of the <u>o. pulmonalis</u>. So much for the direct therapeutic measures. If however, an excessive loss of perspiration has already occurred, the active energy above (i.e. in the <u>o. cardialis</u>) is already depleted, and <u>ardor structivus o. renalis</u> ("structive glare repelled from the renal orb") flares up (as a manifestation of the qualities of the E.P.) Water. If one tried to quell this flaring up (<u>ardor</u>) by cold or cool medicines, it would flare up all the more strongly. Only by copious use of radix Ginseng and radix Aconiti as principal drugs, guided through <u>demittentia</u>[38] and salty <u>sapors</u> like urina puerum or concha Ostreae, will the medicine directly reach the lower calorium[39], hence the <u>yang merum</u>. By such medication, <u>ardor structivus o. renalis</u> is reduced (i. e. "led back") to its origin and perspiration will stop."[40]

The interdependence of energetic qualities manifests itself very strikingly in the symptoms occurring with the total loss of any kind of energy. If structive energy is completely spent, we notice symptoms indicating an excess of active energy: replete or flooding pulses, red body of the tongue, etc. But closer investigation will reveal the subjacent exhaustion symptoms such as critical pedal pulses, exhausted or racing pulses (<u>pp. inanes sive concitati</u>). If active energy is completely spent, the first impression of the patient may be that there is an excess of yin: cool skin, paleness of complexion, of the lips and the body of the tongue etc. Yet here the weak pollicar pulses which at first may be superficial, but later will become minute or even evanescent, will direct us to the correct diagnosis.

---

[35] Cf. op. cit. p. 127.

[36] The technical term <u>qing</u>, literally 'to clear up', has the precise pharmacodynamic connotation of 'refrigeration', 'to refrigerate'.

[37] Cf. Porkert, Theoretical Foundations... p. 138.

[38] As for the salty <u>sapor</u>, cf. the iconography of the renal orb, as well as Porkert, <u>KLinische chinesische Pharmakologie</u>, p. 53.
The term <u>medicamenta demittentia</u>, <u>jiangyao</u>, designates drugs or prescriptions "pushing down", "leading back" active energies into the inner orbs (<u>intima</u>). Cf. Porkert, op. cit. pp. 53 f.

[39] I.e. the <u>oo. renalis et vesicalis</u>.

[40] Xu Lingtai: Treatise on the Total Loss of Yin and Yang.

BASIC CONCEPTS OF DIFFERENTIAL DIAGNOSIS 39

Species AND intima

Application of the guiding criteria species and intima permits us to lend precision to statements as to whether disease develops within or outside, at the surface or in depth. The Chinese terms biao (Latin: species) and li, (Latin: intima) literally designate respectively the outward aspect ("surface") and the inner side ("lining") of a garment. The metaphorical, technical meaning of the terms in Chinese medicine occurs from the very beginning in its Classics. Also, at a very early stage[41], certain slight differences in the definitions of the terms occur - which must be kept in mind, viz.

1. species is a synonym of "outer orb" (= o. aulicus, "aulic orb", fu), and intima is used as a synonym of inner orb, yin orb (= orbis horrealis, "horreal orb", zang); or
2. species designates the functional periphery comprising the skin, the hair and the conduits (sinarteriae); intima designates the inner, central functions, comprising the horreal orbs as well as the aulic orbs and, in addition the para-orbs of bone and marrow (paraorbes ossum et medullae).

The first of these two meanings is the more ancient one, closer to theory, and exclusively advocated in the Inner Classic (Neijing) and the Shanghanlun; the second corresponds to the more pragmatic distinctions of pathologists. We should note, however, that to this day in the signifcant domain of algor laedens-diseases[42], consistent use of the former (first given) meanings is made. Independent of these distinctions, the criterium species, as a rule, points to a superficial, hence a light, recent or receding disease, the criterium intima, by contrast, to a deep seated, prolonged, chronic disease. Naturally, transitory stages between these two may be observed and must be expressly defined.

Species and Intima Symptoms

Within the context of Chinese inner medicine and pathology, disease is essentially induced through heteropathies of the six climatic excesses[43], on which species as well as intima-symptoms may be distinguished, as the following table shows.

---

[41] Since the development of the morbi varii (zabing) theory, i.e. of the principal pathology upon which inner medicine is founded. Cf. below p. 100.

[42] Cf. below pp. 100 ff.

[43] Cf. below pp. 57 ff.

Species-Symptoms	Intima-Symptoms
Fever with shuddering, headache, diffuse pains of the trunk and extremities, stopped up nose, superficial pulses, thin and whitish coating of the tongue.	High temperature, dazedness, restiveness, thirst, pains in the breast or abdomen, constipation or diarrhea. Urine reduced in quantity and/or reddish in colour; submerged pulses, yellow, grey or black coating of the tongue.

The following classical quotations develop further the distinctions given in the table: "The discrimination of species- and intima-diseases may indeed be made by noting whether fever occurs intermittently and with moderate intensity or persistently and at high intensity, whether the patient complains of shuddering or of oppressive heat, of headache or abdominal ache, whether the coating of the tongue is missing or present, whether the nose is closed up or the mouth is dry, whether the pulses are superficial or submerged. When fever is accompanied by shuddering, when the head aches and the nose is stopped up, when the coating of the tongue is missing or reduced in thickness, when superficial pulses occur, this points to a species-(disease). When fever rises and falls periodically, when the patient complains of pains in the abdomen and of a dry mouth, when the coating of the tongue is yellow or even black and when the pulses are submerged, this is an intima-(disease)."[44]

"Intima-symptoms indicate that disease is rampant within, in the orbs. Diseases arising from within, be it by one of the seven emotions or from stress, wrong diet or sexual or alcoholic excesses, produce intima-symptoms[45]. Their quality is easy to determine. But their discrimination becomes more difficult with diseases induced partly by inner lesions, partly by exterior influences showing vague symptoms. Here one may be in doubt whether to class them as intima or as species – thus opening the way to grave therapeutic errors. Hence, a painstaking diagnosis is required. If for example a patient with slightly elevated temperature perspires continuously, his slight temperature does not constitute a species-symptom even if no abdominal pains or spasms and no twisted or accelerated pulses (pp. intenti sive celeri) have been found."

"Or (in another case) it may be that general symptoms give the impression of an exogenous disease. But the absence of shuddering and the fact that the patient, instead, asks to be

---

[44] Cheng Zhongling, op. cit., chapter "On the Distinction of algor and calor, inanitas and repletio, Yin and Yang".

[45] This view put forth during the Ming era (16th century) by one of the most famous physicians, is at the bais of a more comprehensive etiology of intima-symptoms which, since then, has been generally accepted in Chinese medicine.

cooled[46] indicate conclusively that this is no species-symptom but, instead, calor ("heat") powerfully developing in the intima."

"It may be said that all diseases limited to species-symptoms, and where the disease has not yet penetrated within, are accompanied by plentiful light-coloured urine. When species-symptoms are accompanied by good appetite and normal ingestion of drink, when the eliminations go forth unimpeded, the intima should not be affected. If, however, vomiting, fetid breath, feeling of fullness in the stomach and loss of appetite occur, what at first was a species-disease gradually penetrates into the intima. Further signs indicating that the intima has indeed been touched are restiveness, sleeplessness, dry mouth, thirst, raving, pains in the abdomen, diarrhea etc."[47]

The Combination of Species- and Intima-Symptoms with Algor and Calor, Inanitas and Repletio

In practical diagnosis, it usually makes sense to immediately apply to a diagnosis of species and intima the additional guiding criteria of algor and calor, inanitas and repletio. Thus, typical symptoms of

algor speciei are fever with shuddering, headache but no perspiration, stiff neck, ischiatic pains, pains in the joints, superficial or tense pulses (pp. superficiales sive intenti), thin, white coating of the tongue.

Calor speciei: shuddering[48], headache, sometimes perspiration and thirst. superficial or accelerated pulses, white coating of the tongue not extending to tip of the tongue.

Inanitas speciei: increased sensitivity to cold, fitful or constant perspiration, weak, superficial or languid pulses, pale body of the tongue.

Repletio speciei: fever with shuddering, pains throughout the body, no perspiration, superficial and replete or superficial and tense pulses; thin white coating of the tongue.

Algor intimae: cold extremities, aggravation by cold, abdominal pains with diarrhea, nausea, vomiting, no thirst; submerged or slowed down pulses (pp. mersi sive tardi), white or slippery coating of the tongue.

Calor intimae: no shuddering but, instead, oppressive heat, perspiration, thirst, red

---

[46] In Chinese wure, literally "abhors heat".

[47] Chapter 1/28 of the Jingyue quanshu ("Complete Works of Zhang Jiebin").

[48] Chinese wufeng, literally "abhorrence of wind"; cf. also p. 179 below.

scleras, deep red lips; accelerated pulses; bright red body of the tongue, yellow coating of the tongue.

Inanitas intimae: general weakness, weak low voice, reluctance to speak, reduced appetite, dizziness; cold extremities, diarrhea, incontinence of urine, incontinence of semen, even uncontrolled release of urine or faeces; pink body of the tongue, colourless or whitish coating of the tongue, sometimes not covering the centre of the tongue.

Repletio intimae: fever with restlessness, panting respiration, constipation, bloating, hard abdomen, in extreme cases raving, madness; submerged, replete pulses; yellow and dry coating of the tongue.

Symptoms of Part Species, Part Intima

We mention this qualification for the sake of completeness. It is essentially limited to the pathology of algor laedens where we shall revert to it[49]. Its symptoms are: alternation between fever and cold, feeling of fullness and pressure in the breast and below the small ribs; restiveness, nausea, anorexia, bitter taste, dry mouth, murky sight; stringy pulses (pp. chordales).

Combination and Interference of Species- and Intima-Symptoms

In everyday medical practice, cases where different energetic qualities are ascertained at the surface and in depth are rather the rule, either because an external disturbance gradually tends to penetrate, or because an inner factor gradually tends to surface; or because exterior and inner agents simultaneously attack the orthopathy. Here again, diagnosis must combine all six criteria viz. species-intima with the criteria of algor/calor and inanitas/repletio. Thus the following combinations result:

1. Calor intimae et speciei (when an endogenous fever disease meets with an exogenous infection :morbus temperatum[50]): At the beginning red face, headache, oppressive heat, thirst, dry throat and dry tongue, later on restiveness and raving.

2. Algor intimae et speciei (when an exogenous algor-heteropathy combines with a

---

[49] Cf. p. 107 below.

[50] Cf. p. 57 below as well as pp. 113 ff.

BASIC CONCEPTS OF DIFFERENTIAL DIAGNOSIS

structive congestion): Here we observe at first sudden abdominal pains, vomiting and diarrhea, cold extremities, later on shuddering without perspiration, headache and pains throughout the body.

3. Calor speciei combined with algor intimae (when algor inanitatis which at first developed in the oo. lienalis et stomachi, in addition combines with a ventus-heteropathy inducing fever): Fever without perspiration, headache, cough; diarrhea, light to colourless urine, swollen body of the tongue, yellow, moist, murky coating of the tongue[51].

4. Algor speciei with calor intimae: Shuddering, fever, no perspiration; pains in the head and throughout the body; panting, restiveness, thirst; superficial or tense pulses (pp. superficiales aut intenti).

5. Repletio speciei et intimae: Fever with shuddering, no perspiration, headache, pains in the body; abdominal pains aggravated by pressure; retention of urine and faeces; replete pulses.

6. Inanitas speciei et intimae: Cold induced by ventus; spontaneous perspiration; dizziness, disturbed vision, angina pectoris-like sensation; diarrhea; infirm pulses (pp. invalidi).

7. Inanitas speciei + repletio intimae: Cold induced by ventus, spontaneous perspiration, constipation, hard and painful abdomen sensitive to pressure; thick, murky coating of the tongue.

8. Repletio speciei + inanitas intimae: Shuddering, perspiration; headache and diffuse pains througout the body; nausea, hard abdomen, alternation between stomachache and diarrhea; no thirst.

In Chinese medicine, the transition from species- to intima-diseases has been particularly well explored on algor laedens-diseases (shanghan), where we shall deal with it in detail[52]. To start with, two typical examples must suffice.

First, a disease develops from the species into the intima. It is accompanied by symptoms of copious clear urine at first (pure species-symptom), followed by nausea, bitter taste, pressure on the chest, and loss of appetite (transitory symptoms), and it finally ends with restiveness, insomnia, thirst and sticky palate, raving; constipation or abdominal pain accompanied by diarrhea (intima-symptoms).

---

[51] Chinese zhuo, literally 'turbid', 'opaque'.

[52] Cf. below p. 107 as, more in general, pp. 100 ff.

Second, a disease develops from the intima to the species: At first there is inner heat, restiveness, irritation inducing cough, pressure on the chest; then there is fever with perspiration, also exanthemas.

Algor AND Calor ("COLD" AND "HEAT")

A diagnostic statement as to whether there are algor- or calor-symptoms is not simply a statement referring to the thermic nature of disease. In fact, these sensory thermic symptoms constitute only accidents and partial data on deviations classified as algor or calor. Consequently, as stated in the introductory lines, after having qualified symptoms by these criteria, we are already well on the way to defining therapy. This permits us to understand a passage of the Inner Classic[53]: "Where there are cold (i.e. algor-)heteropathies, we apply 'heat', where there are hot (i.e. calor-)heteropathies, we apply 'cold'." In other words, we shall apply warm remedies in the case of algor-symptoms and cold remedies in the case of calor-symptoms.

Of course, just as with other disturbances, the criteria of algor and calor rarely may be applied with the exclusion of all others; as a rule, they must again be combined with other criteria, and distinguished with respect to the topology. Finally we should take note that classical theory here particularly stresses occasions for error described as algor falsus or calor falsus (false 'cold' or 'heat').

Pure Symptoms Either of algor or of calor

At	we define as algor-Symptoms	calor-Symptoms
INSPECTION	The patient lies in bed rolled up with legs drawn to his body, showing great prostration; he has a pale or greenish complexion, clear or tearing eyes, the desire to close these; he has sometimes pale or bluish violet lips and nailmoons the same colour; the coating of his tongue either is lacking or is white and slippery, and definite-	The patient lies in bed on his back with legs extended, moves easily and often, shows restiveness; his complexion is red, his scleras are reddish also, the eyes are wide open and look about with curiosity. The lips are dry or cracked or red and swollen; the nail flesh is red to violet. The coating of the tongue is increased in thickness, yellow to black, sometimes showing pointed eminences; the body of the tongue

---

[53] Chapter 74/802.

BASIC CONCEPTS OF DIFFERENTIAL DIAGNOSIS

At	we define as algor-Symptoms	calor-Symptoms
	ly moist; the body of the tongue is pale or pink, if expectoration occurs, it is copious and thin, clear to whitish.	seems to be shrunken, hard, and looks like leather; there is copious expectoration of yellow colour of thick consistency.
AUSCULTATION	The patient is quiet and reluctant to speak	The patient is loquacious and noisy.
INTERROGATION	The patient shows no thirst but may ask for warm food; he produces much saliva, clear and copious urine and liquid faeces.	He shows thirst and the desire for cold food, has reduced saliva, little urine, which is dark yellow to reddish, and there is constipation.
PALPATION	Submerged, minute, slowed down pulses, sometimes languid, and always weak. His extremities are cold.	Flooding, accelerated, racing and strong pulses; the extremities are warm.

The Combined Occurrence of Algor- and Calor-Symptoms

As the foregoing table should have made impressively clear, the diagnostic differences between the symptoms of algor ("cold") and calor ("heat") are striking. Yet it should be kept in mind, that in practice, such symptoms almost always occur in combinations, in other words one and the same patient shows different symptoms which have partly to be qualified as algor and partly to be qualified by calor; in addition, very often other guiding criteria also apply. Thus it often happens that we observe calor-symptoms above the diaphragm (e.g. pressure, oppression, panting) and algor-symptoms below the diaphragm (e.g. pain combined with nausea, noises in the abdomen, diarrhea). And each must be given adequate and different treatment[54].

Therapy based upon such differential diagnosis will not only take into account whether the different thermic qualities occur above or below the diaphragm[55], whether they occur in the species or in the intima, but also whether certain symptoms seem to prevail over others.

---

[54] The corresponding Chinese prescriptions can be found in Sections 157 and 173 of the Shanghan-lun.

[55] It should be recalled that the diaphragm marks the division between presumed orbs connected to conduits of the hands and conduits of the feet, respectively.

Algor falsus, calor falsus

When we have to deal with light or medium disturbances, the symptoms occurring offer hardly any difficulties when they are to be classed by algor or calor. When a certain disease, however, enters upon a critical stage and, consequently, calor or algor develop with extreme intensity, so-called "false symptoms" may occur. If these false symptoms are misjudged, there is the danger of therapeutic error immediately jeopardizing the life of the patient.

The physician Zhang Jiebin writes: "When symptoms of "false heat" (calor falsus) occur, the effect of Water[56] has attained its apogee, at which point it assumes the outward signs of the E.P. Fire. This may occur in the case of illness as the consequence of algor laedens or in general with morbi varii, when the patient, by his constitutional setup, is predisposed to inanitas and algor, and when this (constitutional predisposition) is struck by a heteropathy. (The false symptoms) may however also be induced by any of the other pathogenic factors such as stress, alcoholic or sexual excesses, extreme release of the seven emotions; in fact, it may even occur in somebody who never had shown any calor-symptoms when cold or cool medicine was erroneously administered. What in such a case produces confusion is that calor merus ("true heat") induces fever, but calor falsus ("false heat") does also; and also that in both cases all other symptoms seem to be congruent, such as red face, restiveness, constipation, reduced reddish urine, panting, painful swollen throat, accelerated or tense pulses (pp. celeri aut intenti). Now, if in such a case a physician without experience simply diagnoses calor and consequently applies cold or cool remedies, the patient may die immediately after having taken the medicine. What had been overlooked was that, although the body showed an elevated temperature, it was algor intimae which had produced this, releasing an exhausted yang. What should have put the physician on guard was that, in spite of calor-symptoms such as dry mouth and thirst, the patient was unable to take any cold liquid or, if he did accept it, only in very small quantities; also that there was no constipation or, instead, that the retention of urine was accompanied by diarrhea (an algor-symptom!); or that frequent micturition of clear urine occurred, sometimes alternating with small quantities of yellow or reddish urine, that the patient at once was short of breath and reluctant to speak, showing a dark complexion and great prostration, or that even if he at first shows extreme restlessness, he will keep quiet if he is only slightly restrained. His case, hence, is in no way comparable to that of a patient with an irrepressible urge to move about, to swear and to cry (as with "true heat"); the same holds true

---

[56] This refers to energies qualified by the E.P. Water and, within the concert of all orbs, being represented by the renal orb.

BASIC CONCEPTS OF DIFFERENTIAL DIAGNOSIS 47

of widely scattered, pale red spots the size of insect bites. They constitute a marked contrast to the purplish or scarlet exanthema accompanying high fever of <u>calor merus</u>.

Similar distinctions obtain for the pulses of "false heat": They are always submerged, minute, slowed down, and infirm (<u>pp. mersi, tardi, minuti, invalidi</u>); and if, for some reason, there ever should occur a superficial, a flooding or an accelerated pulse (<u>pp. superficialis, exundans, celer</u>), the latter will be weak, without configurative force (<u>shen</u>) – for with <u>calor falsus</u>, the heat is only in the skin, at the surface, whereas in depth, within the orbs, there is cold (<u>algor</u>). And the saying goes: 'The abhorrence of "heat" (<u>wure</u>)' does not constitute "heat" (<u>calor</u>); indeed it constitutes a yin-symptom. Every time when signs of collapse or oppression of the <u>intima</u> appear and one cannot think of anything better than of attacking the heteropathy, one will surely kill the patient. What is required instead is a rapid completion and support (<u>suppletio et sustentatio</u>) of the <u>yang merum</u>[57] by which we shall reduce "glare" (<u>ardor</u>) to its origin. By gradually effecting the return of the <u>qi primum</u>[58], we will of necessity make <u>calor</u> withdraw and will heal the disease. In brief, if in a feverish patient, we diagnose an accelerated pulse without tension or force[59], this is a sure sign that a vigorous yin pushes yang into the <u>species,</u> and that there is no real <u>calor</u>[60]."

"(We have a case of) "false cold" (<u>algor falsus</u>) when manifestations of the E.P. Fire reach their apogee, and take on the outward signs of the E.P. Water. If for example in the case of an <u>algor laedens</u>-disease, there was high fever at first which the doctor had erroneously treated by (excessive) diaphoresis and purgation, the result will be that the <u>calor</u>-heteropathy, after prolonged ravages, will assemble within and will then advance through the yang conduits into structive (yin) energies. The result of this will be that despite high temperature, the extremities will grow cold, the patient will become listless, will abhor cold – all these yin-symptoms. Now it is true that both, <u>algor merus et falsus</u> ("true and false cold"), similarly induce an abhorrence of cold (<u>wuhan</u>), and that a flexus[61] increases or decreases parallel with fever; nevertheless, in this case extreme heat has changed into its opposite. What lets us perceive the difference is that in this case of false cold, the voice of the patient will be strong; his lips may be cracked,

---

[57] Cf. p. 36 above.

[58] This refers to the structive aspect of the <u>qi nativum</u>, in other words to the structive aspects of the energy potential present at birth.

[59] Literally "is not felt as a forceful beat, when pressed".

[60] <u>Jingyue quanshu</u>, Chapter 1, section 8: <u>De algore et calore meri et falsi</u> ("On True and False Heat and Cold"), pp. 27 f.

[61] This technical term designates an inversion of the flow of energies, leading to cold extremities.

his tongue black: he will show thirst and the desire to have cold beverages; his urine will flow sparingly and be of red colour; there will be constipation. And even if the administration of remedies should have produced liquid diarrhea, the faeces will contain dry clots and be extremely malodorous. And there will be strong submerged or slippery pulses (pp. mersi sive lubrici). All these[62] are yang-symptoms."

"Similar remarks hold true for algor falsus ("false cold") occurring in connection with morbi varii[63]. Here also we shall either see abhorrence of cold or even shuddering − induced by heat culminating within − with cold affecting the species; hot and cold energies do not mingle, hence the shuddering. In such cases we have algor in the skin and calor in the bones and marrow. That is why the classical saying goes: 'Shuddering (indicating abhorrence of cold) are not algor[64]'; no doubt, these are calor-symptoms. For if one examines the inner symptoms, one will either ascertain the desire to have cold beverages; or there will be constipation, urine of dark colour and reduced in quantity, bad breath, restlessness − and certainly strong slippery or replete pulses (pp. lubrici aut repleti). This kind of diagnosis makes us apply medicines sustaining the yin (medicamenta sustinentia sive rigantia yin) and cooling glare (mm. refrigerantia ardoris). After having eliminated calor intimae, the outward cold will disappear by itself.'[65]

"When a patient enjoys hot drinks in spite of calor-symptoms, this may be described as 'like attracts like'; if, however, a patient showing algor-symptoms tries to ingest cold beverages but does not succeed, this is a symptom of "false thirst". If there are calor-symptoms, yet these are accompanied by thin diarrhea, we call this a heat diarrhea induced by endogenous or exogenous influences. If there are calor-symptoms yet the extremities show flexus-cold, we should reflect upon the fact that there is a direct relationship between the intensity of a flexus and the intensity of heat."

"If one ascertains algor-symptoms on a restive patient who desires to sit or lie in loam, this symptom is called 'structive restiveness'. If despite perspiration, repletion symptoms occur, we must conclude that a calor-heteropathy has penetrated into the intima. If there is lack of perspiration accompanied by inanitas-symptoms, we must conclude that the fluids (= yin

---

[62] The pronoun "these" must not be taken as a general reference to all submerged pulses. Cf. p. 210 below.

[63] Cf. with this pp. 66 ff. following below.

[64] In Chinese, there is a play of words here, since it is possible to pronounce and interpret one and the same Chinese character in two different ways, viz. ehan or wuhan. In the first case, we must interpret: "bad cold" = shuddering, in the second case: "abhorring cold".

[65] P. 28 of the Jingyue quanshu.

BASIC CONCEPTS OF DIFFERENTIAL DIAGNOSIS

energies) are deficient.

If the patient showing intima-symptoms shudders, this indicates that he is affected by an algor-heteropathy. If he abhorrs heat, is thirsty and shows species-symptoms, this indicates that an exogenous morbus temperatus sive febrilis emerges on the surface from within[66]."

"In order to determine whether the patient will be adversely affected in the case of algor falsus by hot remedies or in the case of calor falsus by cold remedies, one should make him drink a small quantity of cold water. In the case of calor falsus he will not swallow it at all or will vomit it immediately after having drunk — which indicates that he must be treated with warm or hot remedies. If there is a case of algor falsus, however, he will eagerly ask for the cold water and feel improved after having swallowed it; and he will not vomit it. In this case, he must be treated with cold or cool remedies[67]."

Inanitas AND repletio

The guiding criteria of inanitas (xu, "exhaustion") and repletio (shi, "repletion") constitute not only semantic complements; it should be recalled and underscored once more that they refer to different elements of pathology. Inanitas refers to an energetic deficiency, to an exhaustion of the orthopathy (in the singular!), i.e. of the capacity of the individual to maintain its functional integrity. By contrast, repletion (repletio) designates a redundancy, an energetic excess of one or more heteropathies, i.e. of deviating factors, detached from the orthopathy and disturbing, endangering this orthopathy. As the classical saying goes: "If heteropathic energy is vigorous, there is repletion, if the structive potential is impaired, there is inanitas".[68] In therapy, repletion symptoms require the dispersion (dispulsio, xiao, xie or san) of energy, whereas inanitas-symptoms must be treated by completing or sustaining (bu, suppletio, sustentatio), in other words by using mm. supplentia, rigantia, adiuvantia.[69] We already met with examples where these guiding criteria may be combined with the aforementioned ones, also where both, inanitas and repletio may occur in one and the same patient.

---

[66] Op. et loc. cit.

[67] Op. et loc. cit.

[68] Huangdi neijing Suwen, Chapter 28/278.

[69] The former therapeutic effect may be achieved either by prescriptions or by acupuncture, the latter by the prescription of drugs and moxibustion. Acupuncture cannot compensate a true and generalized deficiency of energy.

The Symptoms of inanitas and repletio

For practical reasons it is useful to subdivide the symptoms of inanitas and repletio, depending on whether they affect active individually specific energies (qi) or structive individually specific energy (xue); also, certain affinities with the orbs may be taken into account. The former distinction is related to the fact that in a medical theory based upon an essentially functional view, a fundamental distinction is made between energy emanating from a given source and spreading throughout the system (yang), and the the energy making up that system (yin, structive energy). The former may bear a qualitative determination indicating its origin; the latter makes up the system and, consequently is tied to that system[70]. The following symptoms may be distinguished:

1. Inanitas qi: Exhaustion of active, individually specific energy

a. inanitas qi pulmonalis: asthma, shortness of breath, spontaneous perspiration, weak voice;

b. inanitas qi medii (= depletion of the qi lienalis et stomachi): reduced vital warmth in the extremities, intermittent bloating of the abdomen, abdominal pains improved by pressure; loss of appetite, collapsed digestion; stools: diarrheic or fluid; limpness and numbness of hands and feet; and

c. inanitas qi primi (= inanitas qi renalis): welling up of the depleted active energy, consequently red spots on the cheeks; raucous voice; sore throat; tinnitus, temporary deafness because of exhaustion, dizziness, palpitations, slow speech, drooling; alternation between dilated and conctracted pupils, twitching eyelids, twitching of the extremities, and especially of the hands; irregular breathing.

2. Repletio qi: Repletion of the active individually specific energy

a. Repletio qi pulmonalis: tense, hard thorax; dizziness, great quantities of sputum, impeded breathing which may may reach the point where the patient cannot bear a horizontal position; the patient breathes through the mouth, pulls up his shoulders;

b. repletio qi stomachi: obstructed centre, noises and rumbling in the stomach, foul or sour eructations; in extreme cases the refusal of all food, convulsions and vomiting;

c. repletio qi intestinorum: slowed down functions in the abdomen, bloated, distended

---

[70] We shall meet again with these distinctions in modified form when dealing with pulse diagnosis: There the qualities of a given orb are reflected a. by the specific quality of the pulse independent of the site of its occurrence; b. independent of the quality of the pulse and the changes observed at one or several sites of the pulse. Cf. below pp. 248 ff.

BASIC CONCEPTS OF DIFFERENTIAL DIAGNOSIS 51

abdomen; pains around the navel; stools either dry and hard or diarrheic, of reddish or white colour; in extreme cases the patient gasps for breath, cannot lie down, raves, and has intermittent fevers; finally

   d. repletio qi hepatici: headache, dizziness.

3. Inanitas xue: Exhaustion of the structive individually specific energy

   Pale lips, pale complexion, nervous restiveness, insomnia, mental exhaustion; deficiency of the juices, hence dry tongue, cracked lips, nocturnal fever with heavy perspiration during sleep; twitching muscles; in extreme cases convulsions and tic convulsifs.

4. Repletio xue: Repletion of the structive individually specific energy

   Hematomas; painful, tense muscles, lancinating pains in the thorax, the mediastinum, the shoulders and the arms; heat sensations emanating from the centre; pains and bloating of the midriff region; lancinating pains around the navel or in the abdomen; purple or dark-red body of the tongue with purple spots on its margin; black stools; grating or fixed pulses (pp. asperi aut fixi).

5. Inanitas orbium: Exhaustion of the energies of the orbs

   a. inanitas orbis cardialis: despondency, sadness; tense thorax and abdomen; pains around the small ribs, exhaustion;

   b. inanitas orbis hepatici: blurred vision, shrunken scrotum; convulsions, timidity; lack of initiative and imagination;

   c. inanitas o. lienalis: paretic extremities, depressed digestion, hard and tense abdomen; depressed mood;

   d. inanitas o. pulmonalis: shortness of breath, shallow breathing; dry skin; and

   e. inanitas o. renalis: dizziness, forgetfulness; stiff back; pain in the extremities or inability to move these, especially the lower extremities; morning diarrhea or inability to defecate; retention of urine or enuresis; uncontrolled loss of semen.

6. Repletio orbium: Repletion of the energy of the orbs

   a. repletio o. cardialis: whimsical ideas; convulsive laughter;

   b. repletio o. hepatici: pains in the flanks and in the centre of the abdomen, choleric mood;

c. repletio o. lienalis: tense, hard abdomen, feeling of repletion, constipation; turgid body;

d. repletio o. pulmonalis: contravective[71] energy, shortness of breath, panting, irritated throat; and

e. repletio o. renalis: congested lower abdomen with pains and swellings.

The outer orbs (aulic orbs, orbes aulici) indirectly participate in the symptoms and disturbances of all horreal orbs discussed here[72].

The Combined Manifestation of inanitas- and repletio-Symptoms

If the same patient concurrently manifests inanitas-symptoms in one system and repletion-symptoms in another, this is called the combined manifestation of inanitas and repletio. To cope with such a situation, therapy must combine suppletive and dispelling measures. The correct dosage of competing and sometimes antagonistic medication requires special consideration.

The Chinese physician Yu Genchu states: "(Suppose that) among a great number of inanitas-symptoms, suddenly signs of repletion occur. In this case, even if throughout the individual we had hitherto observed only inanitas-symptoms, if repletion manifests itself only in only one or two spots, the latter will require most urgent attention. Also (inversely), if among a great number of repletive symptoms suddenly signs of inanitas manifest themselves, these latter will require the most urgent attention, even if inanitas is limited to one or two spots only. We should here keep in mind what Zhang Jingyue expressed thus[73]: 'In the solitary traveller there lurks treachery.'

To illustrate, let us first look at the case of a woman showing all signs of "dry stressful depletion of the xue"[74]. Her face looks haggard and shrunken, her body is emaciated, her flesh shrunken, her skin dry; she is restive and filled with inner heat, her appetite is reduced – all this constituting striking inanitas-symptoms. If, under these conditions, suddenly the body of the tongue shows a purple and dark tint and congestive spots on its margin, if her menses

---

[71] Contravection, in Chinese ni, designates a movement contrary to the general or normal flow of energy, sometimes contrary to the movement of the orthopathy.

[72] Cf. above pp. 77 f.

[73] Quoted from p. 112 of the Zhongyi zhenduanxue jiangyi - cf. my Bibliography below.

[74] Cf. on this p. 115 below.

BASIC CONCEPTS OF DIFFERENTIAL DIAGNOSIS   53

stagnate for a prolonged time, if her weak pulse shows signs of roughness (grating, <u>asperitas</u>) this means that within her <u>inanitas,</u> repletive symptoms appear, and that in treatment one must pay close attention to the latter.

Then there is the case of an emaciated patient whose body bloats immediately after the ingestion of food or beverage. His complexion shows a greenish, yellowish or dark tint, his body and his face are haggard, his extremities are swollen; his excretions are stagnant, the body of his tongue is dark red or scarlet, the coating of the tongue appears to be dry, rough, yellowish or sticky; among his pulses there are frail or languid (<u>pp. lenes, languidi</u>) or submerged, minute, stringy, accelerated ones (<u>pp. mersi, minuti, chordales, celeri</u>). All these signs are indicative of the fact that in the midst of numerous repletive symptoms, <u>inanitas</u> appears. Consequently, in therapy very cautious purgation must be combined with generous suppletive measures.

Finally, we should visualize two contrary eventualities, first that a weak and instable patient who, by his constitution, inclines toward <u>inanitas,</u> is affected by some disease that produces repletive symptoms, e.g. as the consequence of an <u>algor laedens</u>-heteropathy or after the ingestion of unwholesome food; second that a strong and robust patient contracts some disease that produces <u>inanitas</u>-symptoms, e.g. as the consequence of massive loss of blood or of extreme bodily exhaustion."

False <u>inanitas</u> and False Repletion (<u>inanitas falsa et repletio falsa</u>)

While considering <u>calor</u> and <u>algor,</u> we learned that when in any energetic process an extreme is attained, a reversal of direction, hence the appearance of the opposite or complementary quality will be observed. Similar phenomena may occur when dealing with <u>inanitas</u> and <u>repletio</u> in diagnosis. And here again, we are confronted with the problem of true and false symptoms. Thus we should be on guard against <u>repletio falsa</u> and <u>inanitas falsa</u>

<u>Repletio falsa</u> ("false repletion") is present "if the disease has been induced by an emotion, by irregular intake of food, by alcoholic or sexual excesses or if some constitutional weakness is at the root of the disturbance; here we observe a hot body, constipation, a red face, tympanites, delpletion madness, spurious exanthema. Such signs seem to indicate some kind of energetic redundancy but, in fact, are the result

of a deficiency[75]"; also, "if there are pains in the stomach as if there were a lump[76]", and "if these pains are improved by the application of pressure, when there is a sunken face, if the voice appears to be weak, the pulses are feeble, all this indicates inanitas; but when the disease enters upon an extreme stage, symptoms like tympanites, anorexia, laboured breathing, constipation appear. This is so because extreme exhaustion produces symptoms of vigorous energy."[77]

Reliable signs for false repletion are that the feeling of surfeit in the patient does not persist: It disappears and reappears; also that pressure exercised upon a distended and painful abdomen alleviates the pain or makes it disappear; finally, besides submerged or slowed down pulses (pp. mersi sive tardi) stringy pulses (pp. chordales) may be observed.

Inanitas falsa ("False Exhaustion").

"When exogenous heteropathies have not been eliminated and continue to lurk in the conduits; when food and beverages have not been digested but have collected in the oo. intestinorum et stomachi and burden the patient; when contravehend congested energies have not been dispersed (cf. the iconography of the pulse), when consequently, persistent pituita ("phlegm") and congested xue stagnate in the orbs, and if such burdens upon the individual persist chronically, the patient may show symptoms of energetic deficiency"[78].

"When there exists a structive concretion within, sensitive to pressure, when the patient shows a red face, rough breath as well as powerful pulses, these are signs of repletion. If repletion comes to an extreme, we shall observe that the patient becomes quiet or minces his words, and if he speaks, he does so with a loud, resonant voice, breathing audibly; also that he is reluctant to move, feels dizzy, has blurred vision and diarrhea... – all these are symptoms of exhaustion accompanying extreme repletion of energy."[79]

Reliable signs of false exhaustion (inanitas falsa) are a loud, sonorous voice and breath in a patient reluctant to speak; diarrhea which gives relief to the patient; a patient without appetite, who sometimes takes and digests food; a patient feeling tired and exhausted, yet who is

---

[75] Jingyue quanshu, chapter on inanitas and repletio, pp. 25 ff.

[76] The Chinese term pi, 'plexus region', describes what is meant by the Chinese xinxia, "below the heart", indicating the centre of the body.

[77] Gushi yijing quoted after Zhongyi zhenduanxue jiangyi, p. 112.

[78] Jingyue quanshu, loc. cit.

[79] See note 77.

BASIC CONCEPTS OF DIFFERENTIAL DIAGNOSIS

improved by moderate movement; a patient with a swollen, distended abdomen, sensitive to the slightest pressure; fixedly localized and uninterrupted abdominal pain."

The authenticity of <u>inanitas</u> or <u>repletio</u> must be determined individually, taking into account the data of tongue inspection, interrogation and pulse diagnosis. But we must never overlook

1. the relative force of the pulse, whether it shows configurative force[80], whether it is closer to the surface or submerged;
2. whether the body of the tongue is lightly coloured and tender or deeply coloured and leatherlike;
3. whether the voice of the patient sounds loud and clear or low and indistinct;
4. whether the body of the patient looks well nourished or emaciated;
5. whether the disease is recent or has lasted for a long time, finally
6. the precise nature of previous therapeutic measures.

---

[80] Cf. below p. 123 and pp. 244 ff.

THE AGENTS OF DISEASE *(bingyin)*

Any medicine, to the extent that it justifies the qualification of "rational science", does not directly combat disturbances defined empirically, i.e. their symptoms, their symptomatic anomalies. Instead, it strives to isolate and define general or basic postulates producing these disturbances.

In Chinese medicine, as in all Chinese science primarily concerned with function, movement, vital manifestations, every pathological anomaly corresponds to an impairment of orthopathy, in other words to a "biassing", running askew, deviation (xie) of the straight or correct direction of function. By extension, any factor producing such an anomaly termed "biassing", "heteropathy", xie must be defined as a factor or influence liable to directly induce or provoke such a deviation. By individually defining the one or more factor(s) provoking or inducing the momentary deviations, clear and precise instructions are implicit as to their compesation or correction.

In Chinese medicine the factors inducing functional deviations - underlying any disease - are termed "agents", (yin[81] or bingyin), agents of disease.

For the sake of linguistic clarity and rational precision, we do well to underscore here the basic affinity and, at the same time, difference between those agents and the resulting heteropathies.

The agents correspond either to exogenous – climatical, social or cosmic – or to endogenous – i.e. emotional, constitutional – factors favouring or producing a deviation of function.

The heteropathy in turn is the result, the pathological response of the individual towards these agents of disease. Thus ira, wrath, irascibility is a propensity constitutively present in an individual and possibly exacerbated under some, dampened under other momentary social or climatic conditions. Ventus ("wind"), stringently linked to ira "wrath", by the common conventional standard of Wood, may be the heteropathic response of the individual personality which becomes manifest in diagnosis.

Occasions for confusion are even more numerous if a term like ventus ("wind"), at different levels designates basically different entities. In common speech, "wind" is a meteorological or, better still, a sensory phenomenon. Under certain conditions, this phenomenon is liable to induce a deviation of biological function. Under these circumstances, "ventus" is considered

---

[81] It should be recalled that this term, completely homonymous with yin meaning 'structive', is again written with a different character, and is without semantic affinity to the former, as well as to the following term yin, (Cf. next note) again written with a different character.

BASIC CONCEPTS OF DIFFERENTIAL DIAGNOSIS

and treated as an agent of disease, viz. a climatic excess (yin[82]). If this climatic excess calls forth a <u>specific</u> pathological response in a particular individual, the result will be a heteropathy, again termed <u>ventus,</u> "wind".

So one and the same term really is used for three different concepts, viz. first a sensory phenomenon, second a logically relatively abstract postulate ("agent") and third a complex pathological situation defined according to very precise criteria (a "heteropathy").

Some of the major fallacies about Chinese medicine are due to the fact that self-styled experts and interpreters of Chinese medicine are utterly oblivious of these distinctions.

In Chinese medicine, the agents of disease, according to conventions established since the Sung[83], may be classed into three categories, viz.

1. Inner or endogenous agents (<u>neiyin</u>);
2. exterior or exogenous agents (<u>waiyin</u>) and, finally
3. (neither inner nor outer, hence) neutral agents.

According to a more ancient theory[84], inner agents are factors inducing heteropathies within the conduits and the orbs, and exogenous agents are those which provoke heteropathies in the exterior (active) distribution of energy, in the active manifestations, at the surface of the body and in the extremities. The third category is left over for the consequences of sexual excesses as well as for the consequences of mechanical accidents.

A more recent theory[85] attempts greater stringency by stressing the active aspects of the endogenous agents, which here are equated to the Seven Emotions viz.

1. pleasure (<u>voluptas</u>), 2. wrath (<u>ira</u>), 3. anxiety (<u>sollicitudo</u>), 4. sorrow (<u>maeror</u>), 5. fear (<u>timor</u>), 6. excessive reflection (<u>cogitatio</u>) and 7. fright (<u>pavor</u>).

Or of the exogenous agents comprising the Six Climatic Excesses (<u>liuyin</u>) viz.

1. <u>ventus</u> ("wind"), 2. <u>algor</u> ("cold"), 3. <u>aestus</u> ("oppressive heat of summer"), 4. <u>humor</u>

---

[82] This term <u>yin</u> is in the second tone and, aside from this difference, completely homonymous with the two other terms mentioned in the former note. Of course, it is written by a character having nothing in common with the two former ones.

[83] More precisely in 1171 by Chen Wuze.

[84] This is usually attributed to Zhang Zhongjing of the 2nd century (whose <u>Shanghanlun</u> I quote frequently), in his <u>Jinkuei yaolue</u>, with close reference to clincal data.

[85] Chen Wuze mentioned in note 83 first formulated this theory in his <u>Sanyin ji yibing yuanlun</u> ("How the Three Kinds of Agents Serve to Explain the Rise of All Disease").

("humidity"), 5. ariditas ("dryness, drought") and 6. ardor ("glare").

Here again a category of neutral agents exists, into which fall dietetic or sexual irregularites as well as the consequences of mechanical accidents. This more recent interpretation has remained valid to this day without completely obliterating the more ancient view. What follows is, however, essentially a summary of the modern systematization.

THE SIX CLIMATIC EXCESSES (liuyin) AND THEIR SYMPTOMS

Ventus ("Wind", feng)

Ventus is qualified by the Evolutive Phase Wood, thus defining its particular affinity to spring and to the oo. hepaticus et felleus[86] ("liver and kidney orbs"). This is not the only reason why it heads the enumeration; for, moreover, it is the only excess which may combine with the five others to account for complex symptoms, thus: algor venti, aestus venti, calor venti, ariditas venti, ardor venti.

A ventus-heteropathy affecting the surface, the species, produces symptoms such as: fever with shuddering, daze, headache, stuffed-up nose, hoarse voice, tearing eyes, sore throat, superficial or languid pulses, a thin white coating of the tongue.

A ventus-heteropathy developing in depth (in the intima) produces symptoms such as: delocalized, wandering sudden pains in all joints; local, very painful bumps or indurations directly below the skin; fever accompanied by pustule exanthema (rubella), by exanthema venti (fengzhen); also in the guise of ventus internus, flexus (cold extremities) with revolving dizziness and unconsciousness; pareses, dumbness or numbness of parts of the face; partial paralysis of the eyelids or the facial muscles; [tetanus].

Algor ("Cold", han)

The qualification of algor by the E.P. Water indicates its particular affinity to Winter and to the oo. renalis et vesicalis ("kidney and urinary bladder orbs")[87]. Needless to say, just like other excesses, algor may occur during any season and in any other orb.

---

[86] Cf. these iconograms on the folding table.

[87] Cf. ibidem.

BASIC CONCEPTS OF DIFFERENTIAL DIAGNOSIS

What should be kept in mind in connection with this qualification, however, is that an excess corresponding to extreme structivity: the E.P. Water - actual structivity! - is highly liable to produce lesions or the diminishing of the active energies (yangqi).

If algor affects only the surface (species), symptoms may occur such as: fever without perspiration but with shuddering and gooseflesh; pains in the neck, in the head, in the back, in the loins, also diffuse pains throughout the body; superficial or tense pulses (pp. superficiales sive intenti); whitish, moist coating of the tongue.

If the algor-heteropathy has penetrated into the conduits, convulsions, painful spasms of the extremities may be observed; also purple colouring of the skin, flexus algoris (cold-induced lowering of the temperature of the hands and feet), evanescent pulses.

An algor-heteropathy affecting the depth, the orbs, may produce abdominal pains, noisy rumbling in the intestines, diarrhea, vomiting, as well as a pale body of the tongue with white coating and submerged and slowed-down or submerged and tense pulses (pp. mersi et tardi sive mersi et intenti).

Aestus ("the Oppressive Heat of Summer", shu)

The qualification of aestus by the E.P. Fire indicates its particular affinity to the oo. cardialis, pericardialis, intestini tenuis et tricalorii ("orbs of the heart, pericardium, small intestine, tricalorium").
The most striking symptoms produced by aestus are fevers accompanied by their corollaries such as dazedness, heavy breathing, extreme lassitude, heavy perspiration, sallow complexion, thirst, reduced secretion of reddish urine; exhausted pulses (pp. inanes), red body of the tongue, thin yellow coating of the tongue. In extreme cases called percussio aestus [heat shock], sudden unconsciousness, rapid breathing and profuse perspiration may be observed.

Very often aestus, combining with other climatic excesses, may induce complex heteropathies such as e.g.

(a) a patient exposed to extreme heat, who has been suddenly chilled, may contract what is called percussio algoris mensum aestus (shuyue zhonghan) or aestus structivus (yinshu), accompanied by symptoms of constant perspiration, shuddering, headache, dazedness, sometimes with abdominal pains, vomiting and diarrhea. These symptoms are indicative of the fact that structive cold has inhibited the unfoldment of active energies.

(b) Aestus and humor-excesses may combine to affect the oo. intestinorum, producing dysentery with red and white faeces and even cholera, all these accompanied by vomiting and diarrhea, intense abdominal pains and convulsions.

(c) A syndrome called aestus subreptus ("hidden aestus", fushu) is attributed to an infection contracted during the extreme heat of the summer, but only manifesting itself after prolonged incubation toward the end of autumn in symptoms reminiscent of malaria: oppressive feeling in the plexus solaris, sluggish digestion, thirst increasing in the afternoon and strongest in the evening; relief after a flush of perspiration setting in at dawn.

(d) Malaria.

Humor ("Humidity", shi)

The qualification of humor by the E.P. Earth expresses a particular affinity to the oo. lienalis et stomachi ("spleen and stomach orbs"). The effects of this climatic excess are re-enforced if the patient wears wet garments, if he spends much time in damp surroundings, if he is addicted to eating very "humid" food (such as melons) and sweets (which latter put a particular strain on the active energy of the o. lienalis).

Depending on the propagation and particular direction of the symptoms, four kinds of humor-heteropathies may ensue:

(a) humor superior producing dazedness, stopped-up nose, yellowish complexion, heavy breathing;

(b) humor inferior leading to a swollen nose, gynecological ailments with murky evacuations;

(c) humor externus: perspiration utterly independent of the surrounding temperature, great prostration, painful joints, swellings;

(d) humor internus: oppressive feeling in the thorax, turgid plexus solaris, loss of appetite, nausea; icterus, diarrhea.

Ariditas ("Extreme Dryness", zao)

The qualification of ariditas by the E.P. Metal indicates its particular affinity to Autumn and to the oo. pulmonalis et intestini crassi ("lung and large intestine orbs"). Among the heteropathies developing under the influence of this excess, we may

BASIC CONCEPTS OF DIFFERENTIAL DIAGNOSIS 61

distinguish

(a) <u>ariditas frigidula</u> ("cool <u>ariditas</u>-symptoms") such as light headache, shuddering, no perspiration, cough, sore throat, stopped-up nose, dry, whitish coating of the tongue.

(b) <u>ariditas temperata</u> ("warm <u>ariditas</u>") with symptoms such as fever accompanied by perspiration, sore throat, thirst, intensive irritation and cough, pains in the breast; in extreme cases blood-streaked mucous expectoration, dry nose, superficial or flooding pulses (<u>pp. superficiales sive exundantes</u>); yellow, dry coating of the tongue.

Ardor ("Glare", huo)

<u>Ardor,</u> like <u>aestus</u> is qualified by the E.P. Fire; yet unlike the latter, it may develop from any of the other climatic excesses. The resulting heteropathy produces intensive processes and dangerous symptoms, resulting especially from the loss or diminishment of the fluids, hence of all structive energy.

Typical symptoms of <u>ardor</u> are: high temperature with extreme restiveness, thirst, sore throat, red face, red skleras, accelerated pulses, dry, yellow coating of the tongue with pointed protuberances and a red or deep-red body of the tongue.

THE SEVEN EMOTIONS (<u>qiqing</u>) AND THEIR SYMPTOMS

1. Pleasure (<u>voluptas, xi</u>)

Pleasure may be considered a normal manifestation of the functions of the <u>o. cardialis,</u> indicating a healthy development of imagination and of the constructive and defensive energies. If developed in excess, it will produce exhaustion (<u>inanitas</u>) of the energies of the <u>o. cardialis</u> and, consequently, lead to a scattering of the configurative force and to an accroachment of the <u>o. cardialis</u> by the energies of the <u>o. renalis</u>[88]. As a consequence, symptoms may occur such as impaired consciousness, disrupted, incoherent speech, erratic movements and erratic demeanour.

2. Wrath (<u>ira, nu</u>)

Wrath shows a specific dependence upon the individually specific structive energy (<u>xue</u>) stored in the <u>o. hepaticus.</u> Consequently, all irascibility, wrathful or uncontrolled

---

[88] Cf. Porkert, <u>Theoretical Foundations...</u> pp. 52 - 54, and p. 127.

demeanour has repercussions on the energy level of the oo. hepaticus et felleus and indirectly on that of the o. cardialis et renalis[89]. Repletion of energy in the named orbs favours explosions of wrath which, in turn, redounds upon these orbs, in particular on the o. hepaticus, then producing symptoms such as contravections (i.e. counter-current flow) of the qi hepaticum, with red face and, in extreme cases, unconsciousness and stroke.

3. Anxiety (sollicitudo, si)

Anxiety predominantly affects the functions of the oo. pulmonalis et intestini crassi. If one anxiously dwells upon troublesome ideas, eventually the o. pulmonalis and its function of rhythmic distribution of energy in all orbs will be affected, in retrograde manner also the function of the o. lienalis - thus producing symptoms such as: general loss of tonus, shallow breath, cough, shortness of breath, much expectoration, feeble extremities, turgescent abdomen, reduced appetite, diarrhea.

4. Reflection (cogitatio, si)

Reflection is the normal function of the integrative o. lienalis ("spleen orb") responsible for the assimilation of all external influences, starting with food and beverages, and comprising social, cosmic or psychic inputs. Excessive reflection (induced by an excess of active impulses and excess of activity in general[90]) will eventually produce lesions of the functions of the o. lienalis, manifesting themselves through symptoms such as fatigue, loss of appetite, forgetfulness, palpitation, extreme lassitude, perspiration during sleep, and emaciation.

5. Sorrow (maeror, you)

Sorrow somewhat resembles anxiety (sollicitudo) in affecting primarily the o. pulmonalis, and indirectly the o. cardialis. Prolonged influence of sorrow will produce symptoms such as a pale, fallen face, listlessness, reduced mental alertness.

6. Fear (timor, kung)

Fear corresponds to tension induced by supposed or expected danger; it is primarily induced by energetic deficiency of the o. renalis, indirectly sometimes by a deficiency

---

[89] Cf. op. cit. p. 119 as well as p. 84.

[90] Op. cit. p. 132 as well as 128 f.

BASIC CONCEPTS OF DIFFERENTIAL DIAGNOSIS

of the energies of the o. cardialis. Inversely, persistent fear will produce identical disturbances indicated by symptoms such as: despondency, irresolution, restiveness, persecution mania and the desire to shut oneself off from other people.

7. Fright (pavor, jing)

Fright corresponds to the tension induced by an unexpected real or supposed danger. The disposition to fright primarily results from an energetic deficiency of the o. cardialis; in turn, frightful events will primarily affect the o. cardialis. Then symptoms will occur such as: irregular accelerated breathing, restlessness, incoherent or contradictory actions, raving speech and erratic behaviour.

NEUTRAL AGENTS AND THEIR SYMPTOMS

1. Unwholesome Diet

Incorrect or unwholesome diet may produce symptoms such as the feeling of a lump in the stomach, turgidness and pains, sour or foul eructations, vomiting of undigested food; in extreme cases (when the o. lienalis has also been affected) alternation between constipation and diarrhea.

2. Excessive Bodily Stress

Excessive bodily stress may impair the qi primum, in other words, the structive potential and/or the resources of constitutionally inborn energies deposited in the o. renalis. Then symptoms such as extreme prostration and enfeeblement, shortness of breath, tachycardia, inner heat, spontaneous perspiration and restiveness will appear.

3. Sexual Excesses

Sexual excesses may induce symptoms such as cough, bloody sputum, recurrent slight rise in temperature, tachycardia; perspiration during sleep. If the active energies of the o. renalis have been exhausted, atrophy of the penis, ejaculatio praecox, clammy hands and feet, weakness in the hips and loins and lower extremities, loss of semen during sleep may result.

ADDENDA

Epidemic Infections (Epidemics)

In spite of the excellent accomplishments of modern Western medicine in the diagnosis and treatment of epidemics, we should not completely loose sight of what Chinese medicine has to say about them. The infectious nature of epidemics, in other words the fact that these are transmitted by contact with a sick person, is already explicitly discussed in the Inner Classic of the Yellow Sovereign[91]. The expediency of a prophylactic inoculation of healthy people was known in China as early as the 12th century, at least as far as smallpox is concerned[92]. Besides, there were essentially two factors to which the outbreak of epidemics was attributed, viz.

(a) the development of "perverse" meteorological situations (sudden cold in summer, hot days in late autumn etc.) affecting certain regions and putting an excessive stress on the orthopathy of a considerable number of individuals. (Because of this dependence upon a pernicious temporal configuration, epidemics are also called "chronodemic" diseases, i.e. diseases spreading at certain times: shiqibing).

(b) Bad hygienic conditions in a crowded population. (It was the latter consideration which in China, already in the 2nd century of our era, prompted edicts concerning the cleaning of public streets and the establishment of public toilets in cities.) Aside from these notions, the diagnosis and therapy of infectious diseases conforms to the basic rules given here.

Diseases Developing After a Time of Latency (qi subreptum), i.e. Hidden Disease Configurations"

Whenever diseases are developing gradually and the diagnosis of present or recent factors does not produce any conclusive evidence, it is thought that in an individual with a weak orthopathy, already a very weak biassing influence may have induced a heteropathy. Because of its relative insignificance, it was not immediately noticed by the subject or by those who came into contact with him. Only when the latently affected orb was destabilized and increasingly sensitized during a corresponding season, did the heteropathy become manifest.

---

[91] Chapter 72, compiled in the 3rd century B.C. at the earliest, in the 7th century A.D. at the latest.

[92] Cf. Willy Hartner's essay on Chinese medical history: "Heilkunde im alten China", published in the journal SINICA 16/1941 pp. 242 - 265 and 17/1942 pp. 27 - 89.

Chapter Three: Pathology

In practically every medical system, pathology represents a section whose divisions and terminology are preponderantly determined by habit and convention rather than by stringent logical arguments - rightly so because the purpose of pathology is to put the salient characteristics of different diseases within the reach of practicing physicians by the use of handy and impressive concepts and models. After the factors thought to cause or to induce these diseases have been defined, in Western medicine by fundamental disciplines such as biochemistry, physiology, bacteriology, in Chinese medicine by orbisiconography, it is left to the discretion of pathologists to class certain symptoms separately or to lump them together into a syndrome, to attribute certain peripheral symptoms to one pathological complex or to another, and so on.

All this must be kept in mind if one wants to get the correct perspective on what Chinese pathology has arrived at after sifting its postulates for more than 2000 years, and grouping its diseases within three overlapping categories, viz.

> 1. the description of "varied diseases" (morbi varii, zabing) - closely related to orbisiconography;
> 2. the description of so called "damaging cold" diseases (algor laedens-diseases, shanghan) closely related to a terminology thought to be derived from the qualification of the conduits; and
> 3. the description of so called "temperate diseases" (morbi temperati, wenbing) closely connected with medical energetics.

Anyone having gained some familiarity with these systems will perceive that the preference of one of these three keys for assessing and grouping symptoms, today as in former times, predominantly depends upon geographical and personal preferences and, at worst, will affect therapeutic choices, but will never lead to discrepancies in prognosis and therapeutic effectiveness.

THE PATHOLOGY OF THE ORBS *(morbi varii, zabing)*

To describe diseases with direct reference to orbisiconography furnishes the most comprehensive and most widely used framework for pathology in traditional Chinese medicine. It is the most comprehensive framework because, without exception, all "inner" diseases can be described rationally by using this paradigm; and it is the most widespread system because in China inner medicine (neike) has predominantly used this formula since the 2nd century of our era.

The foundations of orbisiconography were laid in the Inner Classic of the Yellow Sovereign (Huangdi Neijing Suwen)(3rd century B.C.). The clinical and pathological applications of these insights were first developed by Zhang Zhongjing (flourished in the 2nd half of the 2nd century of our era) in his 'Treatise on "Damaging Cold" and Varied Diseases'(Shanghan Zabinglun). The criteria used for describing those "varied diseases" (morbi varii, zabing) constituted the basis for inner medicine which evolved thereafter until the 17th century.

DISEASES OF THE orbes hepaticus et felleus ("LIVER AND GALL-BLADDER ORBS")

Orbisiconographic Data

The functional yoke uniting the oo. hepaticus et felleus has its specific unfoldment (perfectio) in the nervus (i.e. in the muscles and sinews constituting the motive organs of the locomotive apparatus); the eyes constitute its sense organs; its sinarteries ("conduits") touch the ocular plexus and the top of the skull. This is why the o. hepaticus, on the one hand, is responsible for the mobility of the individual, for the production and employment of locomotive force, for the active projection of the personality in general, and on the other hand for the storage and dosage of individually specific structive energy (xue). Presence of mind, the capacity to make decisions, to develop initiative and alertness as well as courage, are dependent upon the healthy functioning of the oo. hepaticus et felleus[93].

b) Data of Pathology

The orbs here discussed may be affected by depletion or by repletion; it is symptoms of the latter which prevail in practice.

---

[93] Here, as in subsequent sections, the reader should consult the folding table and, if he is curious for more details, the corresponding iconograms in Porkert, Theoretical Foundations...

PATHOLOGY

For example, the disease mechanism of ventus internus ("internal wind") may be defined as follows: Lesions of the o. hepaticus produced by emotions[94] impair the normal outflow of energy from the o. hepaticus, producing congestions eventually leading to "glare" (ardor) o. hepatici. As a consequence of this ardor, the storage (and control) of active energies may be impaired - which then will produce the symptoms of ventus internus. In connection with these, depending upon the gravity of the disease, signs of calor repletionis such as congestion of energy in the o. hepaticus, flaring up of the yang o. hepatici or erratic movement[95] of the yang o. hepatici may be observed.

Another disturbance observed rather frequently is that kind of repletion which had been induced by algor externus retained in the conduits of the o. hepaticus, there producing congestive symptoms.

Quite a different etiology ensues if, because of deficiency of the structive energies in the o. renalis ("kidney orb"), the structive potential (jing) is not sufficiently transformed into xue ("individually specific structive energy") so that the functions of the o. hepaticus receive insufficient energetic support. In this case we may observe deficiency of yin o. hepatici and, as a consequence, inanitas-symptoms because of interference effects from an upflaring yang hepaticum. These mechanisms may be summed up in the following table:

Disease Mechanisms of the orbis hepaticus

Agent	Differential Diagnosis	Symptoms	
Emotion	Congestion of the o. hepaticus -- ardor	ardor hepaticus flares up erratic movement of the yang o. hepatici	Repletion
algor-heteropathy	Penetration of an algor-heteropathy into the conduits -- algor -- algor blocks the conduits of the o. hepaticus --	Insufficient deployment of the energies in the conduits of the oo. hepaticus et felleus	
Deficiency of the yin o.renalis	Insufficient maintenance of the functions of the o.hepaticus --	Deficiency of the structive energies of the o. hepaticus Interference from the uncontrolled yang hepaticum	Depletion

---

[94] This refers primarily to the emotion corresponding specifically to the orbis hepaticus, viz. ira, wrath; yet it may include any other sudden eruption or pent-up feelings.

[95] Chinese: wangdong, literally an "erratic movement" or an "incalculable move".

Clinical Symptoms of Disturbances of the oo. hepaticus et felleus

Vento percussio [stroke], vertigo oculorum [vertigo], headache, spastic pareses, epilepsy, flexus occaecans [syncopes with cold extremities], concretiones et congelationes [neoplasias and indurations], tinnitus, deafness, chordapsus [hernias and other abdominal disturbances], epistaxis, hemoptoea, excitability, insomnia, loss of sensitivity or atrophy, tremor.

Differential Diagnosis

a - Symptoms of Repletion

1. Congestion of the Active Energies of the Hepatic Orb (qi orbis hepatici)

a) Disease Mechanism: Suppressed wrath or similar emotions have affected the total function of the o. hepaticus. As a consequence, the energetic quality defined by the E.P. Wood and, manifesting itself through imagination, inventiveness, initiative and resoluteness, cannot develop harmoniously. Instead, encroachments or contravections of the qi hepaticum (i.e. of the active energies of the o. hepaticus), general lack of force and drive, pains and congelationes [indurations] will appear; indirectly, hematomas and congestions, spastic tensions, tympanites, constipation and finally concretiones [neoplasias] may ensue.

b) Special Symptoms: Painful flanks, eructations, abdominal ache accompanied by diarrhea which brings no relief; concretiones aut congelationes [palpable indurations in the regions of the abdomen and the plexus]; thin coating of the tongue; stringy pulses (pp. chordales). The patient complains of pains in his flanks which prevent him from lying on his side. This kind of pain is induced by congested energy, due to repletion. Contravections in the digestive tract may lead to the vomiting of bile.
The unusual symptom of abdominal pains combined with diarrhea producing no relief, is due to the suppressed or misdirected emotions.

Localized indurations (concretiones) may appear below the small ribs whereas congelationes may be observled sporadically and intermittently; but both are accompanied by pains of turgescence, by lancinating pains. In addition, there may be symptoms of irascibility and loss of appetite.

c) Therapy: Dispulsio of heteropathies in the o. hepaticus, normalization of the energy flow, cracking the concretiones, dispersing the congelationes.

PATHOLOGY

2. Flaring up Glare of the o. hepaticus (ardor o. hepatici)

a) Disease Mechanism: The energy flow from the oo. hepaticus et felleus is drastically reduced so that subsequent congestion leads to ardor ("glare"). This "glare" is transported by the qi to the different body sites, possibly even to the top of the skull.

b) Special Symptoms: Pains below the small ribs as a consequence of ardor. Bitter or bilious vomiting. Vertigo, hot head accompanied by piercing, more rarely by dull headache; uncontrollable twitching of the muscles, pulsations in different parts of the body. Intense tinnitus and deafness, decreasing and increasing intermittently, not relieved by pressure on the foramina of the ear. Intensely red borders of the eyelids, very painful, sometimes swollen; intense, profuse sudden hemorrhage from the nose and the mouth. Difficulty of urination, yellow or reddish urine; hot red face; dry mouth, bitter taste; fits of wrath; intensely coloured tip and margins of the tongue; yellow or dry or sticky coating of the tongue; stringy and accelerated pulses (pp. chordales et celeri).

c) Therapy: Dispulsio oo. hepatici et felleus, refrigeratio caloris.

3. Erratic Movement of the yang o. hepatici

a) Disease Mechanism: If the qi hepaticum (i.e. the active energy of the liver orb) changes into "glare" (ardor), a dramatic expansion of yang, of active energy, will ensue. "Glare" will spread with active energy throughout the individual and will rush uncontrolled through the conduits. This will eventually start the xue ("individually specific structure energy") also, moving upwards until it strikes the top of the skull. This syndrome is called "ventus hepaticus rising within".

b) Special Symptoms: Flexus occaecans [Sudden syncope with cold extremities, spastic twitchings, phlegm flowing from the mouth]; spasms with stiff neck or contracted extremities; pareses, loss of sensitivity, sometimes pricking sensations in the hands, feet, the face and lips; vertigo in the wake of piercing headache. After awaking from the syncope, sometimes unilateral paresis or paralysis of the extremities and of the facial muscles; oscillating tongue, blurred speech. Red body of the tongue, yellow coating of the tongue, stringy pulses (pp. chordales).

c) Therapy: Pacactio o. hepatici ("Sedation of the active energies of the liver orb"), pacatio venti hepatici.

4. Algor ("Cold") Blocks the Conduits of the o. hepaticus

a) Disease Mechanism: An exogenous algor-heteropathy has penetrated into the conduits of the o. hepaticus, i.e. the sinarteriae yin flectentis pedis, there reducing or completely blocking the energy flow.

b) Special Symptoms: Tension or pain in the abdomen which may radiate into the scrotum and testicles; swelling of the testicles, contraction of the scrotum. White coating of the tongue; glistening, slippery tongue; submerged as well as stringy or slowed down pulses (pp. mersi aut chordales et tardi).

c) Therapy: Tepefactio orbis et cardinalium hepatici ("Application of warm remedies to the liver orb and its conduits").

b - Inanitas ("exhaustion")-Symptoms

1. Deficiency of the Yin o. hepatici

a) Disease Mechanism: The o. hepaticus, as indicated by its qualification by means of the E.P. Wood, indirectly constitutes a yang orb[96], hence, for its structive part requires that its energy level be maintained from aqua renalis, i.e. the energy emanating from the o. renalis. A deficiency of the structive energy in the o. renalis consequently will affect the transformation of structive potential (jing) into xue ("individually specific structive energy"). And the latter is indispensable for maintaining the material, i.e. structive part of the o. hepaticus. Thus a deficiency of the yin hepaticum may ensue, and as a consequence of this, encroachments of the yang hepaticum will be observed.

b) Special Symptoms: Headache with vertigo oculorum; tinnitus, gradually setting in and of moderate intensity, cannot be influenced by covering the ears; deafness, pareses, paresthesias of the extremities; twitching muscles of the extremities, improved by massage; night blindness and reduced secretion of tears; hot, red face and red spots on the cheeks in the afternoon; dry mouth and throat; little sleep, numerous dreams. Red body of the tongue, dry or almost dry; reduced coating of the tongue; minute, stringy, accelerated pulses (pp. minuti, chordales, celeri).

---

[96] Cf. the general remarks made in Porkert, Theoretical Foundations... pp. 111 ff as well as the corresponding iconogram of the hepatic orb, pp. 117 ff.

PATHOLOGY 71

c) Therapy: Softening[97] of the energies of the o. hepaticus (Compensation of its yang [hard quality]); rigatio (suppletive moistening, replenishing of the structive energies) of the o. renalis; sustentatio yin; demissio yang ("pushing down the active energy").

c - Complex Symptoms

1. The Energy of the o. hepaticus Affects the o. stomachi

a) Symptoms: Pain or the feeling of a lump in the stomach; radiating pains below the small ribs; digestive block, malodorous or sour eructations. Thin and yellow coating of the tongue; stringy pulses (pp. chordales).

b) Therapy: Dispulsio (Dispelling) redundant energies from the oo. hepaticus et stomachi.

2. Disharmony between the o. hepaticus and the o. lienalis

a) Symptoms: Poor appetite, no thirst; distended abdomen, noisy rumbling in the intestines; diarrhea; white and sticky coating of the tongue; stringy or languid pulses (pp. chordales sive languidi).

b) Therapy: Compositio (harmonization) of the energies of the o. hepaticus et lienalis.

3. Restive Functions of the oo. hepaticus et felleus

a) Symptoms: Restiveness and exhaustion, insomnia, also nightmares with terrified awakening; the patient is timid and easily startled; he is short of breath, easily exhausted, has impaired vision, bitter taste in the mouth. The coating of his tongue is thin and white, his pulses are stringy or minute (pp. chordales sive minuti).

b) Therapy: Sustentatio (conservation) of the energies of the o. hepaticus and refrigeratio of the o. felleus; sedation of the shen (the configurative force).

4. Inanitas of the Structive Energies in the o. hepaticus et renalis

a) Symptoms: Exhausted, tired physiognomy, faintly pink cheeks; dizziness, pains in the eyes because of reduced secretions; weak and painful back and knees; dry and

---

[97] The Chinese term rou expresses that its yang quality ("hardness") is to be conpensated, mitigated.

painful throat; tongue of deep red colour without coating; minute pulses.

b) Therapy: <u>Rigatio yin, refrigeratio ardoris</u> ("Moistening, replenishing structive energy and cooling the glare").

5. Glare (<u>ardor</u>) in the <u>o. hepaticus</u> Affects the <u>o. pulmonalis</u>[98]

a) Symptoms: Sharp pains in the chest and flanks, fits of coughing; coughing up light red blood; increased irascibility and irritability; the patient feels oppressive heat, has a bitter taste in the mouth, is seized by vertigo, has red-bordered eyelids, the body of his tongue is intensely red; the coating of the tongue is reduced in thickness; there are stringy and accelerated pulses (<u>pp. chordales et celeri</u>).

b) Therapy: <u>Refrigeratio o. hepaticus, dispulsio o. pulmonalis.</u>

Synthetic Table of the Symptoms related to the <u>orbis hepaticus</u>

Diagnosis	General Symptoms	B. & C. of Tongue	Pulses	Relations with Other Orbs
Ardor ("Glare") in the o. hepaticus	Red, swollen and painful eyelids, feeling of heat in the thorax, palpitations, great irritability. Restive sleep, bitter taste, dry mouth; yellow or reddish urine.	Deep red colour of the margins and tip of the tongue	Striny and accelerated (pp. chordales et celeri)	Danger of inducing glare in the o. cardialis
The yang ("active energy") of the o. hepaticus flares upwards	Vertigo, great irascibility, heavy head and feet; also numbness of the fingers and hands, tension in the ribs and lower chest, headache in the temples.	Body of the tongue red to crimson red	Stringy or tense (pp. chordales sive intenti)	These symptoms may be due to a deficiency of the structive energy of the o. renalis.
Ventus hepaticus	Disturbed vacillating vision; numbness or twitching of the muscles in different parts of the body; also convulsive cramps of the hands and feet; tetanic distortions.	Vibrating tongue or tongue pulled to one side; white coating of the tongue	Stringy and exhausted (pp. chordales et inanes)	Factors producing these symptoms may be a deficiency of the energy of the o. renalis or an inanitas xue ("exhaustion of the individually specific structive energy"), as the consequence of which ventus may result from excessive heat.
Congested energy in the o. hepaticus	Headache and vertigo, tension or pains in the flanks; also distension of the abdomen and menstrual troubles	Slightly red body of the tongue, thickly coated.	Stringy, accelerated, also submerged and stringy	

---

[98] According to the "violation sequence" of the E.P.s; cf. Porkert, <u>Theoretical Foundations...</u> p. 53.

PATHOLOGY

Diagnosis	General Symptoms	B.& C. of Tongue	Pulses	Relations with Other Orbs
Algor in the o.hepaticus	Piercing pains in the lower abdomen, tense or convulsed nervus ("muscles and sinews") and conduits; hence radiating pains into the scrotum; also pains at the top of the skull and vomit- of transparent mucus.	Bluish or purple body of the tongue, humid and slippery coating of the tongue	Submerged and stringy or slowed-down (pp. mersi et chordales aut tardi)	

DISEASES OF THE orbes cardialis et intestini tenuis ("HEART AND SMALL INTESTINE ORBS")

a. Orbisiconographic Data

The specific unfoldment (perfectio) of the functions of the yoked oo. cardialis et intestini tenuis are the sinarteries (= conduits)[99], more exactly the conduits (xuemo, xuemai) carrying the individually specific structive energy (xue). The corresponding sense organ is the tongue.

The o. cardialis is considered the seat and storehouse of configurative force (shen), consequently of the influence or force lending each personality its individual qualities and ensuring its cohesion and integration; thus the o. cardialis is compared to the "prince" among all orbs, from which emanates clear insight and all orienting influences.

There is a close interrelationship between the functions of the oo. cardialis et intestini tenuis on the one hand and those of the o. pericardialis and tricalorii on the other.

b. Pathological Data

As may be deduced from the data of orbisiconography, disturbances of the oo. cardialis et intestini tenuis directly affect the flow of structive energy and the emotional projection of the personality. In the case of contravective encroachments of heteropathies due to morbi temperati[100] [infectious diseases], the o. pericardialis

---

[99] Cf. op. cit. p. 126.

[100] On the Chinese term wenxie cf. pp. 113 ff. below.

usually is affected first as the "outer defence"[101] of the system. By contrast, if the o. cardialis is directly affected, its disturbance is due to inner lesions (neishang)[102] or to constitutive inborn weakness; it may also occur in the wake of very serious general disease, or as the consequence of exaggerated cogitatio[103]. No matter whether in such cases the structive or the active part of the energies of the o. cardialis has been more seriously impaired, there will always be repercussions on the configurative force (shen), consequently on the cohesion of the personality, on its self-confidence and self-assertion, on its coherence and consistency.

If the orbis cardialis is affected by congested emotions, sticky mucus may result as the consequence of "glare" (ardor) - and penetrate upwards. The result will be congestions and blocks of the energy flow in the cardinal and reticular conduits and repletive symptoms of all kinds.

Disease Mechanisms of the o. cardialis

Agents	Differential Diagnosis	Symptoms	
Constitutional weakness Energetic deficiency of the orb Malfunction as the consequence of disease	Deficiency of the qi cardiale, Deficiency of the xue cardiale	Deficiency of the shen, of the configurative force	→ inanitas
Excessive cogitation (intellectual stress) ↓ Congestion, Agglutination ↓ obstructio qi	Pituita-heteropathy ("mucus"-heteropathy) ardor ("glare") --→ sticky pituita ("mucus") penetrates upwards and blocks the o. pericardialis	Obstruction of the yang cardiale Congested flow of energy→ Hematomas etc.	→ repletio

---

[101] The Chinese term waiwei, 'outer defense', is sometimes applied to the pericardial orb; cf. Porkert, Theoretical Foundations... p. 147.

[102] The reader should always keep in mind that by lesions (shang), Chinese medicine designates any kind of noxious effect. Consequently, the significance of the term is not restricted to mechanical lesions; in fact it does not even apply to these preponderantly.

[103] If it is true that cogitation primarily affects the lienal orb, by indirectly depleting the cardial orb, the latter, too, becomes depleted of energy.

PATHOLOGY 75

Clinical Symptoms Accompanying Malfunctions of the oo. cardialis et intestini tenuis

Palpitations, heartache; forgetfulness; insomnia; loss of semen; dementia, mental disease; laboured breathing, asthma; hemoptoea, epistaxis; ulcers on the tongue and apthae; hematuria etc.

Differential Diagnoses

a - Inanitas-symptoms

1. Inanitas yang cardialis ("Exhaustion of the Active Energy of the Heart Orb")

a) Disease Mechanism: Deficiency, induced by excessive cogitation and its concomitant, unproportional use of energy in the oo. lienalis et cardialis.

b) Special Symptoms: Palpitations; asthmatic states; acute heart pains. Colourless to whitish coating of the tongue; minute or infirm pulses (pp. minuti et invalidi) or large and exhausted pulses (pp. magni et inanes).
The palpitations are accompanied by precordial fear and the fear of imminent heart failure; they are aggravated by movement; asthma attacks, aggravated by movement; intense heart attacks with cold extremities, racing or accelerated pulses (pp. concitati sive celeri) or even dispersed (diffundentes) pulses; in extreme cases, increasing cyanosis of the tips of the nose and of the lips or waxen physiognomy, spontaneous perspiration, cold skin.

c) Therapy: Tepefactio yang cardialis, suppletio qi cardialis (the administration of warm or suppletive remedies bolstering the active energies of the heart orb.)

2. Inanitas yin cardialis ("Exhaustion of the Structive Energies of the Heart Orb")

a) Disease Mechanism: Identical emotional factors as under 1., yet a different constitutional situation, have brought on a deficiency of all kinds of structive energy, hence of xue (individually specific structive energy, practically identical with ying, "constructive energy", and also of jing, "structive potential"). Thus active energies of the o. cardialis have an insufficient basis and are dispersed uncontrolled.

b) Special Symptoms: Palpitations accompanied by fear and nervousness; sleep fleeting and shallow, disturbed by nightmares; nausea accompanied by burning pains or hunger pangs; also forgetfulness, loss of semen, perspiration during sleep; very often a distrustful yet easy to deceive person.

c) Therapy: <u>Rigatio yin, suppletio xue orbis cardialis; pacatio shen</u> (the use of remedies to humectate and complete the structive energies of the yin, and in particular of the yin of the heart orb, the use of sedatives - in the sense of Chinese pharmacology - to contain the configurative force.)

b - Repletion Symptoms

1. Irritation of the <u>orbis cardialis</u> by <u>ardor</u>-induced pituita ("Mucus" induced by "Glare")

a) Disease Mechanism: Emotions violently suppressed have produced inner glare (<u>ardor</u>) which in turn leads to the formation of tough mucus (<u>pituita, tan</u>) affecting the functions of the <u>orbis pericardialis et cardialis,</u> and pushing out the configurative force (<u>shen</u>) from its regular system, the <u>o. cardialis.</u>

b) Special Symptoms: Continuous palpitations, accompanied by stabbing pains in the heart and hot flushes; disturbed mind with raving speech, in extreme cases crying and laughing without reason; insomnia accompanied by excitation and nightmares. The patient may further show a red face, thirst and the desire to have cold drinks; there may be hemoptea, epistaxis, reddish urine, even hematuria with troubles of micturition. The body of the tongue is intensely red or scarlet, sometimes dry and cracked, with reduced coating. The pulses are slippery and accelerated (<u>pp. lubrici et celeri</u>).

c) Therapy: <u>Refrigeratio o. cardialis, exstillatio humoris, demissio ardoris</u> (thus the use of cooling remedies, of remedies drawing off mucus, of remedies "pressing down" (<u>zhen</u>) the glare).

2. A <u>Pituita</u>-heteropathy Checks and Obstructs the Deployment of the Yang of the <u>orbis cardialis.</u>

a) Disease Mechanism: Congested or deeply hidden <u>pituita</u> ("mucus") formed in the thorax region and obstructing the deployment and the distribution of active energies of the <u>o. cardialis.</u>

b) Special Symptoms: Palpitations accompanied by oppressive feeling in the thorax and laboured breathing; vertigo, sometimes accompanied by nausea; vomiting of mucus and saliva; sometimes also shuddering, feeling of a lump in the plexus regions, noisy rumble in the intestines. White and sticky coating of the tongue; slippery or submerged and tense pulses (pp. lubrici sive mersi et intenti).

c) Therapy: Transformatio et exstillatio pituitae (the use of remedies affecting the transformation or evacuation of sticky mucus.)

3. Stagnation of the xue cardiale ("Individually Specific Structure Energy of the Heart Orb")

a) Disease Mechanism: The o. cardialis has been affected by excessive stress; thus its (active) energies are not deployed to the extent required - leading to stagnation of the energy flow of the structive energies in the conduits. The result is a breakdown of the harmonious flow of energy in the complete system of cardinal and reticular conduits.

b) Special Symptoms: Palpitations with nervousness, lancinating pains in the chest, the flanks, the back and the shoulders. The body of the tongue is intensely red, sometimes showing blue-red stripes or spots. The coating of the tongue is reduced. There are grating pulses (pp. asperi).

c) Therapy: Animatio xue (revival of the movement of the xue through the use of appropriate drugs), restitution of the energy flow in the reticular conduits, breaking up the stagnation.

c - Complex Symptoms

1. Inanitas in the orbis cardialis as well as in the orbis lienalis

a) Symptoms: Sallow complexion, reduced appetite, intense fatigue; the patient is short of breath, nervous and easily upset, forgetful, complaining of palpitations and disturbed sleep, irregular menses. The body of the tongue is pale, the coating is white. The pulses are minute, frail or infirm (pp. minuti, lenes, invalidi), and weak in all cases.

b) Therapy: Suppletio et augmentatio oo. cardialis et lienalis (completing and bolstering the energies of the affected orbs).

2. Insufficient Coördination between the o. cardialis and the o. renalis[104]

a) Symptoms: Insomnia induced by inanitas-nervousness; loss of semen during sleep; periodical fevers rising at the same time each day; perspiration during sleep; dry throat, dizziness, with wide open eyes; tinnitus, loins and legs feeling weak, sometimes painful; polyuria during the night. Body of the tongue intensely red, no coating; accelerated and exhausted pulses (pp. celeri et inanes).

b) Therapy: Re-establishing the rapport between the oo. cardialis et renalis.

d - Special Symptoms Related to the o. intestini tenuis (the "Small Intestine Orb")

The function of the o. intestini tenuis, within an integrate organism, is to receive and transform all food and to seperate it into clear and murky elements - passing on the first to all orbs and the latter only into the orbes intestini crassi et vesicalis. In its function as an outer complement (orbis aulicus) of the o. cardialis, it partakes of all disturbances affecting the o. cardialis; in particular it is affected by diseases accompanied by calor-symptoms.

1. Algor inanitatis intestini tenuis ("Exhaustion-induced algor of the Small Intestine Orb")

a) Symptoms: Dull pain in the lower abdomen, improved by applying pressure; rumbling noise in the intestines, diarrhea; frequent evacuation of small quantities of urine; pale body of the tongue, white and thin coating of the tongue; minute or languid pulses (pp. minuti atque languidi).

b) Therapy: Tepefactio et patefactio o. intestini tenuis (applying warm and opening remedies to the affected orbs).

2. Calor repletionis intestini tenuis ("Heat in the Wake of Repletion of the Small Intestine Orb")

a) Symptoms: Nervousness, palpitations; aphthae; sore throat; hardness of hearing; diminished, reddish urine, pains in the penis; abdominal tension and distension, slightly improved after defecation; intensely red body of the tongue, yellow coating of the

---

[104] According to the conquest sequence of the E.P.s the renal orb physiologically checks the cardial orb.

PATHOLOGY

tongue; slippery and accelerated pulses (pp. lubrici et celeri).

b) Therapy: Refrigeratio et laxatio caloris repletionis (the administration of cooling and laxative remedies to draw off and compensate the heat symptoms due to repletion).

3. Pains as the Consequence of Active Energy Blocked in the o. intestini tenuis

a) Symptoms: Intense abdominal pains, radiating into the loins, the back, the testicles; white coating of the tongue; submerged or stringy pulses (pp. mersi atque chordales) or stringy and slippery pulses (pp. chordales atque lubrici).

b) Therapy: Imparting motion to the qi, dispersal of blocked energy.

Synthetic Table of the Symptoms Related to the oo. cardialis et intestini tenuis

Diagnosis	Symptoms	Tongue	Pulses	Relations with other orbs
Inanitas o. cardialis	Palpitations, anguish; insomnia, spontaneous perspiration, reduced power of concentration and of memory.	Pale body of the tongue, reduced coating	Minute and infirm pulses pp. minuti et invalidi)	Very often the symptoms are induced by inanitas o. lienalis and by weakness of the digestive functions.
Calor o. cardialis	Oppressive feeling and heat in the thorax; thirst, secretion of diminshed reddish urine	Intensely red body of the tongue, tip of the tongue crimson to scarlet; some times red spots on the tongue	Accelerated (pp. celeri)	Induced by redundancy of the energies in the o. hepaticus
Calor extends to the o. pericardialis	Restiveness accompanying high fever, daze, confused speech	Intensely red body of the tongue	Flooding and accelerated (pp. exundantes et celeri)	Often induced by exogenous heteropathies provoking calor-symptoms
Thick pituita impairs the configurative force and the sensorium	Impaired senses and emotions	Coating of the tongue very thick and dirt coloured	Flooding and replete or submerged and slippery	1. Induced by inner lesions of erratic emotions; 2. Induced by fever diseases or ventus internus.
Algor inanitatis o. intestini tenuis	Pains in the abdomen, diarrhea; faeces mixed with chunks of undigested food; frequent evacuation of small quantities of urine	Body of the tongue pale to red; coating thin or white	Minute, with a tendency to infirmity (pp. minuti, invalidi,) particularly in evidence at the left pedal site.	

Diagnosis	Symptoms	Tongue	Pulses	Relations with other orbs
Calor repletionis o. intestini tenuis	Nervous restlessness; diminished reddish urine; pains in the penis; turgidness or tenseness around the navel, improved by the evacuation of faeces	Body of the tongue crimson; yellow coating of the tongue	Slippery and accelerated, in particular at the left pedal site	May be due to calor in the cardinal conduit of the o. cardialis thus transmitting it to the o. intestini tenuis.
Pains induced by the congestion of active energy within the o. intestini tenuis	Tension and pain in the abdomen which may radiate into the loins and hips region or into the scrotum and the testicles.	White coating	Submerged and stringy or stringy and slippery (pp. mersi et chordales sive chordales et lubrici.	

DISEASES IN THE orbes lienalis et stomachi ("SPLEEN AND STOMACH ORBS")

a) Data of Orbisiconography

The functional yoke uniting the o. lienalis and the o. stomachi has the specific unfoldment of its functions ("perfectio") in the flesh (caro), i.e. those tissues which determine the outward shape of the body; their specific body opening is the mouth. The most evident function of the oo. lienalis et stomachi is the assimilation, transformation and distribution of the energies entering the body as food (which may briefly be stored there); more important, however, the function of these orbs, in particular that of the orbis lienalis, clearly indicated by its qualification by the E.P. Earth, is the integration and harmonization of all energetic processes within the individual, i.e. the exchange between different orbs as well as the integration of outward stimuli and influences, be these of intellectual, psychic, social or cosmic origin. The o. lienalis thus maintains the balance between all energies and functions qualified by peripheral E.P.s and is considered the "seat of the constructive energy" (ying) and the "root of the acquired constitution"[105].

b) Pathological Data

The orthopathic functions of the oo. lienalis (et stomachi), consequently, may be

---

[105] Cf. Porkert, Theoretical Foundations... pp. 128 - 136.

PATHOLOGY

impaired by malnutrition (in excess or in deficit), by excessive cogitatio, by climatic excesses, in particular humor (excessive humidity) and, of course, by excessive emotional stress overtaxing the integrating faculty of the individual. As is the case with other orbs also, disease of the o. lienalis may also be due to a constitutional weakness or to heteropathic factors transmitted from other orbs. The result of the pathogenic influences enumerated first, usually is repletion, that of the latter, almost always exhaustion.

Disease Mechanisms of the orbis lienalis

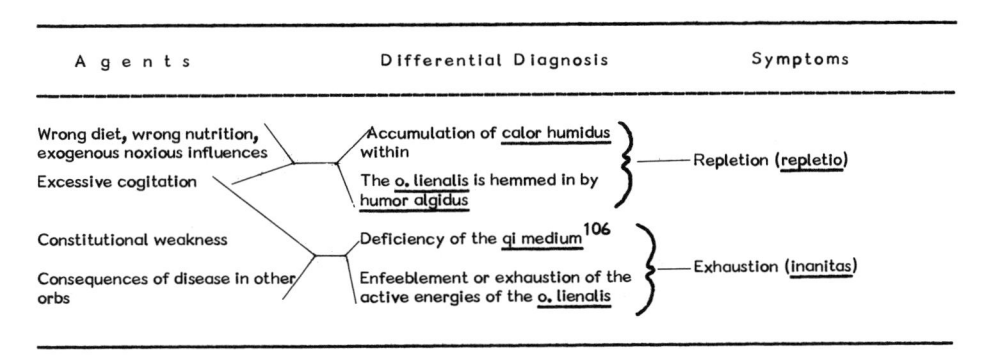

Agents	Differential Diagnosis	Symptoms
Wrong diet, wrong nutrition, exogenous noxious influences	Accumulation of calor humidus within	Repletion (repletio)
Excessive cogitation	The o. lienalis is hemmed in by humor algidus	
Constitutional weakness	Deficiency of the qi medium[106]	Exhaustion (inanitas)
Consequences of disease in other orbs	Enfeeblement or exhaustion of the active energies of the o. lienalis	

c) Clinical Symptoms Indicating Disturbances of the o. lienalis et stomachi

Fluid stools and diarrhea; cholera; icterus; stomachache; vomiting, eructations; ascites, tympanites; pituita ("phlegm"), hemoptea; miscarriage.

d) Differential Diagnoses

a - Symptoms of Exhaustion (inanitas)

1. The Active Energy of the o. lienalis is Exhausted and Enfeebled (yang lienale inanis et dilabens)

a) Disease Mechanism: Due to the absorption of unboiled (raw) cold, sweet or fat food, as the consequence of the excessive use of cold or cool remedies[107], or as the

---

[106] In this term 'medium', 'central', refers to the E.P. Earth, qualifying the o. lienalis.

[107] I.e. drugs which, due to their pharmacodynamic quality, reduce calor - so-called medicamenta refrigerantia. Cf. Porkert, Klinische chinesische Pharmakologie, pp. 144 - 210.

consequence of protracted illness impairing the active energy of the o. lienalis, these energies have become decrepit - thus enfeebling the integrative and distributive functions of the orb.

b) Special Symptoms: Pale, bloodless complexion; feeling of coldness or of splashing fluid in the stomach; tympanites, weak digestive function, desire to absorb hot beverages; diarrhea, plentiful light urine; sometimes general emaciation, always cold extremities; laboured breathing, reluctance to speak; pale body of the tongue, white coating of the tongue; frail or infirm pulses (pp. lenes aut invalidi).

c) Therapy: Tepefactio et animatio yang medii (the application of warm or dynamizing remedies acting upon the active energies of the oo. lienalis et stomachi).

2. Deficiency of the qi medium (Deficiency of the Active Energies in the Central Orbs, i.e. the "Spleen and Stomach Orbs")

a) Disease Mechanism: Either as the consequence of a constitutional inanitas or of prolonged illness, the active energies of the oo. lienalis et stomachi have been reduced; as a consequence, the separation of clear and murky energies takes place without vigour.

b) Special Symptoms: Reduced appetite and weak digestion; halting, faltering speech; general lack of vigour; rumbling noise in the intestines, tumescent abdomen, frequent defecation or diarrhea; sometimes general emaciation and rapid exhaustion; prolapsus ani. Pale body of the tongue, white coating of the tongue; languid or frail and minute pulses (pp. languidi or pp. lenes et minuti).

c) Therapy: Elevatio yang, suppletio qi (the application of remedies lifting up, exteriorizing activity, completing the active energies).

b - Repletion Symptoms

1. The Function of the o. lienalis is Hemmed in by humor algidus ("Cold Humidity")

a) Disease Mechanism: As a consequence of prolonged, unwholesome contact with water, e.g. when fording a river or after having been drenched by rain, or after prolonged sojourn in humid places, the active energies of the central orbs (i.e. the oo. lienalis et stomachi) have gradually been hemmed in as the result of the excessive

PATHOLOGY 83

presence of (structive) humidity. The consequence is a notable impairment of the functions of these orbs.

b) Special Symptoms: The patient abhors the smell of food; he feels satiated, has a sweetish taste in the mouth, a sticky tongue; he feels dazed, greatly fatigued; his faeces are soft or diarrheic; white and sticky coating of the tongue; frail and minute pulses (pp. lenes et minuti).

c) Therapy: Restoration of the dynamics of the energy of the affected orb and transformation of the "humidity" (transformatio humoris).

2. Calor humidus ("Humid Heat") has Accumulated Within

a) Disease Mechanism: The functions of the oo. lienalis et stomachi have either been affected by an exogenous heteropathy or by the excessive ingestion of alcohol. Consequently, the energy circulation has been impaired because the combination of "humidity" and "heat" (humor & calor), and the flow of structive energies, i.e. of the fluids, has been slowed down. Therefore, the structive energies of the o. felleus will not follow its normal path but, instead, impregnate the flesh, i.e the perfectio of the o. lienalis.

b) Special Symptoms: Complete loss of appetite, with turgescence and pressure in the stomach region and flanks; extreme fatigue; yellow colour of the scleras, of the complexion and of the body; itching skin; urine reduced in quantity and of reddish colour; yellow and sticky coating of the tongue; frail and accelerated pulses (pp. lenes et celeri). - Occasional symptoms are also: thirst, bitter taste, diarrhea, fever.

c) Therapy: Refrigeratio caloris, exstillatio humoris (the application of cooling remedies to combat calor, of diuretic remedies to evacuate excessive humidity).

c - Complex Symptoms

1. Lost Harmony Between the oo. lienalis et stomachi

a) Symptoms: Feeling of a lump in the stomach, persistent tensive, slight pain; weak digestion; hiccup, eructation, even vomiting; thin white coating of the tongue; minute pulses.

b) Therapy: <u>Augmentatio qi, compositio</u> (applying remedies increasing the active energies in the affected orbs, re-establishing the circulation of energy, harmonizing the exchange of energy).

2. <u>Inanitas yang orbium lienalis et renalis</u> ("Exhaustion of Yang in the Spleen and Kidney Orbs")

a) Symptoms: Laboured breathing; reluctant speech; the patient feels cold, with cold hands and feet; great propensity to perspire; soft faeces and diarrhea, also diarrhea including undigested food. Pale red body of the tongue, thin whitish coating of the tongue. Submerged and minute pulses (<u>pp. mersi et minuti</u>).

b) Therapy: <u>Suppletio o. lienalis, tepefactio o. renalis</u> (applying remedies strengthening the <u>o. lienalis</u> and re-enforcing the active function of the <u>o. renalis</u>).

3. <u>Humor lienalis</u> Affects the <u>o. pulmonalis</u> ("Humidity in the Spleen Orb Affects the Function of the Lung Orb")

a) Symptoms: Cough with sticky or clear sputum, pressure on the chest, shortness of breath; reduced appetite; white, somewhat sticky coating of the tongue; slippery pulses (<u>pp. lubrici</u>).

b) Therapy: <u>Tepefactio, transformatio pituitae</u> (applying remedies absorbing the humidity and transforming the phlegm).

4. <u>Inanitas orbium cardialis et lienalis</u> (For this cf. the cardial orb above)

d - Particular Symptoms of the <u>orbis stomachi</u>

One of the functions of the <u>o. stomachi</u> is to act as a regulating reservoir (<u>mare, hai</u>) for all energies absorbed from food and beverages. In its role as yang-complement (<u>orbis aulicus</u>) of the <u>o. lienalis</u>, it is qualified as <u>humus aridus</u> ("dry E.P. Earth") - which in turn expresses the particularity that the <u>o. stomachi</u>, unlike the <u>o. lienalis</u>, requires humidity and abhors dryness. If symptoms of congested or dry heat occur, these very often are a hint of a disturbance of the <u>o. stomachi</u>.

1. <u>Algor stomachi</u> ("A Cold Heteropathy in the Stomach Orb")

a) Symptoms: Feeling of satiety, tension, persistent pain in the region of the

PATHOLOGY

stomach, improved by the application of warmth or pressure; eructation of clear fluid, hiccup, white and slippery coating of the tongue; slowed-down pulses (pp. tardi).

b) Therapy: Tepefactio o. stomachi, dispulsio algoris (the application of warm remedies acting upon the o. stomachi, and effecting the dispersion of the cold-heteropathy)

2. Calor stomachi ("A Heat Heteropathy affecting the Stomach Orb")

a) Symptoms: The patient is thirsty and asks for cold drinks; his digestion is good, his appetite is increased; noisy vomiting or immediate vomiting of ingested food; bad smell from the mouth; toothache, painful, swollen, ulcerated, bleeding gums; reduced secretion of saliva; scarlet body of the tongue, yellow coating of the tongue; slippery and accelerated pulses (pp. lubrici et celeri).

b) Therapy: Refrigeratio o. stomachi, dispulsio ardoris (the application of remedies cooling the "heat"-heteropathies in the o. stomachi and dispelling the "glare").

3. Inanitas stomachi ("Exhaustion of the Energies of the Stomach Orb")

a) Symptoms: Feeling of satiety or of a lump in the stomach; sluggish digestion, sometimes eructations, loose stools; reduced coating of the tongue; frail pulses (pp. lenes).

b) Therapy: Augmentatio qi, suppletio qi medii (using remedies completing and increasing the energetic resources of the central orbs, i.e. the oo. lienalis et stomachi).

4. Repletio stomachi ("Repletion in the Stomach Orb")

a) Symptoms: Satiety, reluctance to eat, surfeit; constipation; bad smell from the mouth and foul eructations; also vomiting; yellow coating of the tongue, slippery pulses (pp. lubrici).

b) Therapy: Dispulsio (dispersion) of the congested energies.

THE ESSENTIALS OF CHINESE DIAGNOSTICS

Synthetic Table of the Symptoms Related to Diseases of the oo. lienalis et stomachi

Diagnosis	Symptoms	Tongue	Pulses	Relations
The qi lienale is exhausted (inanis) and without vigour (invalidus)	Reduced appetite, turgid abdomen, diarrhea, weak extremities; there may also occur emaciation, swellings, hematuria, gynecological hemorrhages.	The body of the tongue is pale, the coating is thin and slippery	Exhausted or languid pulses (pp. inanes sive languidi)	
The yang lienale is not deployed	Persistent tensive pains in the abdomen, diarrhea with watery stools, cold extremities; retention of urine	The body of tongue is pale and turgid, also very sensitive	Submerged, slowed down pulses (pp. mersi et tardi)	This situation is frequently induced by deficiency of the yang renale or by a loss of vigour in the porta furtunae.
Humor ("Humidity") hems in the specific energies of the o. lienalis: humor lienalis	Heavy, dazed head, fatigue, great prostration of the body and of the limbs; depressed breathing and reduced appetite. There may also occur ikterus - with much sticky phlegm in the mouth and on the tongue.	Gluey, sticky coating	Frail and languid (lenes et languidi)	
Algor o. stomachi	Pains in the stomach, improved by applying warmth or pressure; expectoration of clear phlegm; during seizures of pain: cold extrmities.	White and slippery coating	Submerged and slowed down, especially at the clusa of the right hand – which will become recondite (subreptus) during heavy seizures of pain.	
Calor o. stomachi	Thirst and the desire to absorb huge quantities of beverage; frequnt hunger, with rumbling noise in the stomach; bad breath; painful and swollen gums.	Scarlet colour-ed body of the tongue; reduced secretion of saliva	Slippery and accelerated (lubrici et celeri)	
Inanitas orbis stomachi	Feeling of a lump in the stomach, sometimes loud eructations; loss of appetite; loose diarrheic stools.	The body of the tongue is pale; the coating is reduced, or it may be totally lacking in the centre.	Infirm pulses (pp. in-validi); there may also be a soft (mollis) infirm pulse restricted to the clusa of the right hand.	These symptoms are related to the weakness or exhaustion of the active energies of the o. lienalis.
Repletio orbis stomachi	Surfeit, tension and pain in the stomach region, improved by the application of pressure; there may also occur sour, foul repletion, the vomiting of sour food; constipation.	Yellow and thick coating	Slippery, large or or submerged and replete (lubrici, magni sive mersi et repleti)	These symptoms are connected with calor repletionis o. intest. crassi

PATHOLOGY

DISEASES OF THE oo. pulmonalis et intestini crassi ("Lung and Large Intestine Orbs")

a) Orbisiconographic Data

The o. pulmonalis is linked with the orbis intestini crassi in a functional yoke. The body opening as well as the sense organ corresponding to this is the nose and its olfactory faculty. The skin and the body hair are considered the 'specific unfoldment' (perfectio) of the functions of the o. pulmonalis Since the defensive energy[108] is essentially deployed in the skin, the o. pulmonalis has an eminent role within the defense system of each individual. The specific function of the o. pulmonalis within the concert of all other orbs is that of a "Governor of all rhythm", in other words, it gives the rhythmic cue for the deployment of energy at all levels of the personality.

b) Pathological Data

The kind of disturbances we meet with in connection with the o. pulmonalis may be directly deduced from the orbisiconographic data[109]. Irregular life habits, disruption of the rhythm between day and night, extremes of cold or heat, abrupt changes of temperature, chemical or mechanical agents affecting the respiratory system and, not to be forgotten, extreme gradients of energy between certain orbs, put a particular strain on the rhythm-imposing system of the o. pulmonalis, and may impair its functions. Such impairment may become manifest as energetic exhaustion, accroachment, or congestion in the wake of algor or pituita.

c) Clinical Symptoms Accompanying Disturbances of the o. pulmonalis (et intestini crassi)

Influenza-type affections, cough, panting, shortness of breath [phthisis, phthisic affections; bronchitis, bronchopyelitis; ulcers of the lungs]; loss of voice, hemoptea, epistaxis; piercing pains in the thorax etc.

---

[108] On the Chinese term weiqi = qi defensivum cf. Porkert, Theoretical Foundations... pp. 188 ff.

[109] For this iconogram cf. op. cit. pp. 136 - 140.

Disease Mechanism of the orbis pulmonalis

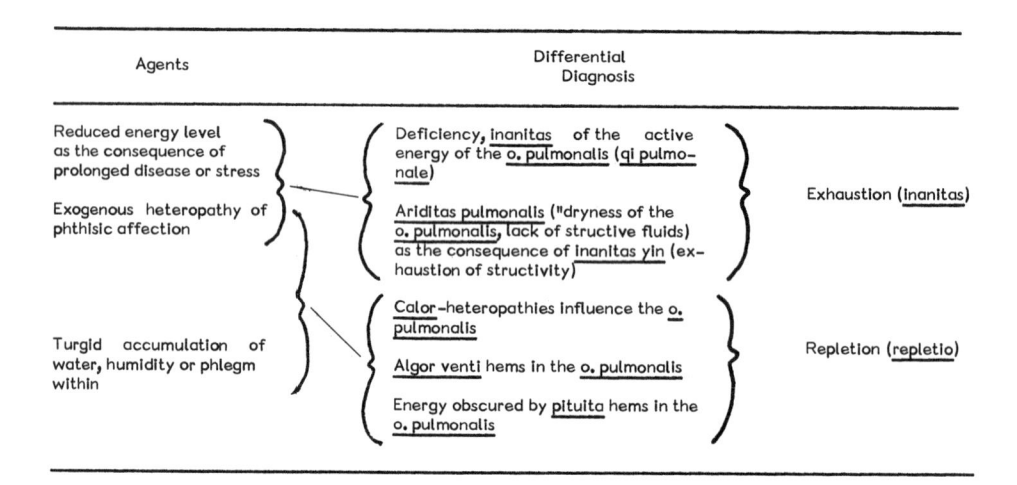

Agents	Differential Diagnosis	
Reduced energy level as the consequence of prolonged disease or stress Exogenous heteropathy of phthisic affection	Deficiency, inanitas of the active energy of the o. pulmonalis (qi pulmonale) Ariditas pulmonalis ("dryness of the o. pulmonalis, lack of structive fluids) as the consequence of inanitas yin (exhaustion of structivity)	Exhaustion (inanitas)
Turgid accumulation of water, humidity or phlegm within	Calor-heteropathies influence the o. pulmonalis Algor venti hems in the o. pulmonalis Energy obscured by pituita hems in the o. pulmonalis	Repletion (repletio)

d) Differential Diagnoses

a - Inanitas-Symptoms ("Symptoms of Exhaustion of the Energies of the Lung Orb").

1. Ariditas pulmonalis Induced by inanitas yin ("Depletion of Structive Fluids of the o. pulmonalis as a Consequence of the Exhaustion of Structivity")

a) Disease Mechanism: As the consequence of an exogenous ariditas-heteropathy, by phthisic agents or after chronic cough, all energies of the o. pulmonalis have been reduced, thus resulting in a deficiency of the yin pulmonale. This in turn leads to calor inanitatis ("exhaustion heat") which in turn impairs the potential structivity of the o. pulmonalis.

b) Special Symptoms: Frequent urge to clear one's throat, irritation and cough, after which only a small quantity of sticky phlegm is evacuated; cough with expectoration containing bloody spots or streaks or clumps; periodic fevers with perspiration during sleep; red cheeks in the afternoon; restlessness and insomnia; dry mouth and throat; hoarseness and loss of voice. Intensely red body of the tongue with reduced coating. Minute and accelerated pulses (pp. minuti et celeri).

c) Therapy: <u>Rigatio yin, madefactio o. pulmonalis</u> (the application of remedies bolstering the structive basis and moistening the <u>o. pulmonalis</u>).

2. The Active Energies of the <u>o. pulmonalis</u> are reduced or Depleted

a) Disease Mechanism: If, as the consequence of extreme stress or prolonged disease, the <u>qi primum</u>[110] could not be regenerated, or if chronic cough has impaired the <u>qi</u>, i.e. the active energy of the <u>o. pulmonalis,</u> these energies appear to be reduced or depleted, and the orb lacks warmth.

b) Special Symptoms: Cough and shortness of breath; thin, clear expectoration; whispering voice, reluctance to speak; great prostration; white, waxy complexion; lack of natural warmth, also spontaneous perspiration; pale body of the tongue, whitish thin coating of the tongue; infirm and exhausted pulses (<u>pp. invalidi et inanes</u>).

c) Therapy: <u>Suppletio o. pulmonalis</u> (administering remedies increasing the energy level of the <u>o. pulmonalis</u>).

b - Repletion Symptoms

1. The Function of the <u>o. pulmonalis</u> is Hemmed in by Murky Phlegm

a) Disease Mechanism: As the consequence of unwholesome cooling off of the body, or of the ingestion of cold drinks, <u>pituita</u> ("phlegm") has condensed in the <u>intima</u> (at first of the <u>o. lienalis et stomachi</u>), which finally also blocks the <u>o. pulmonalis</u> and impedes the normal flow of breathing energy.

b) Special Symptoms: Cough, panting, rattle of phlegm, expectoration of thick, sticky phlegm, pains in the chest and flanks, acute shortness of breath when in a horizontal position; sticky and yellow coating of the tongue; slippery pulses (<u>pp. lubrici</u>).

c) Therapy: <u>Dispulsio repletionis o. pulmonalis, demissio yang, exstillatio pituitae, patefactio</u> (administering remedies dispelling the repletive heteropathies, leading down the active energy (into the <u>o. intestini crassi</u>), draining the humidity of phlegm, and clearing the passages of energy).

2. <u>Algor venti</u> Fetters the <u>o. pulmonalis</u>

---

[110] Cf. note 58 on page 47 above.

a) Disease Mechanism: It may happen that either a "cold"-heteropathy induced by wind (algor venti) affects the skin[111] and confines the energies of the o. pulmonalis, or that pituita algoris condensed within, impairs the normal condensating and cooling function of the o. pulmonalis.

b) Special Symptoms: 1. Algor venti active in the species: Fever with shuddering, no perspiration; headache and pains in the body; blocked nasal passages and secretions from these; cough producing thin phlegm; thin whitish coating of the tongue; superficial and tense pulses (pp. superficiales et intenti).
2. Pituita algida affecting the intima: Continuous irritation inducing cough, expectoration of much white, sticky phlegm, impeded breathing; great fatigue, fever with shuddering; white and slippery coating of the tongue; superficial and tense pulses (pp. superficiales et intenti).

c) Therapy: Dispulsio algoris venti sive tepefactio et transformatio pituitae algidae (Dispersion, release of the "cold" heteropathy, or the administration of warm or transformative remedies to eliminate the cold mucus.)

3. Heteropathic calor ("Heat") Encroaches upon the o. pulmonalis

a) Disease Mechanism: If a calor-heteropathy has developed within the o. pulmonalis, this orb loses its capacity to cool other orbs, in particular the o. intestini crassi. Such a heteropathy may have been induced by ventus ("wind"), by algor ("cold") or by pituita ("phlegm").

b) Special Symptoms: Blaring cough, loud panting; expectoration of thick yellow phlegm or malodorous pus; pains on the chest radiating into the back during coughing seizures; dry nose or bloody or pussy secretions from the nose; nostrils move when breathing; the patient feels that his exhaled breath is hot; hot skin, fever, intense thirst; swollen painful throat; dry and solid faeces, red and sparing or entirely retained urine; intensely red body of the tongue, yellow and dry coating of the tongue; accelerated pulses (pp. celeri).

c) Therapy: Refrigeratio o. pulmonalis, dispulsio caloris (the administration of cooling remedies and of dispellants of heat).

---

[111] Refer to the folding table as well as to the iconogram in Porkert, Theoretical Foundations... pp. 136 ff.

PATHOLOGY

c - Complex Symptoms

1. Exhaustion of the orbis lienalis (inanitas lienalis) Affects the o. pulmonalis

a) Symptoms: Dazedness and lethargy, extreme fatigue, weak extremities; diarrhea; cough with copious expectoration; in extreme cases tumescence of the face and of hands and feet; white coating of the tongue; frail or infirm pulses (pp. lenes sive invalidi).

b) Therapy: Suppletio transvectus humi ut producit metallum (remedies applied to develop the energetic potential of the o. lienalis qualified by the E.P. Earth, in order that it may produce Metal, i.e. deploy the energies of the o. pulmonalis).

2. Deficiency of Energy in the o. pulmonalis et o. renalis

a) Symptoms: Cough, aggravated during the night; movement immediately entails an acceleration of respiration; loins and lower extremities painful and weak; perspiration during sleep; loss of semen; intensely red body of the tongue, reduced coating; minute and accelerated pulses (pp. minuti et celeri).

b) Therapy: Rigatio yin, sustentatio o. pulmonalis (the administration of remedies enhancing the structive energies and sustaining those of the o. pulmonalis).

d - Special Symptoms of the orbis intestini crassi ("Large Intestine Orb")

The principal function of the o. intestini crassi is the transport and transformation of food. This is why in its pathology, constipation is a very frequent symptom, induced by the insufficient availability of fluids, as a consequence of calor-heteropathies. These heteropathies may either impede the cooling influence of the o. pulmonalis to reach the o. intestini crassi; or they may provoke a deficiency of the aqua renalis - which has indirect repercussions on all orbs, but especially on the oo. intestinorum et vesicalis ("intestinal and urinary bladder orbs"). A third factor inducing constipation may be a weakness of the energies of the oo. lienalis et stomachi with which the o. intestini crassi is systematically linked in sequence I of the E.P.s, and by their common sinarteries.

1. Algor intestini crassi ("Cold Heteropathy in the Large Intestine Orb")

a) Symptoms: Stomachache, rumbling noise in the intestines, diarrhea; clear urine; white and slippery coating of the tongue; languid pulses (pp. languidi).

b) Therapy: Dispulsio algoris, asperatio profluvii (dispersion of the "cold" and control of the diarrhea by appropriate remedies).

2. Calor intestini crassi ("Heat Heteropathy in the Large Intestine Orb")

a) Symptoms: Dry mouth, cracked lips; constipation; very malodorous stools; anus inflamed, swollen, painful; reddish, sparing urine; yellow and dry coating of the tongue; accelerated pulses (pp. celeri).

b) Therapy: Refrigeratio caloris, dispulsio of the congestion (the application of cooling remedies to combat "heat", dispersion of the congested energies.) If the symptoms of "heat" in the large intestine orb occur during a dysentery attack, with bloody or purulent faeces and symptoms like fever, extreme prostration, yellow sticky coating of the tongue, slippery, accelerated pulses (pp. lubrici et celeri), this is called a calor humidus dysentery, which must be treated by refrigerantia et laxantia (cooling and laxative prescriptions).

3. Inanitas intestini crassi ("Exhaustion of Energy in the Large Intestine Orb")

a) Symptoms: Persistent diarrhea, prolapsus of the anus, cold extremities; pale body of the tongue, thin coating of the tongue; minute or evanescent pulses (pp. minute sive evanescentes).

b) Therapy: Stabilization or concentration of the energies of the affected orb by the administration of appropriate remedies.

4. Repletio intestini crassi ("Repletion of Energy in the Large Intestine Orb")

a) Symptoms: Stomachache aggravated by pressure; fever, vomiting, constipation; defecation does not bring relief to the patient; yellow coating of the tongue; submerged and replete pulses (pp. mersi et repleti).

b) Therapy: Refrigeratio caloris (the administration of cooling remedies) and breaking up the block.

PATHOLOGY

Synthetic Table of the Symptoms Related to Diseases of the oo. pulmonalis et intestini crassi

Diagnosis	General Symptoms	Tongue	Pulses	Relations
Exhausted active energy of the o. pulmonalis (inanitas qi pulmonalis)	Shortness of breath, asthmatic symptoms, weak voice, waxen complexion, spontaneous perspiration	Pale body of the tongue	Minute or infirm pulses (pp. minuti sive invalidi)	These symptoms may have been induced by a deficiency of the qi medium, i.e. the energy of the oo. lienalis et stomachi.
Ariditas (= lack of fluids in the o. pulmonalis)	Dry cough without expectoration, sore pharynx and throat; dry mouth and nose; hemoptea and loss of voice.	Dry and rough; reduced secretion of saliva.	Superficial, minute and grating (pp. superficiales, minuti et asperi)	These symptoms may be due to a deficiency of the yin renale.
Calor o. pulmonalis	Cough and expectoration of thick, yellow, sometimes blood-streaked phlegm, accelerated respiration, movement of nostrils when breathing; red, swollen throat; dry and lumped faeces.	Intensely red body of tongue, dry and yellow coating.	Flooding and accelerated or exhausted and accelerated (pp. exundantes et celeri sive inanes et celeri.	Symptoms either induced 1. by vigorous "glare" (ardor) in the oo. cardialis et hepaticus or 2. by a lesion or deficiency of the yin renale.
Algor o. pulmonalis	Cough accompanied by the expectoration of thin phlegm; patient shivers from feeling cold on the chest and back; in extreme cases difficult respiration, especially when lying down.	Swollen, tender and pale body of the tongue; white thin and slippery coating.	Slowed down, sometimes stringy (pp. tardi, chordales)	Symptoms usually induced by an exogenous algor-heteropathy, fixing thin pituita in the intima.
The active energy of the o. pulmonalis is not deployed	Impeded respiration, difficult respiration with shoulder movements; little or no perspiration at all; in extreme cases, retention of urine.	White coating.	Superficial and tense or superficial and languid pulses (pp. superficiales et intenti sive superficiales et languidi).	
Algor inanitatis o. intestini crassi ("Exhaustion cold fo the Large Intestine Orb")	Stomachache, rumbling or splashing noise in the intestines; diarrhea, sometimes sudden watery stools; after prolonged dysentery the evacuation of mucus.	Pale body of the tongue; white and slippery coating; sometimes slippery yet very thin coating.	Submerged and slowed down or minute and grating pulses (pp. mersi et tardi sive minuti et asperi)	These symptoms may be conditioned by algor inanitatis oo. lienalis et stomachi.
Calor repletionis orbis intestini crassi ("Repletion Heat in the Large Intestine Orb")	Constipation, stomachache aggravated by pressure; sometimes very malodorous diarrhea; excretion of purulent or bloody faeces.	Body of the tongue intensely red or crimson red; coating usually yellow and thick, sometimes dry	Slippery and accelerated or submerged and replete (pp. lubrici et celeri sive mersi et repleti)	These symptoms very often appear because calor or calor repletionis have been transmitted from the o. stomachi

DISEASES OF THE oo. renalis et vesicalis ("KIDNEY AND URINARY BLADDER ORBS")

a) Orbisiconographic Data

The o. renalis ("kidney orb"), together with the o. vesicalis ("urinary bladder orb"), forms a functional yoke. The specific unfoldment of the functions of these orbs is the bones and teeth. Their corresponding body openings are those for urine and faeces; their corresponding sense organs are the ears.

The basic function of the o. renalis is "potentiation of power". It thus is at the root of technical capacities and/or the deployment of directed emotions. The o. renalis stores structive potential (jing) and is consequently considered the root, seat or foundation of the inborn constitution or as the root of an individual's life[112].

The qualification of the o. renalis by the E.P. Water ("actual structivity") expresses the influence ascribed this orb upon the individual economy of fluids and liquids, which constitute an essential part of structive energies.

Finally, we must not forget that the oo. renalis et vesicalis comprise not only all sexual and reproductive functions but also what Western medicine categorizes as the nervous or neurological functions[113].

b) Pathological Data

Dysfunctions of the o. renalis essentially arise when its storage capacity of energies received at birth (the yin merum and the yang merum[114], which, according to Chinese medical theory, must never be dispersed) is affected. The consequence is a constitutional deficiency produced by prolonged, serious disease, by abnormal stress or by sexual excesses.

---

[112] Cf. the iconogram in Porkert, Theoretical Foundations... pp. 140 - 146.

[113] For the rational argument behind this correspondence, cf. op. cit. p. 163, as well as in the present book, pp. 110 f. below.

[114] For these terms cf. pp. 35 f. above.

PATHOLOGY

Disease Mechanism of the orbis renalis

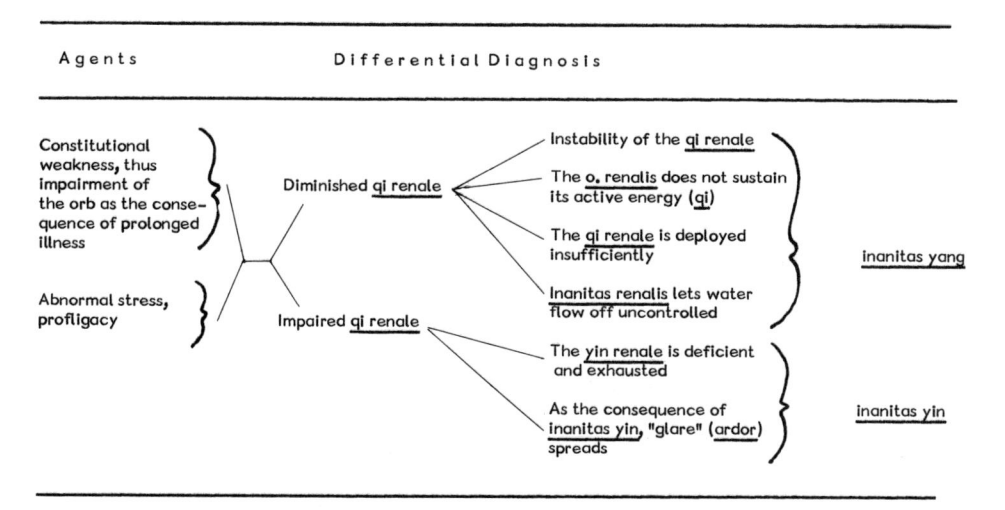

Agents	Differential Diagnosis	
Constitutional weakness, thus impairment of the orb as the consequence of prolonged illness	Diminished qi renale → Instability of the qi renale / The o. renalis does not sustain its active energy (qi) / The qi renale is deployed insufficiently	inanitas yang
Abnormal stress, profligacy	Impaired qi renale → Inanitas renalis lets water flow off uncontrolled / The yin renale is deficient and exhausted / As the consequence of inanitas yin, "glare" (ardor) spreads	inanitas yin

c) Clinical Symptoms of Disturbances of the oo. renalis et vesicalis

Sitis diffundens, variatio inferior [diabetes mellitus]; paralysis, pareses; ascites, asthma; hematuria; sandy urine; rentention of urine, enuresis; loss of semen, impotency, pains in the loins etc.

d) Differential Diagnoses

a - Symptoms of Exhausted Yang of the o. renalis (inanitas yang renalis)

1. Instability of the Active Energies of the o. renalis (qi renalis)

a) Disease Mechanism: Congenital weakness of the yang renale, extraordinary strain and prolonged illness may reduce the store of active energy in the o. renalis - as a consequence of which the orb loses its power of concentration and control.

b) Special Symptoms: Pale, sallow face; weak and painful loins and back; reduced acuity of hearing; continuous impulse to urinate, clear urine; in extreme cases incontinence of urine and, after urination, dripping urine; ejaculatio praecox. Pale body of the tongue, thin whitish coating of the tongue; minute or infirm pulses (pp. minuti sive invalidi).

c) Therapy: Consolidation and concentration of the active energy in the o. renalis by the administration of supplentia yin, rigantia yin.

2. The o. renalis ("Kidney Orb") Does not Contain its qi ("Active Energies")

a) Disease Mechanism: If the qi renale has suffered a lesion by extraordinary strain or as the consequence of prolonged disease, the feedback upon the structive potential (qi primum) contained in the o. renalis is affected. And, as a consequence, again the o. renalis loses its concentrating and regulative power.

b) Special Symptoms: Shortness of breath, laboured breathing, exacerbated by movement; nervous cough accompanied by perspiration and enuresis; in extreme cases rattle of phlegm, diaphanous white face; thin, whitish coating of the tongue; exhausted or infirm pulses (pp. inanes sive invalidi).

c) Therapy: Reduction of the qi into the o. renalis by the administration of medicamenta demittentia ("reductive" prescriptions, leading back the energies into the o. renalis).

3. The yang renale is Deployed Insufficiently

a) Disease Mechanism: Congenital weakness, strain or chronic disease, in some cases also sexual profligacy, may produce a lesion of the o. renalis leading to a withering of vital resources.

b) Special Symptoms: Pale complexion, aching loins, weak legs; impotency, dazedness, tinnitus, cold skin, continual urge to urinate; pale body of the tongue; submerged and infirm pulses (pp. mersi et invalidi).

c) Therapy: Tepefactio et suppletio yang renalis (the administration of remedies warming and completing the active aspects of the o. renalis).

4. Water Flows off Uncontrolled Because of inanitas renalis ("The Specific Energies - Qualified by the E.P. Water - of the o. renalis are Dispersed Because of Basic Exhaustion of this Orb.")

a) Disease Mechanism: Because of a feeble constitution or prolonged illness, the yang renale has been reduced and become insufficient to warm and transform the fluids (=

PATHOLOGY

yin). Consequently the latter will condense as heteropathies and move controvehently ("in a wayward, pathological direction") upwards or into the flesh.

b) Special Symptoms: Liquid infiltrations throughout the body; swollen, turgid appearance; ascites, especially in the legs; soft tissues like slime; distended abdomen; little urine; sometimes cough with the expectoration of great quantities of thin watery phlegm; panting breath after slight movement; whitish body of the tongue; submerged and slippery pulses (pp. mersi et lubrici).

c) Therapy: Tepefactio yang, transformatio humoris (the administration of remedies warming, thus bolstering, the yang and transforming water (the liquids)).

b - Symptoms of the Exhaustion of Structive Energies (Inanitas yin Symptoms)

1. Deficiency and inanitas ("Exhaustion") of the yin renale

a) Disease Mechanism: By alcoholic or sexual profligacy or as the consequence of excessive cogitation [nervous stress], or also in the wake of very serious disease, the yin merum has withered.

b) Special Symptoms: General weakness of the body, dizziness, tinnitus; bad sleep, forgetfulness; aching loins, weak legs, loss of semen and dry mouth; intensely red body of the tongue, reduced coating of the tongue; minute pulses (pp. minuti).

c) Therapy: Rigatio et sustentatio yin renalis (the administration of bolstering and nutritive prescriptions sustaining the yin renale).

2. Ardor ("Glare") Spreads Uncontrolled as the Consequence of inanitas yin renalis

a) Disease Mechanism: Indulgence in profligate habits or a severe fever disease has drastically reduced the structive energies of the o. renalis. Because of the depleted antagonist, the heat within (ardor, "glare") flares upward and outward.

b) Special Symptoms: Intensely red cheeks, scarlet lips, hot flushes, perspiration during sleep; painful back and loins; exhaustion, excitement and insomnia; voluptuous dreams and loss of semen during sleep; dry and sore throat; irritation stimulating cough; yellow urine, constipation; intensely red body of the tongue with little coating; minute and accelerated pulses (pp. minuti et celeri).

c) Therapy: Rigatio yin, demissio ardoris (the administration of remedies augmenting the structive energy and leading the glare back down to its source).

c - Complex Symptoms

1. Inanitas renalis cum humo[115] dilabente ("Exhaustion of the o. renalis Concomitant with Weak Functions in the oo. lienalis et stomachi")

a) Symptoms: Diarrhea containing undigested food, uncontrollable urge to defecate; distended abdomen, reduced appetite; lassitude and shivering; weakness of the limbs; pale body of the tongue, thin coating of the tongue; submerged or slowed down pulses (pp. mersi sive tardi).

b) Therapy: Suppletio ignis to produce Earth (the administration of nourishing, suppletive remedies acting upon the o. cardialis in order to bolster the energies of the o. lienalis, produced by the former according to sequence I of the E.P.s).

2. The aqua renalis Shocks the o. cardialis ("Spurious Repletion of Yang in the o. renalis Affects the Energy in the o. cardialis)

a) Symptoms: Palpitations and restiveness, ascites; feeling of congestion in the thorax and abdomen; cough with short breath; the patient cannot bear to lie down; cyanosis of lips and nails; cold extremities because of flexus; thin, colourless coating of the tongue; exhausted, accelerated pulses (pp. inanes et celeri).

b) Therapy: Tepefactio et demissio aquae (the administration of warm and regulating reductive remedies to control the energetic situation in the o. renalis).

d - Special Symptoms of the o. vesicalis ("Urinary Bladder Orb")

As yang complement of the o. renalis, the o. vesicalis operates in close dependence on the latter, especially as far as the storage and transformation of liquids and fluids is concerned. Consequently, the particular disturbances in the o. vesicalis essentially consist in irregularities of urination.

1. Algor inanitatis o. vesicalis ("Cold Heteropathy from Exhaustion of Energy in the Urinary Bladder Orb")

a) Symptoms: Continuous and uncontrollable urge to urinate; enuresis; pale body of the tongue, glistening, wet coating; submerged, minute pulses (pp. mersi, minuti).

b) Therapy: Consolidation and concentration of the qi renale (administration of remedies collecting and bolstering the active energies in the o. renalis)

---

[115] The Latin humus, Chinese tu points to the E.P. Earth, the qualifier of the oo. lienalis et stomachi.

PATHOLOGY

2. <u>Calor repletionis o. vesicalis</u> ("Repletion Heat Affecting the Urinary Bladder Orb")

a) Symptoms: Infrequent, diminished urination, reddish urine; sometimes yellow or murky urine; urination is accompanied by the feeling of heat and pain in the penis; in extreme cases retention of urine or purulent, bloody admixtures or urinary sediments; intensely red body of the tongue, yellow coating of the tongue; accelerated pulses (<u>pp. celeri</u>).

b) Therapy: <u>Refrigeratio caloris et exstillatio humoris</u> (the administration of remedies clearing the "heat" and aiding the diuretic elimination of excess water).

Synthetic Table Showing the Symptoms Related to Diseases of the <u>oo. renalis et vesicalis</u>

Diagnosis	General Symptoms	Tongue	Pulses	Further References
<u>Inanitas yin renalis</u>	Loss of semen, painful and weak loins and legs; impaired potency, tinnitus, deafness; vertigo or mouches volantes, perspiration during sleep; cough and hemoptea	Body of the tongue intensely red or crimson; reduced coating.	Exhausted, minute or accelerated (<u>pp. inanes et minuti, sive celeri</u>)	Pathological influences from the <u>oo. cardialis, pulmonalis et hepaticus</u>.
<u>Inanitas yang renalis</u>	Cold and watery ejaculation; atrophy of the genitals; feeling of cold in the loins and legs; atrophic tendencies accompanying tumescence. Sometimes morning diarrhea, tense or congested abdomen; cold feet; hiccup and laboured breathing.	Body of the tongue swollen and tender, coating black and moist.	Submerged and slowed down, always exhausted (<u>pp. mersi et tardi, semper inanes</u>)	There are close relations with the <u>oo. lienalis, pulmonalis et tricalorii</u>.
<u>Ardor</u> affects the <u>porta fortunae</u>	Extreme excitation, shallow sleep with many dreams; patient awakes in the middle of the night with a dry mouth; diminished and reddish urine. Faltering and diminished urination, yellow to reddish urine; sometimes murky urine and pains in the penis; in extreme cases complete retention of urine or purulent or bloody admixtures and sediment.	Body of the tongue intensely red; reduced coating, reduced salivation.	Submerged and accelerated (<u>pp. mersi et celeri</u>) especially impressive at the pedal sites.	
<u>Calor repletionis orbis vesicalis</u>	Faltering and diminshed urination, yellow to reddish urine; sometimes murky urine and pains in the penis; in extreme cases complete retention of urine or purulent or bloody admixtures or sediment.	Body of the tongue intensely red; yellow coating.	As a rule submerged and accelerated or submerged and stringy pulses (<u>pp. mersi et celeri sive mersi et chordales</u>)	The symptoms may have been induced by the transmission of a <u>calor humidus</u>-heteropathy from the <u>o. intestini tenuis</u>.
<u>Algor inanitatis orbis vesicalis</u>	Continuous urge to micturate small quantities of clear or cold urine; sometimes retention of urine accompanied by tumescence, dark to blackish complexion or also, on the contrary, enuresis.	In general a pale body of the tongue with strikingly moist coating.	The rule are submerged and minute pulses (<u>pp. mersi et minuti</u>) strikingly weak at the pedal sites.	This syndrome very often is conditioned by deficiency of the <u>yang renale</u> or by an insufficiently deployed <u>qi pulmonale</u>, also by exhaustion of the energy of the <u>o. pulmonalis</u> (= <u>inanitas o. pulmonalis</u>)

PATHOLOGY OF CONDUITS (*algor laedens,* "harmful cold" diseases)

The pathological classificatory convention second in importance in Chinese medicine is that of the so-called algor laedens-diseases. It first appeared in the writings of the famous physician Zhang Zhongjing, flourishing during the 2nd century of our era.

It may be said that Zhang Zhongjing "founded" clinical medicine by writing his classic "Treatises on algor laedens" (Shanghanlun), dealing with the clinical course and treatment of certain common fever diseases. Taking his cue from chapter 31 of the "Ingenuous Questions in the Inner Classic of the Yellow Sovereign" (Huangdi Neijing Suwen) entitled Relun, Tractatus de calore, "Treatise on Heat", he evolved a more subtle scheme for the description of the diseases in question, grouping them into six cyclical categories labelled with the quality standards of the triple yang and triple yin: yang maior ("major yang"), splendor yang, yang minor, yin maior, yin flectens ("yielding yin"), yin minor.

Now to clear up and obviate the confusion arising from this use of these standards, several things must be kept in mind.
1. The sexpartite cyclical convention apparently was already present in the classical version of the Neijing then in use. BUT,
2. to all evidence it seems not to have been primarily linked or exclusively used with one group of theoretical postulates only, e.g. those of sinarteriology. Thus, indeed,
3. Zhang Zhongjing felt free to use these sexpartite conventions for establishing a more stringent terminological and diagnostic scheme, conceived to serve as the premise for pharmacotherapeutic treatment.
4. In the 3rd century of our era, Huangfu Mi compiled his "Systematic Classic on Acupuncture and Moxibustion" (Zhenjiu jiayijing), chiefly from quotations collected from the Neijing. In this compilation, the sexpartite cycle of yin and yang was used to univocally qualify topological data or postulates: the conduits (jing, sinarteriae) linking the foramina (xue) at the surface of the body.
To the extent that this text, to the exclusion of all others, for centuries established itself as the basic authority on acupuncture (thus on sinarteriology), the qualitative conventions of the sexpartite cycle gradually came to be primarily associated with and tied to the sinarteriological theories, hence, in a way, were monopolized by acupuncture.

PATHOLOGY

5. Consequently, since approximately the 7th century - Zhang Zhongjing's as well as Huangfu Mi's texts then were firmly entrenched as classics - the idea spread that Zhang Zhongjing, without having ever referred to acupuncture, still must also have had a sinarteriological concept at the back of his mind. This is why one gradually came to speak of a "jingluoxue": "sinarteries-" or "conduit"-theory applied to pharmacotherapy by Zhang Zhongjing.

6. Further on, this historical confusion eventually led to mixups and arguments in that part of medical literature predominantly dealing with abstract and theoretical considerations. It barely affected clinical applications.

Indeed, the so-called "conduit"-theory of pathology or, more exactly, the "harmful cold" (shanghan) pathology has heuristic advantages and clinical uses. Zhang Zhongjing himself seems to have used it concomitantly with the morbi varii-typology mentioned before, when dealing with certain exogenous factors liable to be qualified as algor laedens ("harmful cold").

It should also be noted that in the revived tradition of Chinese medicine in Japan, the algor laedens-pathology represents the primary and chief mode for the systematization of pathology.

To repeat, when dealing with certain very common heteropathies induced by an exogenous factor called algor laedens (shanghan), "harmful cold", the conduit pathology furnishes additional means for the subtle evaluation of diagnostic data.

It was already stated above, in connection with the guiding criteria of species and intima, that a disturbance limited to the conduits, may be considered a light, recent, acute disease; by contradistinction, an affection that has penetrated into the intima, into the orb, corresponds to severe, prolonged, chronic disease. Now the shanghan-pathology introduces additional criteria for describing the evolution, we may even say the swerve toward the intima or toward the species, of a pathological process. As can easily be seen from the table below, if all observed symptoms are qualified by means of the sexpartite conventions, an evolution of symptoms in clockwise direction may be understood as an outward movement, an improvement or amelioration; a movement in counterclockwise sense as penetration towards the intima, and consequently aggravation and prolongation of the illness.

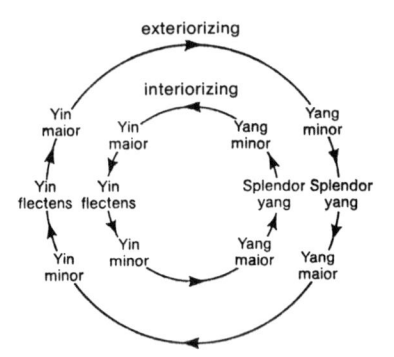

Fig. 5.

Before dealing individually with each of the six aspects of algor laedens pathology, a few more general remarks should be made.

1. In spite of the independent interpretations of the sexpartite terms in acupuncture (sinarteriology) and pathology (pharmacotherapy) at the inception of the theory, the use of identical designations immediately established an additional cross-link between all orbs, complementary to that of the evolutive phases (E.P.s)[116]. Thus we have

Sinarteriae	orbes	orbes	
Yang maioris	intestini tenuis	vesicalis	
Splendoris yang	intestini crassi	stomachi	oo. aulici
Yang minoris	tricalorii	felleus	
Yin maioris	pulmonalis	lienalis	
Yin minoris	cardialis	renalis	oo. horreales
Yin flectentis	pericardialis	hepaticus	

2. Furthermore, it was inevitable that, because of the systematic "pressure" of sinarteriological theory, topological considerations gradually filtered into the algor laedens postulates. In weighing these against arguments resulting from the morbi varii theory, we should keep in mind the more fundamental character of the latter.

---

[116] On this cf. Porkert, Theoretical Foundations... pp. 111 f.

3. Still, there are no basic contradictions either between these two systems or between these and all other more comprehensive qualitative conventions. Thus the precise association of yin (structivity, structure aspect) and yang (activity, active aspect) are perfectly valid in algor laedens pathology also: Diseases qualified by one of the three yang are essentially manifesting symptoms of repletio and calor and call for treatment of heteropathies; diseases qualified by one of the three yin preponderantly manifest algor or inanitas-symptoms and consequently require a bolstering of the orthopathy.

Yang maior (taiyang) DISEASES

1. Sinarteriological Data and Disease Mechanism

The yang maior cardinal conduits (cardinales yang maioris) directly belong to the oo. intestini tenuis et vesicalis and indirectly attach to their complements, the oo. cardialis et renalis. This is why diseases related to yang maior affect the economy of liquids and fluids, the separation of clear and murky (turgid) (liquid and solid) energies and excretions, and the production (: o. cardialis) and control (: o. renalis) of calor ("heat")[117].

The yang maior cardinal conduits cross the forehead and top of the head, pass across the neck and shoulders. Within the system of algor laedens pathology, they are considered the most outward species and thought to determine the harmonious concert of all constructive and defensive energies (ying and wei, qi constructivum et qi defensivum) of an individual. For any exogenous noxious influence, liable to produce a heteropathy, first strikes the defensive energy present at the surface of the body, then enters into the reticular and cardinal conduits (jing and luo), there affecting the constructive energy present in these, and their harmonious movement. In the case of a vento percussio, (zhongfeng) [apoplectic stroke], for example, the conduits of the parts of the body mentioned above are first affected. If, during this first stage, no effective treatment is undertaken, the resulting heteropathy will penetrate into the orbes aulici, i.e. the oo. intestini tenuis et vesicalis - with symptoms such as irregularities of micturition and tense, hard abdomen. If, at this stage, again no treatment or a wrong one is administered, the heteropathy eventually will penetrate into the horreal orbs, i.e. the oo. cardialis et renalis (for the symptoms, cf. below).

---

[117] Cf. the folding table in front as well as the respective iconograms.

2. Clinical Manifestations

If the climatic excesses of ventus and/or algor strike the yang maior conduits with their particular affinity to the complete surface (= species) of the individual, corresponding symptoms will be: fever, shuddering, headache, stiff neck, superficial pulses. In addition other symptoms may arise.

Additional Symptoms of the Cardinal Conduits

These symptoms, depending upon the constitutional reaction of the patient, will result in two perfectly distinct syndromes, viz. vento percussio (zhongfeng) (cardinalis yang maioris) or algor laedens (shanghan) cardinalem yang maiorem ("wind stroke") affecting the yang maior cardinal conduit or "harmful cold" affecting this conduit.

1. Vento percussio cardinalis yang maioris is characterized by pains in the head and neck, stiff neck; fever; great sensitivity to draft; spontaneous perspiration[118]; loud breathing through the nose; empty eructation and retching; superficial or languid pulses (pp. superficiales sive languidi). Because of the spontaneous perspiration and the superficial and languid pulses, these symptoms are usually qualified as inanitas speciei. (It should be noted, however, that such a qualification does not conform to the classical convention given above.)

2. Algor laedens affecting the yang maior cardinal conduits is characterized by intense pain in the head and neck; fever, shuddering, no perspiration; panting, retching, nausea; diffuse pains throughout the body, especially in the joints; superficial and tense pulses (pp. superficiales et intenti). Because of the absence of perspiration[119] and the superficial and tense pulses, these symptoms are classed as repletio speciei.

Symptoms Related to the orbis aulicus

Depending on whether a heteropathy develops within active energies (qi, qifen) or within structive energies (xue, xuefen), two distinct groups of symptoms may arise, viz.

1. Retention of water (retentio aquae). A heteropathy developing within active energies produces fever, perspiration, intense thirst and the desire to obtain water,

---

[118] The agent of ventus ("wind") is an active agent, consequently of "opening", "dispelling", "diffusing" nature, and liable to induce perspiration.

[119] Algor ("cold") is a yin agent, thus favouring a contractive, conservative, obstructive tendency - which explains why the secretion of sweat is impeded or completely stopped.

which, however, is immediately vomited after swallowing; little urine, tense abdomen, superficial and accelerated pulses (pp. superficiales et celeri).

2. Retention of xue (retentio xue). A heteropathy developing within the structive energies (xue), produces intense stabbing pains in the abdomen, a hard abdomen, raving madness, frequent micturition with copious urine, and black, sticky, laquer stools.

Complex Symptoms Related to yang maior

These usually arise as a consequence of constitutional strain or of incorrect treatment. Thus, for example, the symptoms associated with an asthmatic disposition may flare up after a vento percussio in the yang maior cardinal conduit. Similarly, the disposition to have hot flushes or experience inner heat may be accentuated by an algor laedens heteropathy.

3. Therapy

If yang maior is affected, liberantia speciei combined with tepefacientia, transformatoria, regulatoria et asperantia cutis may be administered (in other words, prescriptions opening up the species to permit diaphoresis, prescriptions cautiously warming from within, either transforming excess humidity or excreting it, or economizing the store of structive energy, by preventing excessive perspiration). In the case of retentio xue, the congestion must be broken up.

Splendor yang (yangming) DISEASES

1. Sinarteriological Data and Disease Mechanism

The cardinal conduits of splendor yang directly belong to the oo. stomachi et intestini crassi and indirectly attach to the oo. lienalis et pulmonalis. Hence, heteropathies affecting splendor yang will produce disturbances in the assimilation of food, in the harmonious exchange of energies between all orbs, and in the rhythm of all orbs.

A disturbance related to splendor yang, consequently, endangers, diminishes or destroys the "humidity" qualified by and belonging to the manifestations of the E.P. Earth. Thus, if the heteropathies affect the conduits only, symptoms such as fever with profuse perspiration, thirst, and flooding pulses (pp. exundantes) will result; if moreover, orbs are affected, constipation from dried up faeces, hot flushes, little urine, raving speech, submerged and replete pulses (pp. mersi et repleti) will occur.

2. Clinical Manifestations

a) Additional Symptoms of the Cardinal Conduits: Very high fever, yet no shuddering but, instead, oppressive heat, the desire to be cooled and aerated, profuse perspiration, intense thirst; yellow and dry coating of the tongue; flooding pulses (pp. exundantes).

b) Symptoms of the Aulic Orbs: Temperature rising and falling periodically, confused speech, constipation, tense and painful abdomen; relief after diaphoresis; submerged and replete pulses (pp. mersi et repleti); in extreme cases, aimlessly groping hands, shallow, panting breath, fixed stare.

c) Complex Symptoms: If the unrelieved "heat congestion" of a splendor yang disease meets with a calor humidus heteropathy, the harmony of the energy exchange may be disturbed to the extent that gall fluid extravasates into the flesh (= perfectio o. lienalis) and an icterus occurs (= to the transition into a yang minor stage). If the orthopathy of the patient gives way, a direct transition into a yin maior stage may occur, in which case calor and repletion symptoms are replaced by algor and inanitas symptoms.

3. Therapy

Cardinal conduit symptoms, hence species-symptoms are treated by refrigerantia intimae, hence by prescriptions cooling from within; if orb symptoms are present, purges with cold, bitter, laxatives or, in the case of instability of the o. lienalis, in addition transformatoria humoris, exstillantia humoris, hence diuretics of different affinity, are indicated. If icterus is present, the corresponding refrigerantia caloris must be used, and the o. felleus must be relieved by again using exstillantia humoris ("diuretics").

Yang minor (shaoyang) DISEASES

1. Sinarteriological Data and Disease Mechanism

The cardinal conduits of yang minor directly belong to the oo. felleus et tricalorii, and indirectly attach to their intimae, the oo. hepaticus et pericardialis. Consequently, disturbances qualified by yang minor directly affect the active control and dynamization of the flow of fluids and juices, the availability of (structive) energies, and the communication between below and above.

PATHOLOGY

With respect to pathological criteria, disturbances of yang minor show ambivalent and equivocal aspects: the symptoms may be partly classed as species, partly as intima signs because viewed closely, they partake of both. In this system, yang minor is assigned a "pivot function"[120] because, indeed, disturbances thus defined may with equal facility turn either outward or inward. Yang minor diseases occur as the consequence of wrong therapy of some yang disease, or of a powerful algor venti factor that has penetrated directly into the yang minor.

2. Clinical Manifestations

a) Pure Symptoms of Yang minor: Bitter taste, dry throat, dizziness, alternation of heat and shivering, oppressive feeling or tension in the thorax and ribs; lethargy, lack of appetite, restiveness; retching brings relief; stringy or minute pulses (pp. chordales sive minuti).

b) Combined Symptoms:

1. The combination of yang minor with yang maior produces fever, moderate shuddering, painful or tense joints, moderate eructations, spasms in the central plexus region.
2. yang minor combined with splendor yang produces oppressive pressure in the thorax, retching; temperature rising periodically at dusk; sometimes constipation.
3. yang minor combined with yang maior and splendor yang conditions an outwardly hot patient who abhors draft; stiff neck, repletive feeling around the small ribs; warm extremities, thirst.

3. Therapy

When treating yang minor diseases, therapy must concentrate upon restoring an harmonious flow of energy between species and intima - by the use of regulatoria. By contrast, the use of diaphoretics, purgatives or emetics must be avoided. For the heteropathy at the basis of a yang minor disease is not limited to the species. With diaphoresis, consequently, one would unnecessarily diminish the orthopathic fluids and, as a result, the heteropathy would penetrate even deeper. Nor is the heteropathy of a yang minor disease limited to the intima. If, by incorrect assessment of the situation, purgatives are used, the orthopathy within will be diminished, "glare" (ardor) may

---

[120] Cf. Porkert, Theoretical Foundations... p. 37.

ensue and flare up, and there is the danger of a "terror" (pavor) syndrome. And if an emetic were used, the orthopathic yang would again be diminished, producing palpitations and similar disturbances.

Thus, even if a yang minor disease is accompanied by more complex symptoms, the basic therapy must be compositio, harmonization of the energy flow, by the use of regulatoria qi sive xue, to be completed, as the case requires, by liberantia speciei or refrigerantia intimae.

Yin maior (taiyin) DISEASES

1. Sinarteriological Data and Disease Mechanism

The yin maior cardinal conduits belong directly to the oo. pulmonalis et lienalis and attach indirectly to the oo. intestini crassi et stomachi. Since, among the horreal orbs, the o. lienalis effects the integration and dynamization of the energies assimilated from food (which it makes "rise"), and the o. pulmonalis effects the rhythmic control or moderation of all energies within the individual, yin maior functions are involved in all processes of the transformation of energies. Thus a disturbance of yin maior may ensue if a humor algidus excess has induced a lesion in the active energies of the o. lienalis or if some algor factor disturbs the regulation of the energy flow in the cardinal conduits of the o. lienalis - thus eventually affecting also the oo. stomachi et intestini crassi and all digestive processes.

2. Clinical Manifestations

If exhaustion of the orthopathy of the o. lienalis obtains and a humor-heteropathy may develop vigorously, symptoms appear such as: remarkably warm hands and feet in spite of normal body temperature, feeling of surfeit and vomiting, blocked digestion, diarrhea; no thirst; languid and frail pulses (pp. languidi et lenes).

These kinds of digestive troubles are different from those corresponding to splendor yang. Those of the o. lienalis are marked by exhaustion (inanitas); those of the o. stomachi by repletion.[121]

3. Therapy

To compensate inanitas and algor, mm. supplentia qi or mm. tepefacientia are

---
[121] Cf. p. 106 above.

predominantly required. If, in addition to the yin maior disorder, other heteropathies have been diagnosed, it may be necessary to use also liberantia speciei or mm. regulatoria.

Yin flectens (jueyin, "YIELDING YIN") DISEASES

1. Sinarteriological Data and Disease Mechanism

The yin flectens cardinal conduits directly belong to the oo. hepaticus et pericardialis and indirectly attach to the oo. felleus et tricalorii. These relationships express the particular role of such disturbances in the regulation of the quantitative distribution of energy, and in particular of structive energy. Disturbances qualified by yin flectens consequently manifest themselves as irregularities in the distribution of heat and cold, of active and structive energies, and by symptoms of flexus or contravections[122].

In a healthy individual, the ignis ministri o. pericardialis (the "ministerial fire of the pericard orb") exercises its downward action, the structive energies of the o. renalis ("the aqua renalis, "renal water") may continuously replenish the energies of the hepatic orb. Then, in turn, the regulative function of this hepatic orb is stabilized.

If under pathological conditions, a heteropathy has developed in the cardinal conduits or, worse still, in the orbs of yin flectens, this regulating function of the o. hepaticus is disturbed, and the ministerial fire of the pericardial orb may flare up, manifesting itself as calor, hence the heat of fever on top, and algor, i.e. the cold in the extremities, below. If in such cases yang is vigorous, compared to yin, flexus and calor seem to be in balance; or there is an excess of calor-symptoms. If, on the contrary, yang is enfeebled and yin vigorous, the return[123] of yang produces a redundancy of the latter - with more calor- than algor-symptoms, or again, a return of cold, in spite of the persisting heat. This is called a victory/return situation of flexus and calor.

If a heteropathy has developed in the orbs with the consequence that the harmony between active and structive energies (qi and xue) has been shaken, again all kinds of flexus and contravective symptoms appear. A variety of such flexus is the

---

[122] Let it be recalled that flexus designates a yielding, a collapse of an energy circuit. Contravection designates the "countercurrent" movement, in other words a flow of energy or an evolution of symptoms contrary to their normal interrelationships.

[123] This term explained in Porkert, Theoretical Foundations... p. 104, here refers to a microcosmic process.

accumulation of water in the midriff, due to an insufficiently developing active energy, or the accumulation of pituita above the diaphragm. Contravective symptoms are all kinds of vomiting, diarrhea and the like, induced by algor inanitatis oo. lienalis et stomachi.

2. Clinical Manifestations

a) Symptoms of calor above, algor below (such symptoms very often result from wrong therapeutic measures): Sitis diffundens [Diabetes], heart attacks, heat and pain in the region of the heart; hunger despite the absence of appetite; food is vomited immediately after ingestion; continuous diarrhea.

b) Symptoms of "victory" and "return", of flexus and calor: The extremities are alternately cold or feverish (from the relative duration of each phase one may draw inferences as to the evolution of the disease).

c) Symptoms of flexus and contravection: Cold or painful extremities; perspiration; persistent fever, inattention; diarrhea with shivering; food is vomited immediately after ingestion, also vomiting of worms; palpitations; if there is a pituita flexus, tense pulses (pp. intenti) occur.

d) Symptoms with diarrhea and vomiting:
1. Diarrhea due to calor humidus is very intense diarrhea.
2. Diarrhea due to calor repletionis is delayed for some time because of undigested food blocking the intestines; during this phase, incoherent or raving speech.
3. In the case of diarrhea due to algor inanitatis, the active energies are too weak to assimilate food; consequently, undigested food passes with the diarrhea.

3. Therapy

Because of the great diversity of symptoms associated with yin flectens diseases, particular care must be taken with the differential diagnosis. The only general recommendations are that calor-symptoms must be treated by mm. refrigerantia or sometimes by mm. purgativa, algor-symptoms by mm. tepefacientia et supplentia.

Minor yin (shaoyin) DISEASES

1. Sinarteriological Data and Disease Mechanism

The cardinal conduits qualified by yin minor directly belong to the oo. cardialis et renalis and indirectly attach to the oo. intestini tenuis et vesicalis ("small intestine and urinary bladder orbs"). Yin minor thus has an affinity to the axis of the actuality of active and structive energies[124] representing the pivot (cardo, shu) of the three yin conduits. This is why yin minor has extraordinary significance for the active manifestation and structive constitution of the personality and its qualities, as well as for its subjective well being and contentment, its objective presence, resilience, will power, and stamina.

If a heteropathy produces exhaustion or enfeeblement (inanitas, dilapsus) of the energies of the oo. cardialis et renalis, the balanced and harmonious energy supply is jeopardized throughout the individual. Then signs of deficiency of the active and structive energies appear, the former indicated by an evanescent pulse, the latter by a minute pulse. Also there may be great lassitude and the desire to sleep. But it may also happen that a heteropathy in contact with the energies of the o. renalis changes into an algor-heteropathy, and then pushes out the active energies of that orb, thus producing false symptoms of "heat" (calor), such as hot flushes with red face, restiveness etc. (This syndrome is called the yang-cap-syndrome (daiyang) since, so to speak, only the topmost covering of the individual is affected by it.)

A contrary deviation from the aforementioned takes place if a heteropathy, in contact with the ignis cardialis, produces calor or ardor there, and deteriorates and attacks the structive fluids. Then nervousness, insomnia, sore throat, intensely red tongue and minute pulses appear.

2. Clinical Manifestations

Yin minor diseases represent the ultimate step in the sexpartite pathology of the conduits. They thus correspond to the most severe and most dangerous disease symptoms and stages. Without exception, the orthopathy of the patient, hence his defensive and auto-regulative faculty is impaired. Often he is somnolent or comatose, shows evanescent or minute pulses; during the transition from an algor-heteropathy there is shuddering but no fever, restiveness, or palpitations; we also observe vomiting and, if there is thirst, the desire to absorb small quantities of hot beverages; urine is copious and light coloured, hands and feet are cold. The patient curls up in bed. During the transition to a calor-heteropathy, there is fever, a red face, extreme restlessness,

---

[124] It will be recalled that the cardial orb, qualified by the E.P. Fire, corresponds to actual activity, that the renal orb, qualified by the E.P. Water, corresponds to actual structivity.

diarrhea and thirst.

Because of their pivot nature, yin minor diseases may change into any other syndrome or accompany it.

3. Therapy

Owing to the impaired orthopathy, measures to increase and support the active and structive energies (hence the administration of mm. supplentia qi, adiuvantia yang, sustinentia xue, rigantia yin) are indispensable. In some cases the yang may have additional support from mm. tepefacientia and the yin from mm. refrigerantia caloris. In the case of the yang-cap-syndrome, mm. regulatoria, increasing the exchange of energies between above and below, may be employed.

If a yin minor disease has affected the species (= the conduits), cautious and circumspect use of mm. liberantia speciei, with a diaphoretic effect, may be made. If repletive "heat" symptoms in depth (calor repletionis intimae) occur, mild mm. purgativa, with concomitant suppletio yin may be used.

No matter what therapeutic measures are taken, it will be of paramount importance to keep in mind that the greatest danger of yin minor diseases resides in the lesion or the total loss of yang (of the active energies of the o. renalis et cardialis) - with an inevitably fatal issue. Consequently, in diagnosis and therapy, one must take extreme care to evaluate and maintain the yang.

PATHOLOGY OF THE FORMS OF ENERGY *(morbi temperati,* "tepid diseases," *wenbing)*

We have seen that the pathology of algor laedens deals with a common yet special type of diseases, those induced by "harmful cold" (algor laedens, shanghan). Similar remarks obtain for the particular theory of pathology we now have to deal with, morbi temperati, "tepid diseases". Just as it is supposed that algor laedens-diseases are induced by an algor-factor, first attacking the skin, from there penetrating into the conduits, and from these into the orbes aulici, in the case of morbi temperati, "tepid diseases", it is thought that a "warmth heteropathy" (wenxie) passes into the individual through the respiratory and digestive ducts. The result is an infectious poison affecting all or most forms of energy, and manifesting itself through illness, if concomitant climatic excesses have weakened the orthopathy.

To get the right perspective on this theory, we should keep in mind that in Chinese medicine, the terminology of energetics is not the product of essentially abstract theories and speculations, nor that it represents a terminology coined with constant close reference to physical substratums; instead, these terms constitute a fairly wide and finely graded assortment of designations, derived from the direct positive observation of functional phenomena and conventionally defined with the intent to apply them in medical practice[125].

Although the term of "morbi temperati" (wenbing) already occurs in the Yellow Sovereign's Inner Classic, the form of the theory, as it is applied today, is of comparatively recent date: it was only the physician Ye Tianshi (1666 to 1745) who gave it its present form.

According to this theory, morbi temperati factors first affect the o. pulmonalis, from where they pass on contravehently into the o. pericardialis. The o. pulmonalis, as we may recall, controls the movement of the qi, in other words of the active, individually specific energy; also, the defensive energy, having its seat in the skin (= the perfectio, i.e. "specific unfoldment" of the functions of the o. pulmonalis) is thus indirectly dependent upon this orb. And the o. cardialis - closely linked with the o. pericardialis - controls and regulates the movement of the xue, of the individually specific structive energy, including blood; in turn, the constructive energy (ying, qi constructivum) moving in the specific unfoldment (perfectio) of the o. cardialis, the sinarteries, is

---

[125] The reader is referred to the detailed presentation of energetics in Chinese medicine, in Porkert, Theoretical Foundations... pp. 166 - 196.

indirectly dependent upon the orthopathic reserves of this orb[126]. Defensive energy (wei) and qi (individually specific active energy) are active (yang) forms of energy; constructive energy (ying) and xue (individually specific structive energy) are structive (yin) forms of energy. On the other hand, wei and ying are assigned to the species, that is, the surface of the body and the sinarteries there; and qi and xue are assigned to the intima, that is, the deeper layer of the individual, the orbs.

Moreover, within the context of the morbi temperati theory, the postulate of the tricalorium ("the three heated spaces")(sanjiao)[127], in its literal sense of three distinct "heated spaces" (caloria), is given a new meaning.

DEFENSIVE ENERGY (wei, qi defensivum)

"Defensive energy" designates that kind of active energy which is deployed freely without the conduits, and which gives warmth to the flesh, its normal tonus to the skin, regulating the opening and closing of the pores and all other reactions by which this tegument responds to outward stimuli. Thus the defensive energy may energetically be considered to constitute the foremost defense line of an individual.

If the pathogenic factor of a morbus temperatus meets the defensive energy, the following symptoms may occur: fever, light shuddering, headache, cough, some thirst, little or no perspiration; thin whitish coating of an intensely red body of the tongue; superficial and accelerated pulses (pp. superficiales et celeri)

Qi, THE INDIVIDUALLY SPECIFIC ACTIVE ENERGY

The term qi designates the active aspect of all energies constituting the vital functions of a given individual[128]. An affection of the qi, hence, implies that a disturbance has penetrated deeper and spread further than if it affects only the defensive energy. Involvement of the qi in any pathological process is shown by fever, yet rather than shuddering, the feeling of oppressive heat; perspiration, thirst; white coating of the tongue, increasing in thickness and changing to yellow; accelerated pulses (pp. celeri).

---

[126] As has been pointed out in the book and section just quoted on p. 189, the terms xue (hsüeh) and ying do not designate essentially different aspects of energy, but connote only technical distinctions in an identical energy.

[127] Cf. op. cit. pp. 158 - 162.

[128] For other details on this term of essential and basic significance, cf. Porkert, Theoretical Foundations... pp. 167 f, 175, 195.

PATHOLOGY

Depending upon the constitution of the patient and the kind of pathological factor involved, more specific symptoms may ensue. Thus, if
the o. pulmonalis is involved, we observe panting and yellow coating of the tongue;
if the mediastinum is involved or the thorax region in general, there is heavy breathing, palpitations, morosity;
if splendor yang is involved, high fever, perspiration, and panting occur; yellow to reddish colour of the urine; coating of the tongue yellow and dry; flooding pulses (pp. exundantes);
if the oo. intestinorum are involved, fever rising and falling periodically, constipation, tense, tender, hard abdomen; thick, yellow and dry or parched and black coating of the tongue, sometimes with pointed protuberances; submerged, replete pulses (pp. mersi et repleti) are observed;
if yang minor is involved, malaria-like periodic fevers during which there is more heat than cold; bitter taste in the mouth; pains around the small ribs; the feeling of a lump or of pressure in the stomach, nausea; yellow, slightly sticky coating of the tongue; stringy and accelerated pulses (pp. chordales et celeri); if the disturbance persists, also reduced secretion of urine;
if the o. lienalis is involved, we find adynamic fevers, the feeling of a lump in the stomach with nausea; great lassitude; sticky coating of the tongue; frail or languid pulses (pp. lenes sive languidi).

CONSTRUCTIVE ENERGY (ying, qi constructivum)

"Constructive energy" (ying) is the term designating the aspect of that structive energy which flows within the conduits (sinarteriae), and totally represents the circulation of energy between all orbs, thus contributing to and maintaining the material development and sustenance of the body.
An affection to the constructive energy produces symptoms such as: bad distribution of blood, restlessness and apprehension; high fever during the night, insomnia, moderate thirst; also reduced consciousness, dazedness, confused speech, exanthema; body of the tongue intensely red or scarlet.

Xue, "INDIVIDUALLY SPECIFIC STRUCTIVE ENERGY"

"Constructive energy" (ying) and xue constitute different technical aspects of ultimately the same structive energy. In Chinese medicine xue refers not only to what leaks out from wounds as "blood", but also to the basic form and concept of all liquids, fluids, and secretions. Affections of the xue hence contribute to a serious and even critical state of illness. Notable signs of this are: body of the tongue an intense scarlet or purple red, eventually changing to grey and becoming dry, high fever during the hours of the night, admixtures of blood in the sputum, nasal discharge, urine and faeces; exanthemas; black colour of easily evacuated stools; in extreme cases raving madness, convulsions and coma.

THE Tricalorium ("THREE HEATED SPACES" sanjiao)

The tricalorium, in classical and common theory represents one orb without a specified somatic substratum. Still, the name - "three heated spaces" - quite lends itself to being associated with a topographical model. Thus in the theory of the morbi temperati - with which we are dealing here, and only in this theory -
the calorium superius ("upper heated space") is associated with the cardinal conduits of yin maior of the hand and yielding yin (yin flectens) of the hand (cardinales yin maioris manus et yin flectentis manus = cardinales pulmonalis et pericardialis);
the calorium medium ("middle heated space") is associated with the cardinal conduits of splendor yang of the foot and yin maior of the foot (cardinales splendoris yang pedis et yin maioris pedis = cardinales stomachi et lienalis);
finally, the calorium inferius ("lower heated space") is associated with the cardinal conduits of yin minor of the foot and yielding yin of the foot (cardinales yin minoris pedis et yin flectentis pedis = cardinales renalis et hepatica).

Symptoms of the Calorium superius ("Upper Heated Space")

1. Disturbances in the cardinales pulmonalis yin maioris manus usually do not produce languid or tense pulses (pp. languidi sive intenti), but rather mobile or accelerated pulses (pp. mobiles sive celeri). There may even be flooding pulses (pp. exundantes) at the pollex-sites. Also, attention should be paid to calor-symptoms at the pes-sites and, more generally, to the quality of the pel pedalis, i.e. the skin on the inward side of the lower arm[129]. There also is headache, slight shivering under cold or draft; fever and perspiration. thirst or no thirst accompanied by cough, and a notable rise of temperature in the afternoon.

---

[129] For more details on this term cf. below p. 254.

PATHOLOGY

2. Disturbances in the cardinalis pericardialis yin flectentis manus produce a scarlet body of the tongue; fever rising highest during the night; great restlessness and insomnia; impaired consciousness, confused speech.

Symptoms of the calorium medium ("Middle Heated Space")

1. Disturbances in the cardinales stomachi splendoris yang pedis produce red face and borders of the eyelids; loud, raucous voice, audible respiration; constipation, little or faltering urination. The coating of the tongue is leathery and yellow, in extreme cases black with pointed protuberances. There is oppressive heat; at dusk, aggravation of all symptoms.

2. Disturbances in the cardinales lienalis yin maioris pedis produce symptoms such as a pale to yellowish complexion, dazedness, fatigue and prostration; congested thorax; loss of appetite; rise of temperature in the afternoon; impaired micturition; constipation or diarrhea; yellow and sticky coating of the tongue; stringy or minute and frail pulses (pp. chordales sive minuti et lenes)

Symptoms of the calorium inferius ("Lower Heated Space")

1. Disturbances in the cardinales renalis yin minoris pedis produce fever, flushed face; dry mouth and tongue; in extreme cases, black teeth and cracked lips; nervous restlessness, insomnia; nervous and full pulses are indicative of vigor caloris ("vigour of heat") and a yin deficiens ("a deficient yin, deficient structivity"); flooding and exhausted pulses (pp. exundantes et inanes) are the rule; soles and palms have a higher temperature than the back of the feet and hands; listlessness, hardness of hearing; diarrhea. Sore throat and aching hips and calves are indicative of a diminution of the structive potential, consequently of moderate heteropathic "heat" (calor heteropathicus) and much "exhaustion heat" (calor inanitatis).

2. Disturbances in the cardinales hepaticae yin flectentis pedis produce intense fever, accompanied by strong flexus (drop in temperature in the extremities); scarlet body of the tongue, reduced coating; sitis diffundens [diabetes]; shock, insanity; yellow urine; nausea, vomiting of ascarids; minute or agitated pulses (pp. minuti sive agitati); prickling in the fingers and toes; in extreme cases, flexus spasms, flutter of the heart.

Synthetic Table of the Affections of the Energies

Energy	Disease Mechanism	Symptoms
Defensive Energy (weiqi, qi defensivum)	A calor-heteropathy develops in the species, as a consequence of which the deployment of the energies of the o. pulmonalis is impaired.	Fever, slight shivering, slight thirst, cough; superficial and accelerated pulses (pp. superficiales et celeri), thin white coating, red tip and margins of the tongue.
Qi ("Individually specific active energy")	O. pulmonalis: Heat congestion, congestion of energy.	Panting, fever, heat, yellow coating of the tongue, thirst and other calor-symptoms.
	Mediastinum: Calor congestion, insufficient deployment of qi.	Heat, thin yellow coating of the tongue; palpitations, restlessness, nervousness.
	O. stomachi: Vigour of "heat" (calor vigens), conflict between the orthopathy and the heteropathies.	Intense fever, thirst, perspiration, heavy, audible breathing; yellow, dry coating of the tongue; flooding pulses (pp. exundantes).
	Oo. intestinorum: Calor congestion of energy	Intermittent fever, retention of urine, constipation; perspiration, hard, tender, sensitive abdomen; thick, yellow, dry coating of the tongue; submerged and replete pulses (pp. mersi et repleti)
	O. felleus: Ardor ("glare") from the gall bladder orb affects the o. stomachi; block and congestion in the wake of pituita and excessive "humdity".	Alternation between heat and cold as if with malaria, with preponderance of heat; dry mouth; pains at the small ribs; feeling of a lump in the stomach, nausea; yellow, slightly sticky coating of the tongue; stringy and accelerated pulses (pp. chordales et celeri).
	O. lienalis: "Humidity" is not harmoniously integrated, hence the accumulation of a humor-heteropathy.	Heat congestion, feeling of a lump in the stomach with intermittent nausea, fatigue, listlessness; sticky coating of the tongue; frail pulses (pp. lenes).
Ying ("Constructive energy", qi constructivum)	Calor ("heat") affects the structive energies; disturbed 'configurative force' (shen) of the o. cardialis.	Crimson to scarlet body of the tongue, considerable restlessness, insomnia, hot body; all symptoms aggravated during the night; only slight thirst; exanthemas, sometimes incoherent speech; minute and accelerated pulses (pp. minuti et celeri)
Xue ("Individually specific energy")	The xue is hemmed in due to vigor caloris; the 'configurative force' of the o. cardialis is disturbed.	Intensive scarlet colour of the tongue; blood in nasal mucus, saliva, urine and faeces; general exanthemas; restlessness; in extreme cases, insanity and raving madness.
Yin maior of the hand, corresponding to the pulmonal conduit	A heteropathy affects the defenses of the o. pulmonalis; consequently, the cooling, damping faculty of the orb is impaired.	Heat, shuddering, headache, thirst, cough; superficial pulses (pp. superficiales); white coating of the tongue.
	A calor-heteropathy penetrates into the o. pulmonalis; consequently, the deployment of its energy is blocked.	Heat, fever without shuddering; perspiration, thirst, cough, panting; yellow coating of the tongue; accelerated pulses (pp. celeri).
Yin flectens of the hand: the pericardial conduits	Calor destroys the constructive energy of the o. cardialis and blocks the o. pericardialis.	Body of the tongue crimson to scarlet red; dazedness, incoherent speech; sometimes fainting; lallation; cold extremities.
Splendor yang of the foot: Stomach conduits	Vigor caloris in the stomach orb; discordance between the orthopathy and heteropathies.	Fever and shuddering, oppressive heat, red complexion, red skleras, perspiration, thirst, panting; yellow or dry coating of the tongue; flooding and accelerated pulses (pp. exundantes et celeri).

PATHOLOGY

Energy	Disease Mechanism	Symptoms
Splendor yang of the hand: Large Intestine conduits	Calor constricts the flow of energies in the conduits of the o. intestini crassi.	Intermittent fever, constipation; urination reduced in quantity, also incoherent or faltering speech; yellow to blackish coating of the tongue, sometimes scorched or dry.
Yin maior of the foot: the conduits of the o. lienalis ("spleen orb")	Humor lienalis, i.e. the "humdity of the spleen orb" is not transformed harmoniously. From this an accumlation of a humor-heteropathy results.	Heat congestion, feeling of a lump in the thorax or stomach region; seizures of nausea with fatigue and prostration.
Yin minor of the foot: the renal conduits	Calor ("heat") affects the yin merum; there is danger of the exhaustion of the structive potential (jing).	Feverish body, red complexion; soles of the feet and palms of the hands are hotter than the backs of hands and feet; dry mouth and throat; exhausted pulses (pp. inanes); fatigue and listlessness.
Yin flectens of the foot: the hepatic conduits	Water, the energies of the o. renalis, do not irrigate Wood, the energies of the o. hepaticus; consequently, ventus inanitatis, a ventus due to exhaustion of that orb, arises within.	Flexus (retreat of energies inducing cold) in the extremities, flutter of the heart, trembling hands and feet, in extreme cases, spasms and pareses.

PART TWO — THE PRACTICE OF CHINESE DIAGNOSTICS

What makes Chinese diagnostics unique among comparable methods of ancient and modern times is that it achieves an optimum combination of the following criteria:

1. a primary concern with vital functions;

2. remarkable systematic plainness, hence accurate knowability, easy comprehension, great economy;

3. high rational consistency yet lucid stringency and precision;

4. the independence of exceptional endowment in the diagnostician and of complicated techniques;

5. utter absence of secondary side effects or uncontrolled repercussions on the patient; and, not the least merit,

6. unparallelled length of historical time - an average of 2000 years - taken for testing and developing, hence maturing, the methods applied today.

The first criterium - the primary concern with vital functions - has already succinctly been commented upon above[130]. There we also pointed out that one may hardly overrate the significance which the fulfillment of criterium 2 - systematic plainness and simplicity - and 3 - rational consistency and stringency - contribute toward the achievement of high precision, certitude and objectivity of diagnosis and, of course, therapy.

A point to be stressed here is that Chinese diagnostics, on the part of the physician, simply requires a normal and healthy function of his senses; it does not call for any extraordinary skills or faculties or require intricate instruments. (In admitting this, we do not deny that training and education of the senses involved is indispensable - just as with any other bodily skill.)

Finally, a word should be added on the absolute innocuousness of all Chinese diagnostics. That diagnosis primarily aimed at (and very often limited to) the determination of actual and present functions, cannot have the slightest repercusssions on the very data to be determined, may be of immediate evidence to any one used to

---

[130] Pp. 7 f.

dealing with epistemological problems. On the other hand, this fact may be utterly ignored by Western doctors who, because of their substratum-oriented intellectual training and their practical interests, usually are quite resigned to consider this argument of secondary importance, since precisely such repercussions escape their control and observation anyway.

Functional diagnosis, it has been said[131], cannot but encompass <u>all</u> aspects of an individual - not only the momentary effects of physical or biological factors relevant to a situation, but also all psychological and social ones.

Thus, for example, the Chinese never doubted that clothing, as a medium of screening and autorepresentation of a human being, constitutes an integral part of a personality. It is because of this, not because of prudery or indifference, that in Chinese diagnosis and treatment, the patient is never stripped more than the immediate situation requires. For an interrogation conducted with all required care, together with all the other diagnostic methods, as a rule gives precise information even on such pathological changes, which are part of the sphere of intimacy.

Chinese diagnostics gathers all data of specific relevance pertinent to a rational and specific diagnosis by the <u>joint</u> application of what are called the "Four Diagnoses" (<u>sizhen</u>), viz.:

      1. inspection (<u>inspectio, wang</u>),
      2. auscultation and olfaction (<u>auscultatio et olfactio, wén</u>)
      3. interrogation (<u>interrogatio, wen</u>) and
      4. palpation (<u>palpatio, qie</u>).

---

[131] Cf. p. 15 above.

Chapter One: *Inspectio,* The Diagnosis by Inspection *(Wangzhen)*

Inspection deals with diagnostically ascertaining the form, colour and typical movements of the body, also, more in detail, changes of the complexion and on the tongue; it also registers the colour and form of excretions. Inspection properly carried out, consequently, must furnish positive data on:

1. the configurative force (shen), as it manifests itself in the turgor of tissues, the tonus of muscles, the carriage of one's body, the lustre of eyes and skin, the humidity of mucus membranes etc.
2. the colour of particular parts of the face, of the body of the tongue, of the coating of the tongue and of certain other parts of the body acquiring significance in certain cases;
3. the outward form of the body in its entirety and in detail; finally,
4. the demeanour (tai), i.e. the comprehensive and specific qualities of body movement.

INSPECTION IN GENERAL

INSPECTION OF THE "CONFIGURATIVE FORCE" (wangshen)

In Chinese medicine, the term shen ("configurative force") designates that aspect of active energy producing and maintaining the specific existence and quality of an individual: shen, the configurative force, constitutes the personality[132]. However, shen, configurative force, if taken as an active aspect only, by definition[133], cannot be directly perceived; instead its quality must be deduced indirectly from the changes and manifestations in the body. Thus the strength of the configurative force is reflected in the clear and firm expression of the eyes, in the distinct articulation of speech, in the consistency and continuity of reflection, in the firmness of the flesh, in the balanced harmony of breathing, in the regularity of evacuations. If all these signs of a

---

[132] Cf. Porkert, Theoretical Foundations... p. 127 and pp. 181 f.

[133] Cf. what has been said above on p. 18.

strong and intact configurative force are present, a generally reassuring prognosis seems justified - even if other methods of diagnosis should reveal some critical signs.

Inversely, if a patient's gaze appears weak, unsteady, tired, if his body is decrepit and limp, if his breath comes accelerated, irregulary, panting or spluttering, if he cannot control his evacuations, if he moves unceasingly and without aim, if his speech is slurred and incoherent, if he is absentminded or unconscious, if his eyes are half closed and his mouth remains open, these are signs of a drastically depleted or exhausted configurative force, calling for an unfavourable prognosis even if other signs should be less critical. Thus

	A Sound and Intact Configurative Force Manifests Itself by	An Impaired, Defective Configurative Force Produces Symptoms Such as
Body and complexion	Healthy complexion, firm tissues, skin neither extremely dry nor extremely moist	Emaciation, sallow complexion and skin, very dry or very moist skin
Eyes	Vivid, steady, clear gaze	Indifferent, tired, wavering gaze
Emotions and sentiments	Clear, coherent thinking, distinct speech, presence of mind	Incoherent thinking, apathy, torpidness and aimless movements; extreme restiveness in bed.
Breathing	Regular	Irregular, accelerated or slowed down

Note: Symptoms of False Intactness of the Configurative Force:

In clinical practice it is a frequent occurrence that immediately before death, a short interlude of an intact configurative force occurs. This can be distinguished from true intactness by the fact that this false intactness usually is limited to single, particular functions, e.g. the gaze, speech, thinking, whereas the body as whole remains in critical condition, the pulses show serious disturbances. Chinese doctors call this the "last flare of an exhausted lamp", in analogy to what Western medicine knows as premortal euphoria.

THE INSPECTION OF COLOUR

The colour of the skin on parts of diagnostic relevance, e.g. the face, the tongue, the mucuous membranes, etc. changes significantly, depending upon the actual functions of the individual. When evaluating these changes, the diagnostician must of course distinguish between a basic pigmentation due to race or climate - called "dominant colour" - and its variable tinge changing with function - in Chinese this is

INSPECTIO, THE DIAGNOSIS BY INSPECTION

called the deversant[134] colour. As a rule, the dominant colour is withouth diagnostic significance. On the other hand, the deversant colour <u>may, if viewed jointly with other diagnostic results</u>, give an additional cue or confirmation of a certain diagnosis. The following table shows the classical correlations between colour tinges, evolutive phases, seasons and orbs.

Colour	Evolut. Phase	Season	<u>orbis horrealis</u>	<u>orbis aulicus</u>
Green (blue-green)	Wood	Spring	<u>o. hepaticus</u>	<u>o. felleus</u>
Red (scarlet or crimson)	Fire	Summer	<u>o. cardialis</u>	<u>o. intestini tenuis</u>
White	Metal	Autumn	<u>o. pulmonalis</u>	<u>o. intestini tenuis</u>
Black	Water	Winter	<u>o. renalis</u>	<u>o. vesicalis</u>
Yellow	Earth	All year	<u>o. lienalis</u>	<u>o. stomachi</u>

As for the <u>complexion</u> (the "colour of the face"), on a healthy individual, the basic colour produced by race and climate must show the typical pale pink tint, and at the same time a characteristic tonus. This basic colour of a healthy individual, in turn may be overlaid by a deversant colour, depending upon the season and the momentary functional situation. This overlay may be so weak as to pass unnoticed by an inexperienced diagnostician; or so pronounced that even a layman will be struck by it - according to the intensity of a disturbance within the concert of the orbs.

Also on all colour deversants, a distinction must be made between a reassuring and an unfavourable variety, the former indicating that in spite of an imbalance of functions, the configured energy, i.e. the <u>qi,</u> still circulates, the latter that it no longer circulates properly, but, rather is obstructed in certain sections.

In Chapter 10 of the Ingenuous Question in the Inner Classic of the Yellow Sovereign, the differences between reassuring and unfavourable tints is described thus:
"Greenness like a mat of grass is unfavourable, greenness like the plumes of the kingfisher is reassuring; yellow the colour of a lemon is unfavourable, yellow like the belly of a crab is reassuring; red like dried up blood is unfavourable, red like the comb of a cock is encouraging; white like dry bone is unfavourable, white like pork's grease is favourable; black like soot is

---

[134] 'Deversant' from the Latin <u>deversari</u>, "to be a guest", is the complement of <u>dominari</u>, "to be the master".

126   THE ESSENTIALS OF CHINESE DIAGNOSTICS

unfavourable, black like the feathers of a raven is favourable."

As a rule, any colour variety in which the skin still has a mellow glimmer and pink tinge may be classed as reassuring, and any colour variety where the skin looks faded, flabby, without lustre, and whose colour comes out harsh and undiluted, must be taken as a sombre sign. Flabbiness of the skin indicates a loss of the inner balance of energies called "loss of the stomach-qi"[135]; or, it may appear as the consequence of the total breakdown of an orb. (The Chinese called this faded, lustreless appearance of the skin "colour of early death".

The data obtained by the inspection of colour may concur with or differ from the results obtained by other diagnostic methods. In the first eventuality, the relationships defined by the sequences of the evolutive phases are of particular interest, and here especially sequences I and II ("production sequence", "conquest sequence"). For the production sequence indicates a secundovection ("correct, conforming flow of energy"); the conquest sequence corresponds to a contravection ("incorrect, adverse flow of energy").

To illustrate, if with a disease of the o. hepaticus, a greenish tinge of the complexion, a stringy pulse (p. chordalis), pains near the small ribs, a bitter taste in the mouth and dizziness occur, these symptoms all express agreement of colour, pulse iconogram and other signs – and thus facilitate diagnosis. On these premises, in the case of diseases in the o. hepaticus such as ventus-heteropathies, with dizziness, pains and tensions in the region of the small ribs and, on infants, epileptiform symptoms and convulsions, a bluish-green complexion expresses agreement, hence secundovection; by contrast a pure white complexion "conquest", hence contravection : a contrary evolution of symptoms, a contrary flow of energies. If raving madness, palpitations, anxiousness, apprehension are present, all these disturbances pointing to the o. cardialis, a strikingly red complexion indicates agreement (hence secundovection), a darkish complexion expresses conquest, hence contravection, etc.

INSPECTION OF THE BODILY SHAPE

As has been explained above, orbs and the bodily shape are closely and precisely interrelated. This is why the inspection of the so-called "specific unfoldments"

---

[135] More will be said on this notion below on pp. 243 f.

INSPECTIO, THE DIAGNOSIS BY INSPECTION

(perfectiones, chung) and of the "outward manifestations" (flores, hua, rong)[136] furnishes important data on the general constitution as well as on the momentary function of the corresponding orbs in the patient.

Heavy bones, a wide thorax, firm flesh, a subdued lustre and slight pinkness of the skin are distinct signs of a strong constitution, just as delicate bones, a small thorax, meagreness and lustreless pale skin indicate a weak constitution.

The following correlations are of particular interest:

the sleekness of the shape and bodily form: the economy of juices and liquids;

the wideness of pores: the strength of constructive and defensive energies;

the resilience of flesh: the energy level (inanitas: repletio) of the orthopathy in general, and of the qi stomachi;

the strength of the nervus ("muscles and sinews"): the quantity of the xue (individually specific structive energies) stored in the o. hepaticus;

the largeness of bones: the strength of congenital, constitutional energy resources.

A strong body and good appetite indicate strength of the oo. lienalis et stomachi; a fat body and reduced appetite indicate pituita ("sticky phlegm") and exhaustion (inanitas) of the o. lienalis.

A lean body and strong appetite indicate ardor ("glare") in the calorium medium ("middle heated space") (i.e. in the oo. lienalis, stomachi, hepaticus et felleus); a completely emaciated body indicates that active as well as structive energies have been spent to the extreme.

THE INSPECTION OF MOTIONS AND MOVEMENTS

Continuous twitching of the eyelids, of the mouth, of the fingers or toes, in the case of febrile illnesses, may be a precursory sign of imminent spastic paresis, in the case of inanitas-diseases, the sign of imminent exhaustion of structive energies.

Twitching affecting all extremities or the whole body accompanies ventus internus-affections, in particular epilepsy, also ventus laedens perniciosus [tetanus]; also, they may be observed with infantile spasms etc.

Intense trembling, except in seizures of malaria, is observed when a powerful clash between heteropathics and the qi orthopathicum occurs; on first aid cases it must be

---

[136] Cf. p. 29 above.

determined whether this trembling indicates tetanus or general septicemia.

A restlessly groping hand must be considered an unfavourable sign.

A lowered head and the inability of the patient to raise it, also a fixed stare, are symptoms of a depleted configurative force (due to lesions of the oo. cardialis et renalis).

Affections of the thorax may lead to a bent back and to drooping arms; affections of the hips and lower back to the inability to bend in the back.

A forward bend in standing and walking indicate a disease of the nervus (i.e. of the muscles and sinews); the inability to support long standing, and ceaseless quivering of the body, point to a disease of the bones (i.e. the perfectio of the renal orb).

If a patient in bed faces toward the room, and if he is capable of easily turning on the side, this may be interpreted as yang-symptoms, symptoms of calor or repletion. If a patient prefers to face away from the room, if he feels heavy and unable to turn on his side, as a rule this indicates symptoms of yin, algor and inanitas.

A patient bent up in bed usually is affected by inanitas yang (exhaustion of the active energies), by shuddering or by acute pains.

If the patient lies in bed on his back, with the legs stretched out, this indicates yang-symptoms, an excess of calor ("vigorous heat", calor vigens).

A patient asking to be covered up tightly thus expresses inner or outer cold (algor externus sive internus); a patient trying to throw off his blankets shows symptoms of inner or outer heat (calor).

A patient leaning back when sitting indicates repletio o. pulmonalis ("repletion of the lung orb"); a patient leaning forward when sitting expresses exhaustion of that orb (inanitas o. pulmonalis).

A patient gasping for breath or experiencing contravective movement of qi (contravectio qi) when lying down, exhibits signs of a distension of the pulmonary orb, as the consequence of chronic cough [emphysema].

Dizziness when sitting up and the desire to lie down point to exhaustion (inanitas) of active as well as of structive energies.

A fidgety patient who constantly changes from lying down to sitting up is a highly agitated patient.

INSPECTION OF THE TONGUE ("tongue diagnosis," *shezhen*)

1. Theoretical Considerations

Among the various types of diagnostic inspections (inspectiones), the inspection of the tongue is of exceptional importance because of the subtlety and precision of the data it produces. Out of the perspective of Chinese medical theory, three reasons may be adduced to explain this exceptional role.

1. The tongue constitutes the sense organ (guan) of the o. cardialis ("cardial orb"). Now the cardial orb is the "prince" among all orbs, consequently that orb from which all directive influence and clear insights emanate; it is the seat of the configurative force (shen), the orb that establishes the specific quality of a personality and maintains its cohesion[137].

2. The tongue as the seat of taste (gustatory faculty) and the sense organ within the mouth - the latter corresponding to the opening of the o. lienalis - has a particular affinity to that orb and its species, i.e. the o. stomachi[138]. And these two orbs - qualified by the E.P. Earth - constitute the central positions for the assimilation as well as for the distribution of energy, in other words, of the maintenance of the energetic balance between all other orbs.

3. The following conduits touch the tongue or the root of the tongue:

a) the reticular conduit of minor yin of the hand of the cardial orb (reticularis cardialis yin minoris manus)[139],

b) the cardinal conduit of minor yin of the foot of the renal orb (cardinalis renalis yin minoris pedis)[140],

c) the cardinal conduit of yielding yin of the foot of the hepatic orb (cardinalis hepatica yin flectentis pedis)[141], and

d) the cardinal conduit of major yin of the foot of the lienal orb (cardinalis lienalis yin maioris pedis)[142].

---

[137] Cf. Porkert, Theoretical Foundations... pp. 124 - 128.

[138] Cf. op. cit. p. 132.

[139] Op. cit. p. 305.

[140] Op. cit. p. 251.

[141] Op. cit. p. 271.

[142] Op. cit. p. 233.

From all these correspondences, it is evident that the tongue directly reflects the situation in the most important control and regulative centres of the individual, and consequently indirectly shows the functional situation in all other orbs also.

The quantity and precision of diagnostic information obtained from tongue diagnosis in Chinese medicine is second only to that obtained from pulse diagnosis. Moreover the diagnostician can without difficulty also exercise tongue diagnosis upon himself; and there is no limit to the number of patients per day on whom he may do tongue diagnosis. This is why the practitioner should rather quickly acquire familiarity with this diagnostic procedure and apply the inspection of the tongue without exception to every diagnostic case.

Every inspection of the tongue must determine separately the complementary data on the body of the tongue (corpus linguae, shezhi) and the coating of the tongue (tegmen linguae, shetai).

The shape, the colour and other qualities, such as the moistness of the body of the tongue, correspond to information on the energy levels within the orbs, within the intima - thus permitting determination of an exhaustion of the orthopathy (inanitas) or a repletion of heteropathies.

The colour, the thickness and the particular structure of the coating of the tongue essentially correspond to information on the depth of penetration of a heteropathy (into the species or intima), on algor or calor ("heat" or "cold"), and on the constitution of the qi stomachi[143], i.e. on the general balance of energies among all orbs.

The quality of the constantly and quickly changing coating of the tongue is indicative of the state of active energies, and the quality of the relatively inert, slowly transformed body of the tongue is indicative of the state of structive energies.

If we must decide whether a heteropathy has preponderantly affected the active or proponderantly affected the structive energies, inspection of the tongue is of critical value. For in the first case, the coating shows striking changes whereas the body of the tongue appears to be barely affected; in the second case, the inverse is true.

The fact that the body of the tongue gives information about the state of structive energies in general and about the resources of the qi stomachi in particular explains its critical and decisive importance for prognosis: If a practically normal body of the tongue is covered with an abnormal or striking coating, we must conclude that there is a momentary, superficial

---

[143] Cf. note 135 on page 126 above.

INSPECTIO, THE DIAGNOSIS BY INSPECTION

irregularity in the energy flow; if, by contrast, the body of the tongue, without any trace of redness looks shrunken and parched, one would be greatly reluctant to give a reassuring prognosis.

2. Topology and Correspondences

As with other sites of the body of exceptional diagnostic significance - such as the ostium pollicare in pulse diagnosis[144] - all other regions of the body and all orbs are correlated to the tongue on several levels.

To start with, and to bridge the gap between the substratum-oriented view of Western medicine and the function-oriented view of Chinese medicine, we may draw the attention of otorhinolaryngologists to the striking and highly specific changes affecting the coating as well as the body of the tongue during all pathological processes in the maxilla, nose and all sinuses.

Pathological activity of foci in the maxilla entails clearly defined cut-out sections in the coating of the tongue, changing their size from day to day. Serious septic processes in the sinus maxillaris, moreover, affect the body of the tongue, there producing prolonged unilateral shrinkage of the affected side.

And, of course, any pathological process of the nose or its sinuses entails a permanent increase in thickness of the coating of the tongue radiating out from the root of the tongue. The extension of this coating in the direction of the tip of the tongue changes continuously, depending upon the strength of the orthopathy. And yet, Chinese medicine, it should be stressed, cannot conceive of a purely otorhinolaryngological symptom limited to such a small region: Every affection, even the slightest change of the colour of the coating, affects the entire individual.

Indeed, the region of the head beginning with the pharynx and extending upward to the tip of the nose and the so-called plexus ocularis, is the terminal or the transit of nearly all conduits. Thus this region is connected to the

	by its
orbis pulmonalis	paracardinalis
orbis intestini crassi	cardinalis, reticularis, nervocardinalis
orbis stomachi	cardinalis, paracardinalis, reticularis, nervocardinalis
orbis lienalis	cardinalis

---

[144] Cf. below pp. 205 ff.

	by its
orbis cardialis	cardinalis, paracardinalis, reticularis
orbis intestini tenuis	cardinalis, nervocardinalis
orbis vesicalis	cardinalis, paracardinalis, nervocardinalis
orbis renalis	cardinalis, paracardinalis
orbis pericardialis	paracardinalis
orbis tricalorii	cardinalis, nervocardinalis
orbis felleus	cardinalis, paracardinalis, nervocardinalis
orbis hepaticus	cardinalis, paracardinalis.

In other words, the postulates of sinarteriology amply demonstrate the multiple connections and affinities of all orbs with the region of the sensorium of the head, and in particular that of the sinuses and cavities of nose, mouth and throat – thus explaining why every kind of functional change taking place in the individual must have immediate repercussions upon the tongue.

The second (in classical Chinese theory the first) diagnostic correspondence of the tongue is that with the stomach orb - which, as we just explained, is directly or indirectly connected to the tongue by all four kinds of conduits. On this level

the tip of the tongue may be correlated to the "entrance of the stomach" (shangguan),

the middle of the tongue may be correlated to the "middle of the stomach" (zhongguan), and

the root of the tongue may be correlated to the "exit of the stomach" (xiaguan).

Here again, the reader should be warned not to replace the correspondences of Chinese concepts by current Western anatomical terms[145]. Here, as elsewhere in Chinese medicine[146], the physician must have in mind a functional model in which the "entrance of the stomach" corresponds to the assimilating functional aspects, the "middle of the stomach" corresponds to the integrating, provisionally storing functions[147], the "exit of the stomach" corresponds to the distributive and

---

[145] Such as pars kardiaca or pars pylorica...

[146] Cf. Porkert, Theoretical Foundations... pp. 107 f.

[147] Cf. the iconogram of the orbis lienalis in op. cit. pp. 128 - 136.

transmitting functions of the stomach orb (o. stomachi).

The third and last correspondence level to be considered is the equally significant and useful correlation between the tongue and all orbs, thus between

the root of the tongue and the renal orb (o. renalis directly, also to the oo. intestinorum et vesicalis, indirectly);

the tip of the tongue to the cardial orb (o. cardialis directly) (also to the oo. pulmonalis et pericardialis indirectly);

the lateral margins of the tongue to the hepatic and gall bladder orbs (oo. hepaticus et felleus directly); and

the centre of the tongue to the lienal and stomach orbs (oo. lienalis et stomachi) (Fig. 6)

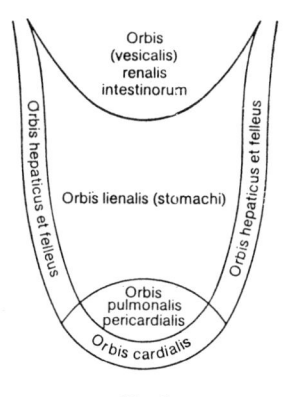

Fig. 6.

When interpreting the data of inspection of the tongue in actual practice, the decision to proceed on one or the other of the "levels" just described is not an arbitrary or accidental one; in fact, it is prompted by the diagnostic context (and clinical experience).

Let us recall that anyone who has advanced more deeply into Chinese medical theory, in the three levels or kinds of topological correlations will not see alternatives excluding each other but rather various aspects of an identical diagnosis merging into each other. Thus, in practice, the availability of other diagnostic data with a clearly circumscribed syndrome will let us begin on level three – and stay there. If, by contrast, all signs point to the hypothesis that the primary affection corresponds to a disturbance of the central controls[148], we shall elaborate on the second level our interpretation of the diagnostic signs obtained by the inspection of the tongue.

Precautions to be Taken When Inspecting the Tongue

1) Lighting

As a rule, the inspection of the tongue should be executed under ordinary daylight conditions or what (in modern cabinets with artificial lighting only) closely reproduces these: Colour temperatures equal to or slightly below 5600° K. Ordinary tungsten bulb lighting, with a colour temperature below 3200° K, would absolutely preclude the quite essential and critical distinction between white and yellow tints of the coating of the tongue.

2. Inquiry into Constitutional Factors and Influences

The typical thickness and tinge of the coating of the tongue on a particular individual may be influenced not only by seasonal changes, but also by inborn constitutional factors. Thus an individual with a higher degree of humor ("humidity") or a higher level of energy in the central orbs (i.e. in the oo. lienalis et stomachi) will, during the greater part of his life span, have a thicker coating of the tongue than other individuals - and still be in perfect health. If, on such an individual, in the wake of a disturbance, a truly "thin" coating is observed, the concomitant disease will be much more serious than on other individuals, normally showing a coating of the tongue of average thickness. If there are doubts in this respect, the patient should be closely questioned.

3) The Traces of Recently Absorbed Food and Drink

If striking modifications of the colour and coating of the tongue are observed, it should be a matter of course that the patient is questioned on the recent intake of food and beverages (spices, fruit juices, alcohol).

4) Cleaning the Tongue

---

[148] Within the context of Chinese medical theory, this implies the orbs qualified by the central E.P. Earth: the oo. lienalis et stomachi.

If a very thick coating of the tongue is present and/or the colour of the body of the tongue can be ascertained only with difficulty, an attempt should be made to wipe the tongue. Such wiping may acquire critical signficance if we must distinguish between "true" and "false" coating. This wiping is best accomplished with a swab of cotton or a small pad filled with cotton and soaked in a very mild disinfectant such as chrysanthemum tea or chamomile tea, and manipulated with a pair of forceps.

4) Diagnostic Inspection of the Body of the Tongue (Inspectio corporis linguae, zhen-shezhi)

As with inspection in general, at inspection of the body of the tongue, its shen ("configurative force"), colour, shape and movement must be registered.

1) Inspection of the Configurative Force of the Body of the Tongue

The presence of configurative force in the body of the tongue manifests itself by its lustre. If the body of the tongue shows lustre and light, bright colours, it is endowed with vital energy and configurative force. On an ill person, such signs justify a reassuring prognosis. If, on the contrary, the body of the tongue looks parched and dried out, or is deprived of lustre or sheen, this indicates a serious deficiency of fluids and suggests a sombre prognosis.

2) Inspection of the Colour of the Body of the Tongue

The body of the tongue of a healthy individual is a vivid and lively neutral red colour. When disease is present, the following deviations may be observed:

a) Deep Crimson Coloured Body of the Tongue (somewhat deeper red than normal): If the body of the tongue shows an intense red, but no other changes, this is a symptom either of calor ("heat") or of repletio ("repletion"). If, moreover, it looks exceedingly dry, it must be inferred that the production of yang fluids in the o. stomachi is impaired. If it is not only dry but, in addition, deprived of a coating, this lesion has progressed considerably (individuals addicted to strong liquor usually show an intensely red body of the tongue).

b) A Pale Body of the Tongue: Paleness is a symptom either of algor ("cold") or inanitas ("exhaustion"). If the body of the tongue, in addition, is deprived of its coating, deficiency, depletion of the active as well as of the structive energies must be inferred.

c) Blood-coloured Body of the Tongue: If fever diseases are present, this is a symptom of calor ("heat"); in the presence of phthisic symptoms, it indicates exhaustion (inanitas) of the structive energies. If, in addition, no coating of the tongue may be observed, we must conclude that ardor ("glare") as the consequence of exhaustion of yin (inanitas yin), i.e. ardor inanitatis yin, prevails; if a blood-red body of the tongue develops pointed protuberances, this must be interpreted as powerful expansion of "heat" of the constructive energy (vigor caloris qi constructivi); if on a blood-red body of the tongue purple strips appear, these are signs for an imminent exanthema.

d) Scarlet-coloured Body of the Tongue: If calor ("heat") in the course of a febrile illness has affected the constructive energy (qi constructivum), the body of the tongue will be scarlet red; if it has affected the xue, i.e. the individually specific structive energy, it shows an intense scarlet colour. If this scarlet tinge of the body of the tongue is preceded by a yellow or white colour of the coating, this lets us conclude that the heteropathy at that stage only deversates in the active energies (qi) and has not yet attained the constructive energy.

If the entire body of the tongue shows a shining scarlet colour, one must consider a disturbance of the o. pericardialis.

If the centre of a scarlet body of the tongue appears to be dry, this indicates that in the wake of "glare" (ardor) in the o. stomachi, the production of yang fluids has been impaired.

If the scarlet colouring is restricted to the tip of the tongue, we may conclude that "glare" is present in the o. cardialis.

If a scarlet body of the tongue shows blood-coloured splashes, this indicates that a calor-heteropathy overlies the functions of the o. cardialis.

If a scarlet-red body of the tongue looks as if lacquer has been applied to it, this indicates that the structive energies of the stomach orb have been dispersed or lost. If, on the contrary, a scarlet body of the tongue is without sheen, even looks dry, this indicates that the structive energies of the o. renalis are about to be depleted.

If a scarlet-coloured body of the tongue looks as if it were dry, yet upon touch proves to be moist, it must be inferred that a "humid heat"-heteropathy (calor humidus) rises to the surface as the consequence of a deficiency of yang-fluids; or a block produced by turgid pituita ("phlegm") may produce this symptom.

If a scarlet-coloured body of the tongue is covered with a sticky coating so that it

INSPECTIO, THE DIAGNOSIS BY INSPECTION

is difficult to determine its quality, this indicates an obscurement of the energies in the calorium medium ("middle heated space").

e) Purple Body of the Tongue: If a purple-coloured body of the tongue looks dry or parched, this is indicative of the presence of a calor-heteropathy; if it is moist or only faintly purple, we may infer an algor-heteropathy. If the intense purple extends over the whole body of the tongue, we may conclude that extreme "heat" (calor, ardor) is present in all orbs. If, however, the purple colour is restricted to certain parts of the tongue, this indicates that the excessive heat is limited to the orb or conduit corresponding to that part of the tongue.

If a faintly purple body of the tongue has a slippery surface, this is an algor-symptom.

If the tongue is moist and the body of the tongue shows a darkish purple colour, this indicates stasis, stagnation of the individually specific structure energies (xue).

f) Blue Body of the Tongue: The blue colour of the body of the tongue is a critical symptom indicating the deficiency both of active and structive energies. If a blue body of the tongue still bears a coating, this indicates that in spite of heavy lesions of the orb functions, a favourable outcome is still conceivable; if this coating, however, has disappeared, the blue colour is an extremely unfavourable sign, pointing to incurable total exhaustion of active and structive energies.

If the blue colour manifests itself only weakly or partially, this, as a rule, is a sign of an acute infectious disease, sometimes also a symptom of an incompletely cured aestus-heteropathy, originally induced by calor humidus.

If the blue colour is limited to the centre of the body of the tongue, and if this tongue is slippery or sticky, we may infer that humor-heteropathies, thus pituita in different stages of maturity, are present.

In conclusion, any kind of bluish tint of the tongue is a critical symptom. However, to assess its importance correctly, we must always compare it with the symptoms showing calor and algor, repletio and inanitas; and, of course, we must also take into consideration the age and the general constitution of the patient according to the data furnished by all other diagnostic processes.

Black Body of the Tongue: If the entire body of the tongue is black, the ancients considered this an infallible sign of imminent death, for this colour implies that the individually specific structive energy (xue) has been entirely corrupted by either extreme "heat" (calor, ardor) or extreme "cold" (algor). In order to decide whether the black colour of the body of the tongue is the consequence of calor or algor, we must ascertain whether the body of the tongue is soft and moist or hardened and parched. The former symptoms then point to algor inanitatis ("cold on the basis of exhaustion"), the latter to ardor ("glare"). Indeed, if a precise and rapid diagnosis is achieved, and immediate treatment undertaken, even a black-coloured body of the tongue does not under all circumstances warrant an unfavourable prognosis.

3) Inspection of the Shape of the Body of the Tongue

When considering the shape of the body of the tongue, we should first correlate it to the general appearance of the individual we are diagnosing. A heavy, thick-set individual, if he is healthy, shows a correspondingly broad and firm body of the tongue; a lean individual in good health, will have a correspondingly lean body of the tongue. Also, there is a correspondence between the abundance of constitutional reserves (corresponding to the inborn resources of the o. renalis) in relation to age: the newborn infant has a broad tongue almost completely filling the space between his gums; an aged person, although quite healthy, because of his relatively depleted resources of the o. renalis, will have a much more slender tongue in spite of the still impressive shape of the body.

Certain degenerative diseases, in particular [multiple sclerosis], produce a typical wedge-shaped body of the tongue.

The massive use of drastic remedies such as antibiotics, if they have severely attacked the congenital or acquired resources of the individual, will produce temporary or lasting shrinkage of the body of the tongue.

When attempting a differential diagnosis of the body of the tongue, note should be taken as to whether it appears to be tender or tough, whether it shows fine pricks, fissures or cracks, whether it looks bloated or, on the contrary, shrunken.

a) Tenderness of the Tongue: The body of the tongue must be called tough or literally "hardened by age", leathery, if, independent of its particular colour - whitish, yellowish, ash-coloured or black - it looks solid and hardened: an impression making us conclude that repletio is present. Inversely, tenderness, i.e. a soft and turgid body of the tongue (sometimes showing imprints of the teeth) is - quite independent of the colour of the coating - always a symptom of exhaustion (inanitas).

b) Pricks and Fissures: Slight roughness of the surface of the tongue was thought by the ancients to indicate that the energy of the o. pulmonalis develops in harmony with

INSPECTIO. THE DIAGNOSIS BY INSPECTION

the inborn energies of the o. renalis[149], in other words, it was taken as a sure sign of the normal functions of the individual. If this slight roughness is barely present or totally absent, this indicates relative exhaustion of the orthopathic energy (qi orthopathicum). On the other hand, prominent pointed protuberances are signs of the accumulation of calor-heteropathies in the individual, and the power of the calor-heteropathy may be directly correlated to the size and number of these protuberances. Moreover, their location on the surface of the tongue may indicate which orbs are particularly affected by the heteropathy.

The pointed protuberances mentioned must also be viewed in connection with the colour of the body and coating of the tongue. If the pointed protuberances appear with a black coating of the tongue, this is a symptom of a more critical stage of a calor-heteropathy than if the same protuberances appeared on a sallow, yellow coating of the tongue. If, on the other hand, the body of the tongue, at the appearance of the protuberances, is scarlet in colour, this implies that a powerful calor-heteropathy has already produced lesions in the store of structive energies.

Fissures and ravines are indicative of "rampant heat" (calor vigens, vigor caloris), either because the individually specific structive energy (xue) shows relative exhaustion, or because structive energies in general are deficient.

If the tongue showing fissures is a lustrous scarlet red, this indicates that the yin-fluids are severely affected; if, by contrast, the fissures appear on a pale-coloured, tender tongue, the depletion of structive energies essentially affects the o. renalis.

c) Puffed Body of the Tongue: A puffed, bloated body of the tongue usually indicates affections of the xue, of the individually specific structive energies, either because pituita is present, or because calor humidus has accumulated within.

A fiery red body of the tongue almost completely filling the mouth is a sign of calor or ardor ("heat" or "glare") in the orbes et cardinales lienalis et cardialis (cardial and lienal orbs and conduits). If, more extreme still, the distended tongue impedes breathing, this indicates extreme ardor in the conduits, in the wake of a block of the energy flow.

A puffed, bluish-green, purple or blackish body of the tongue is a symptom of poisoning, e.g. by alcohol.

---

[149] I.e. a harmonious blending of its energies with the active energies issuing forth from the inborn constitutional reserves of the orbis renalis.

d) Shrunken Body of the Tongue: A body of the tongue must be qualified as shrunken or shrivelled if it looks extremely slender or extremely thin. If such a shrunken body of the tongue has a tender surface and is pale to pale-pink in colour, we must deduce exhaustion of energy in the oo. cardialis et lienalis or sometimes a general deficiency of active as well as of structive energies.

If the shrunken body of the tongue is scarlet to crimson in colour, we may infer an exhaustion of the yin and "rampant heat" (calor vigens), or a critical lesion of active and structive fluids - the latter again critical symptoms.

If the shrunken tongue looks dark, grey or even blackish, and if aphasia is present, the prognosis is unfavourable.

4) Inspection of the Position and Movements of the Tongue (Inspectio positionis motusque corporis linguae)

When considering the position and movements of the tongue at diagnostic inspection, distinctions must be made among

1. an elastic, 2. a stiff, 3. a trembling, 4. a paretic, 5. a side-wise slipping, 6. a drooling, and 7. a retreated tongue, and 8. a tongue oscillating between the lips.

a) An elastic body of the tongue is the rule on healthy persons, indicating normal physiological functions. On a sick individual, an elastic, moist, medium-red tongue of average mobility indicates an harmonious flow of energy throughout all orbs and permits us to conclude that disease in evidence must be slight or at least does not endanger life.

b) A hardened or stiff body of the tongue impeding speech may occur with exogenous disturbances, i.e. those induced by climatic excesses, as well as those resulting from endogenous factors.

Stiffness of the tongue in the wake of an exogenous factor occurs if a noxious influence penetrating through the o. pericardialis eventually affects the configurative force, thus impairing the mobility of the tongue; or if, as the consequence of very high fever, the active fluids have been depleted and the nervocardinal conduits carry an insufficient supply of energy to the tongue. In both cases, the tongue shows an intensely red colour.

Within the frame of morbi varii, a stiff tongue may be the corollary of ventus internus [i.e. states of shock or apoplexy, sometimes accompanied by hemiplegia, disturbed coördination of the muscles of the eyes, mouth and face], sudden collapse. Sometimes stiffness of the tongue is a precursory sign of such an attack of vento percussio [apoplexy]. Finally, the stiffness of the tongue may be due to obstruction of the conduits leading to the tongue by pituita ("phlegm") - such a diagnosis being corroborated by puffedness and a dirt-coloured coating.

c) A quivering tongue indicates exhaustion (inanitas) or ventus of the o. hepaticus. If a quivering tongue is red, and if speech is impeded, there is energetic deficiency in the cardial and lienal orbs; or there may be repletion of structive energies in the wake of profuse perspiration (as part of the symptoms of ventus hepaticus).

If the quivering tongue protrudes from the mouth, this is a symptom of alcohol poisoning. If the quivering tongue is pale red, one may infer the deficiency of structive energies and a welling up of active energies due to ventus hepaticus. If a quivering body of the tongue is purple, this indicates that a calor-heteropathy has developed in the o. hepaticus.

d) A paretic tongue corresponds to an elastic body of the tongue which, however, is incapable of any wilful movement - due to the total deficiency of energy in the nervocardinales.

If a paretic, white tongue occurs after prolonged disease, this is a sign of exhaustion of the active as well as of the structive energies. By contrast, a paresis of a red tongue after recent disease indicates that the yin (structive energies) has been impaired by calor ("heat"). If, after prolonged disease, there is a scarlet, paretic tongue, this is a symptom of extreme deficiency of structive energies.

e) A tongue lolling laterally occurs in the wake of vento percussio [after apoplexy].

f) A protruding tongue essentially points to one of two conditions.
First, if the patient feels relieved when he sticks out his hot puffy tongue, this is a sign of repletion and of calor pituitae orbis cardialis ("heat on the basis of a phlegm-heteropathy in the cardial orb").
Second, a strikingly protruding, insensitive tongue is a symptom of the exhaustion of active energies.

If a protruding tongue cannot be retracted wilfully, or if it is dry and without coating, these are signs of imminent death; if these conditions are absent, there may be room for therapeutic measures.

g) A retracted tongue that cannot wilfully be extended usually represents a critical symptom. If the retracted tongue is white and moist, this indicates algor ("cold") tying up the energy flow in the nervocardinales (muscle conduits). If the retracted tongue is red and dry, a lesion of active fluids from a fever disease must be inferred.

If the retracted tongue has a sticky coating, pituita humida ("phlegm from a humidity-heteropathy") blocks the flow of energy.

If the retracted tongue moreover is stiff, or if the patient is dazed, raves or at the outset had been affected by a pituita-disorder, this combination must be considered a very grave diagnosis.

h) A tongue is said to be oscillating between the lips when the body of the tongue is barely showing between the lips and rapidly withdrawn or advanced or moving rapidly across the lips, appearing and disappearing. Both kinds of movement accompany a serious stage of calor in the oo. cardialis et lienalis.

If the lips are incessantly licked (moistened) by the tongue, this points to ariditas ("dryness") affecting the o. lienalis. If the advanced tongue is purple and painful, calor-heteropathies affecting certain orbs, especially the cardial orb, may be inferred.

The Diagnostic Inspection of the Coating of the Tongue

The coating of the tongue is due to one or several of the following three factors:
1. the radiation of the (active) energies of the stomach orb;
2. the projection of a heteropathy (qi heteropathicum) onto the surface of the tongue; or
3. traces of ingested food and drink.

On a healthy individual, the coating of the tongue is produced by the qi stomachi and is a whitish, sometimes barely yellow, translucent and spotless layer, which is neither dry nor particularly moist, neither slippery nor parched. In summer, the coating of the tongue may have a somewhat increased thickness without completely covering the body of the tongue and without ever forming a solid and brittle layer.

At diagnostic inspection of the coating of the tongue, again a distinction is made between shape and colour.

1) Shape of the Coating of the Tongue and Its Relation to Pathological Disturbances

INSPECTIO, THE DIAGNOSIS BY INSPECTION

When describing the "shape" (xing) of the coating of the tongue, the following criteria must be taken into account:
a) the presence or absence of a coating;
b) the fastness ("trueness") or looseness ("falseness") of the coating;
c) whether the body of the tongue is partly or completely covered by the coating;
d) whether the coating is thick or thin, dry or moist, putrid or sticky.

a') Fast Coating of the Tongue ("True Coating"): A coating which sticks firmly to the surface of the tongue, so to speak growing out of it, and which will not disappear by rubbing or chafing nor change its appearance, is called a fast, sticking or true coating.

A fast coating develops as a consequence of the agglutination of a qi heteropathicum, of heteropathic energy. At the outset or in the middle stage of illness, fast coating indicates a mild course of disease; a loose ("rootless", "unrooted") coating, by contrast, a more profound, more serious course of disease. Also, after a crisis, in the final stage of a disease, a thick, loose coating must be considered a more critical sign than a fast coating. It should, however, be noted that below a thick and apparently "rootless" coating, a fast new coating of different colour has formed - indicating the beginning of recovery.

a") Loose Coating, ("False Coating"): A coating not firmly sticking to the tongue, in a way only painted on, without root, is called a loose or, literally in Chinese, a "false" coating of the tongue. Such a "false" coating, no matter what other characteristics it may show, can be wiped off or rubbed off, thus revealing the naked body of the tongue.

A loose ("false") coating of the tongue corresponds to three kinds of disturbances, viz.

1. If a loose coating has disappeared after a meal, the energy of some horreal orb was momentarily depleted, but there was no serious disturbance.
2. A loose, coloured coating disappearing after the tongue has been wiped, indicates a light disease; a loose coating which can be rubbed off simply by chafing the tongue against the teeth points to a quite superficial disturbance.
3. It is quite a different matter with the third kind of loose coating, which appears after prolonged illness: As a consequence of exhaustion of the active energies in the o. stomachi (qi stomachi), the organism can no longer produce a fast coating. Such a state may occur as the sequel to the prolonged use of cooling prescriptions, which has

impaired the yang or, on the contrary, by the use of hot prescriptions, which has harmed the yin.

b) The Presence or Absence of a Coating of the Tongue: If a patient, at first inspection, shows no coating, but if such a coating suddenly appears during a later stage, this indicates either that the murky energy of the stomach orb extravasates above, or that a calor-heteropathy gradually increases in strength. Inversely, if at the first inspection a coating was present which later on disappears, this disappearance indicates that the structive energies of the stomach orb are approaching exhaustion or, more generally, that the o. stomachi is deficient in energy.

c) Partial or Complete Coating of the Tongue:

A partial coating may be restricted to one side of the tongue, to the centre of the tongue or to the margin of the tongue.

If the tongue of a patient is completely covered by a coating, without corollary symptoms, this indicates that a heteropathy or disturbance affects the complete individual.

If the centre of the tongue is deprived of coating, but if such a coating is present at the margins, it may be inferred that a heteropathy has not yet penetrated into the intima, and that, for the time being, it has only affected the qi stomachi (the active energies of the stomach orb).

If the centre of the tongue is coated, but the margin of the tongue is not, this indicates that a surface-heteropathy may be retreating, that a block affecting the energy flow of the stomach orb persists; or there may be a persistent block affecting the oo. intestinorum; or there may be an accumulation of pituita ("phlegm").

If the coating of the tongue is restricted to one side only, the conclusion to be drawn is that the corresponding heteropathy is partly in the species, and partly in the intima - and that particular diagnostic attention must be paid to the colour of the body of the tongue.

If the centre of the tongue is deprived of coating, this indicates that the yin is exhausted or that individually specific structive energy is exhausted, or that the qi stomachi has been affected.

c') Changes of the coating of the tongue reflect changes in the functional equilibrium of the individual. Thus, after the outbreak of an infectious fever disease (morbus temperatus), the coating very often changes in colour from white to yellow, and in the course of recovery changes back again from yellow to white. However, in

INSPECTIO, THE DIAGNOSIS BY INSPECTION

the course of such a disease, it may also occur that from faulty treatment, the colour of the coating will change from white to yellow, then to dirty yellow or even to black.

If the coating disappears rapidly, this indicates that the heteropathy has sunken into the depth, into the intima, and that the energies of the orthopathy (qi orthopathicum) did not prevail against those of the heteropathy (qi heteropathicum).

c") When a pathological coating disappears, in other words, when it reverts to normal, particular care must be exercised to ascertain whether this represents a true or a false disappearance or a reversal to normal.

A true disappearance of pathological signs on the coating, an amelioration, shows in the gradual thinning out, gradual breaking up, gradual disappearance of the pathological coating, a process which may start at the root of the tongue and gradually reach the tip. Such symptoms indicate a lessening, a resolution of the inner blocks and obstructions. Now if, in addition to the disappearance of the pathological coating, the normal coating, i.e. a thin whitish lustrous coating is formed, this is a most propitious indication showing that the qi stomachi, the harmonizing functions and energies, are recovering and returning and that the energies absorbed from food (qi frumentarium) gradually will be insured normal distribution again.

If, on the contrary, a (pathological) coating suddenly disappears without the formation of a new coating, or if it peels off in spots so that blotches appear on the tongue, or so that a cheese-like pulp sticks to some irregular spots of the tongue, this is a symptom of contravection (i.e. of adverse development and movement of the process). Such may be the consequence of the incorrect use of purging or diaphoretic prescriptions or even of prescriptions opening the surface" (liberantia speciei) - having excessively drained or even impaired the energies and fluids of the o. stomachi.

If a tongue completely covered by a very thick layer suddenly sheds this coating, and if then the body of the tongue remains covered by an insalubrious sticky mucus, or if cinnabar-coloured dots and streaks appear on the tongue, these symptoms indicate a false retreat of the pathological coating. To still warrant a favourable prognosis, the thick coating shed should be reformed within one or two days. If, on the contrary, the surface of the tongue dries out, this is a sombre symptom indicating that the qi stomachi gradually is completely exhausted.

If single clumps break out from an excessively thick coating, producing deep pits with a dry bottom, this is another critical - though not quite so grave symptom. Here again urgent measures must be taken against the complete loss of structive fluids.

d) The Thickness, Moistness and the Putrid or Sticky Quality of the Coating of the Tongue

a) A thin coating indicates either that a disease is in its inceptive stage, that there is the beginning of the development of a heteropathy affecting the surface (species) only, or that there is very mild disease.

b) A thick coating indicates that the heteropathy has already penetrated within, into the intima, that there is serious disease, and that there are blocks or obstructions within the orbs. (Thus, as a disease gains momentum, the thickness of the coating of the tongue may increase).

c) A moist coating of the tongue indicates that the fluids have not yet been seriously affected; a dry coating indicates the contrary.

Moreover, moist coatings of the tongue are also present with affections on the basis of humor ("humidity"); dry coatings occur with diseases accompanied or induced by calor ("heat").

However, it may also happen that a humor-heteropathy affects the active individually specific energy (qi) so that this qi cannot be transmuted into the active fluids (jin) - a situation producing dryness of the coating of the tongue. Inversely, heteropathic "heat" (calor) may strike the individually specific structive energy (xue) and, in a way, make it "disperse", "evaporate" - thus leading to a moist coating of the tongue.

d) A putrid or slimy coating of the tongue that may easily be wiped off indicates an excess of active energy which makes the murky putrid qi of the o. stomachi rise upward.

e) A sticky (pasty) coating of the tongue somewhat thicker at the tip of the tongue, which cannot be wiped or scraped off, indicates that the active energies are restrained, hemmed in by a yin-heteropathy - which may happen when humor-induced pituita or pituita brought on by wrong diet is present.

To sum up: the thickness of the coating of the tongue is related to the seriousness of disease.

The moistness of the coating is related to the quantity of active and structive fluids available.

A slimy or pasty character of the coating of the tongue is related to the humidity (humor) and the degree of refinement of the active energies in the stomach and intestinal orbs.

INSPECTIO, THE DIAGNOSIS BY INSPECTION

2) Colour of the Coating of the Tongue

The colour of the coating of the tongue - white, yellow, ash-coloured, black etc. - is closely connected with the disease present and its evolution. Hence, ascertaining the colour of the coating has great diagnostic significance.

a. White Coating of the Tongue

White is the colour most frequently observed in the coating of the tongue. The normal white coating of the tongue on a healthy individual gives a whitish sheen to the centre and root of the tongue, whereas the margins and the tip look pale red. This coating is moist and shiny.

A more evenly distributed white coating, as a rule, indicates the presence of ventus, algor or humor-heteropathies ("wind", "cold", "humidity"), and an affection of the species. It will be recalled that, depending upon the moistness of the coating and the intensity of the redness of the body of the tongue, combinations between the above heteropathic influences and their qualification by the guiding criteria may occur. Thus, in addition, a white coating precludes the presence neither of algor nor of calor, nor of repletio nor of inanitas.

a^1. Thin, White Slippery Coating of the Tongue: If there is no significant change of the body of the tongue, this may accompany fever, shuddering, superficial pulses, headache, noisy breathing through the nose, cough, stale taste in the mouth and clear urine, and indicates exogenous, ventus-induced algor (algor venti).

If this coating appears on a fiery red body of the tongue, there will be increased fever and shuddering, cough and dry mouth, possibly to such an extent that the patient will be unable to sleep at night: this is a sign that the algor venti just mentioned now is met by "internal heat" (calor internus) symptoms.

a^2. A thick, white, slippery coating of the tongue, accompanied by fever, shuddering and pains in the joints and extremities is a symptom of "external cold" (algor externus) triggered by humor internus.

An identical coating may be found when liquid cold phlegm (pituita) blocks the diaphragm, as well as with obstructions of all kinds, plethora, difficult breathing, laboured breathing, and cough.

a^3. A white slippery to pasty coating of the tongue, accompanied by pains and pressure in the chest and the plexus region, oppressed heartbeat, restlessness, nausea, retching and persistent thirst (yet with immediate regurgitation of water drunk), indicates a calor-heteropathy as the consequence of an accumulation of pituita.

An identical coating is accompanied by symptoms of abdominal plethora and the refusal of all drink, by fatigue, listlessness, cold or only moderately warm body, diarrhea - symptoms concurring in the sense that excessive "humidity" (humor) blocks the unfoldment of the active energies of the lienal orb.

a^4. A white, pasty, sticky coating of the tongue, accompanied by symptoms of light fever, pains in the head and body, and absence of thirst, indicates a humor-heteropathy affecting the active energies.

If the patient ejects thick, opaque phlegm, the diagnosis of "lienal prostration" may be given, corresponding to an accumulation of humor-induced "heat" (calor humidus), which counteracts the spread of the energies absorbed from food (qi frumentarium) and indirectly pushes up murky energy.

a^5. A slippery, hyaline ("glassy") white coating of the tongue, accompanied by slight shivering, superficial and exhausted pulses (pp. superficiales et inanes), slight surfeit, reduced excretion of urine, the feeling of stickiness in the mouth, the evacuation of murky expectorates, and white shiny complexion point toward the diagnosis of inanitas intimae and insufficient transformation of the murky energies (absorbed from food) by the orthopathic energies (qi orthopathicum).

a^6. Thin, dry, white coating of the tongue indicates a lesion or depletion of the active fluids of the o. pulmonalis. If this symptom is accompanied by shuddering, one must, in addition, conclude that there is a superficial (species) heteropathy present.

a^7. A thick, dry, white coating of the tongue indicates the presence of a murky heteropathy. The dryness of the coating corresponds to a lesion of the fluids, either because of the presence of calor ("heat") or because of the inability to correctly integrate or distribute the murky energies derived and obtained from food.

a^8. A white coating of the tongue, looking as if powder has been applied, appears during the initial stage of infectious diseases, when the heteropathy has penetrated into the plexus region.

It can be seen even more often if a humor-heteropathy induced by calor o. pulmonalis ("heat in the pulmonal orb") is rampant.

b) Yellow Coating: As a rule, it indicates one of three disturbances, viz.
1. an affection of the intima, i.e. of the orbs in depth;
2. a calor-heteropathy ("heat-heteropathy") developing in the splendor

INSPECTIO, THE DIAGNOSIS BY INSPECTION

yang-conduits[150]; or

3. calor developing within the active energies.

b[1]. A thin, yellow, slippery coating of the tongue indicates that a ventus-heteropathy ("wind"-heteropathy) is present and has already induced calor, without, as yet, perceptibly depleting the active fluids. (Consequently, it can probably be controlled by the administration of medicamenta liberantia speciei [diaphoretics], re-enforced by mm. refrigerantia). If there is fever yet no perspiration, headache and shuddering, the heteropathy still is limited to the species yang maioris[151]; if headache and shuddering have disappeared, it has already penetrated into the conduits of splendor yang.

b[2]. Thick, yellow, slippery coating of the tongue is a sign of calor humidus ("humid heat") in the o. stomachi.

b[3]. If a sticky yellow coating of the tongue shows only a barely yellow tinge and is pasty, and if there is absence of thirst, one may deduce a humor-heteropathy affecting the active energies.

If the pasty coating is outright yellow, and if the patient complains of feeling a lump in his stomach, of nausea, vomiting, constipation and retention of urine, the calor humidus-heteropathy has affected the calorium medium[152].

It may also happen that the pasty yellow coating of the tongue is the consequence of pituita produced by disturbances of digestion, brought on by overeating.

b[4]. From a thin, yellow, dry coating of the tongue a lesion of the fluids of the o. renalis may be inferred. (In spite of its thinness, suggesting only a slight disturbance, this kind of coating usually is accompanied by constipation.)

b[5]. A thick, yellow, parched coating of the tongue points to calor in the o. stomachi, with concomitant lesion of the active fluids. (Here the application of cooling remedies (mm. refrigerantia) may be sufficient. If, however, the coating looks like cracked old leather, the extreme "glare" (ardor) revealed by this symptom can only be treated with immediate purging.)

b[6]. An almost colourless, faintly yellow coating of a puffed and tender body of the tongue which looks moist and cool, indicates that, from exhaustion of the energies in the o. lienalis (inanitas o. lienalis), a humor-heteropathy spreads within the individual.

---

[150] That is in the conduits belonging to the oo. stomachi et intestini crassi.

[151] Cf. above p. 103.

[152] Here pointing essentially to the oo. lienalis et stomachi.

c) Ashen Coatings. Ashen or ash-coloured coatings of the tongue may accompany either algor ("cold") or calor ("heat") affections of the yin-conduits[153].

c[1]. If a slippery, ash-coloured coating is present, we may infer overpowering (violatio)[154] of the central orbs (i.e. oo. lienalis et stomachi) by the qualities of Water[155]: hence symptoms of algor occur in the conduits of yin maior[156]. This particular syndrome is always accompanied by abdominal pains, vomiting, diarrhea, cold fingers and toes, and submerged and minute pulses (pp. mersi et minuti).

c[2]. A dry, ash-coloured coating of a usually intensely red body of the tongue reveals calor affecting the active fluids.

d) A Black Coating; such a coating of the tongue is always a symptom of serious or critical stages of disease and may accompany inanitas as well as repletio, algor as well as calor.

If it accompanies inanitas (exhaustion) symptoms, the patient will experience clear sensory perception along with great fatigue; if it occurs with repletion, the patient will be confused in his senses, yet speak with a sonorous voice.

A black coating accompanied by significant thirst indicates calor; if there is absence of thirst with a black coating, we may infer algor.

d[1]. A moist, slippery, black coating of the tongue may have varied significance, viz:

a) If it appears on an intensely red body of the tongue, it indicates algor because of the depletion of the active energies (inanitas yang).

b) If it looks like a glaze of diluted ink and is accompanied by cold extremities and evanescent pulses, it indicates exhaustion (inanitas) under all circumstances.

c) If it occurs at the very outset of an illness, accompanied by laboured breathing but no other outward critical symptoms, and covers the entire body of the tongue, a pituita subrepta ("latent phlegm") heteropathy has accumulated in the thorax and centre, and is only now taking effect.

d) If, in addition, pointed protuberances appear on the tongue, and if at first glance it looks dry, although the patient feels no thirst, if at the margin of the tongue the

---

[153] Cf. above pp. 108 ff.

[154] Cf. above p. 24.

[155] I.e. an accroachment by the energies emanating from the renal orb, qualified by the E.P. Water as actual structivity.

[156] I.e. the conduits corresponding to the pulmonal and lienal orbs.

INSPECTIO, THE DIAGNOSIS BY INSPECTION

coating is white or whitish, and if the body of the tongue is pale, this indicates calor falsus ("a symptom of false cold").

d^2. A dry or parched black coating of the tongue may also have varied significance, viz.:

a) If it is fairly thin and develops on a shining red body of the tongue, this is a sign of deficiency of structive energies.

b) If it looks thoroughly parched, this indicates ardor ("glare") has completely exhausted the fluids.

c) If it looks parched, and fissures and pointed protuberances appear, this indicates that ardor has completely evaporated the fluids, that the constitutional, inborn resources of structive energy in the o. renalis (aqua mera yin minoris) are in danger of imminent exhaustion - a very grave symptom.

However, it may also have occurred that this kind of coating (black, dry, with pointed protuberances) develops as the result of algor merus yin minoris ("true cold of minor yin") in the wake of which the active energies of the o. renalis are insufficient to dynamize the secretion of fluids. Since, in such a case, we are confronted by an algor-heteropathy, not by calor[157] (evidenced by the fact that there is no thirst yet the excretion of great quantities of urine), immediate measures must be taken to displace the algor in order to prepare the return of yang.

d^3. A black, parched coating limited to the centre of the tongue, if it is accompanied

a) by blackening of the gums and of the lips, is a sign of imminent collapse of the functions of the stomach orb; otherwise

b) it indicates dried up faeces (provided the patient complains of a hard and tender abdomen).

d^4. A parched, black coating limited to the root of the tongue, indicates calor in the calorium inferius ("heat in the lower heated space"), i.e. in the oo. renalis, vesicalis et intestinorum.

d^5. A parched, black coating limited to the tip of the tongue is a sign of (endogenous) ardor in the cardial orb.

Changes in the colour of the coating of the tongue from white to yellow, from ash-coloured to black, but also the appearance of pointed, black-spotted protuberances are very reliable signs for the advance of a "heat" heteropathy (calor-heteropathy) from the species into the

---

[157] On these terms cf. pp. 44 ff. above.

intima according to the algor laedens-pathology [158].

e) Simultaneous Appearance of Coating of Different Colours

e[1]. White and yellow coating of the tongue: If these two colours combine, as a rule the white portion of the coating may be correlated to species, light and superficial aspects of the affection, whereas the yellow portion of the coating corresponds to an affection of the intima, and to more serious, more profound aspects of the disease. In consequence, transitions from one tinge to the other must be interpreted as corresponding to changes in the disease process.

In practice, the following possibiltiies are frequently met with:

If a coating of initially white colour gradually changes to yellow, this may indicate that algor venti is changing into calor or ardor (a "wind-induced cold heteropathy changes into a heat or glare heteropathy").

If on a white coating yellow spots appear (or if a yellow coating gradually develops), we may conclude that the heteropathy is about to penetrate into the conduits of splendor yang (corresponding to the oo. stomachi et intestini crassi). If the patient showing these symptoms still shivers a bit, this may indicate that the heteropathy is essentially still limited to the surface (species).

If a coating simultaneously shows white and yellow patches, and if the patient complains about a queezy feeling in the stomach, this implies that while an exogenous heteropathy is still present, another one is accumulating independently within (in the intima).

If a white and yellow (or white and ash-coloured) coating of the tongue shows normal moistness in spite of the absence of thirst, it must be concluded that a calor-heteropathy has already formed but is not yet completely present in all symptoms; or that an accumulation of pituita has been present for a long time.

e[2]. A coating of the tongue at the same time white and ash-coloured and slippery points to humor algidus ("a cold heteropathy combined with humidity").

If the transition between white and ash-grey looks vague and washed out, and if the coating looks dirty, we must infer that pituita humoris algidi ("phlegm from a humid cold heteropathy") is present, obstructing the circulation of active energies.

On the other hand, if with a white coating of the tongue, half the tongue shows a dirty white tinge, we may deduce a part species, part intima syndrome.

---

[158] Cf. fig. 5 on p. 102 above.

INSPECTIO, THE DIAGNOSIS BY INSPECTION

e^3. White and black coating of the tongue: If on a white coating of the tongue black spots or streaks appear, and if the coating is sticky, this points to a humor-heteropathy manifesting itself within the active energies of the yin maior conduits.

e^4. A combination of white, yellow and black occurs in the coating of the tongue, combined with a dry tip, a moist root, a parched centre and a slippery margin of the tongue when several independent pathological agents are present, or if calor- and algor-heteropathies compete with each other.

e^5. A white, ash-coloured and black coating either pasty or slippery, indicates the existence of humor in the yin maior conduits.

e^6. A yellow, ash-coloured, parched coating occurring with hard stools indicates calor depleting the structive energies and representing the result of a more or less chronic humor-heteropathy.

e^7. A yellow and black sticky or slippery coating of the tongue indicates a heteropathy of calor humidus operative in the conduits of yin maior. If, with this combination of colours, the margin of the tongue is covered with a yellow coating, the centre is covered with a black one and shows pointed protuberances, and the patient has a tense, hard and painful abdomen, the depth of splendor yang has been affected.

If such a tongue looks singed and leathery, extreme "glare" in the intima prevails. If with a parched yellow coating of the tongue a black zone extends from the centre to the tip, and if malodorous liquid stools are evacuated, this indicates that the functions of the stomach and intestines orbs (oo. stomachi et intestinorum) have been completely ruined.

SUMMARY OF CRITICAL SYMPTOMS THAT MAY BE OBSERVED UPON INSPECTION OF THE TONGUE

Diagnostic inspection diagnosis of the tongue is a very subtle and precise method which, in order to produce results of great reliability, requires prolonged practice. Independent of this, all those symptoms should be especially memorized which indicate critical stages of disease, which, if not treated with dispatch, energy and incisiveness, may end with the death of the patient. The imminent danger of death usually is indicated by signs of depletion - mostly of the structive energies - in one or all orbs, manifesting itself on the tongue by:

Appearance of the Tongue Indicating an Imminent Depletion of Yin (Structive Energies)

A body of the tongue without any coating, bare like the kidney of a pig, indicates severe lesion of the yin in the wake of febrile illness, or the complete loss of the active energies of the o. stomachi: qi stomachi.

A tongue with pointed protuberances like a shark's fin, or parched, deep fissures, indicates depletion of the fluids.

A body of the tongue drastically shrunken in breadth, looking parched, like a dried lizhi [fruit], indicates that extreme ardor has depleted the fluids.

A dry body of the tongue, dark like the liver of a pig, indicates decomposition of the individually specific (structive) energies.

A body of the tongue strikingly reduced in length (occurring with a shrivelled scrotum), indicates imminent depletion of the structive energies of the o. hepaticus (yin hepaticum).

A body of the tongue resembling red loam and showing a blackish tint indicates imminent exhaustion of the structive energies of the renal orb (yin renale).

Appearance of the Tongue Indicating the Imminent Depletion of the Yang (Active Energies):

A body of the tongue white like snow flakes indicates the imminent exhaustion of the active energies of the o. lienalis.

THE DIAGNOSTIC INSPECTION OF DIFFERENT PARTS OF THE BODY
(inspectio topologica partium)

During diagnosis, as circumstances warrant and permit, all parts of the body, especially the face of the patient, must be inspected closely. Such inspection does not aim at registering with great subtlety as many details as possible; instead, the objective of such inspection is to gain a synthetic view of changes, each of which considered separately, would be meaningless, but which acquire diagnostic significance by appearing and being viewed together.

INSPECTION OF THE HEAD (Inspectio capitis)

The head represents, as the saying goes, the conventus omnium yang ("the site in which all yang (conduits) convene"). It is "the hall of brain and marrow" (aula cerebri et medullae), i.e. the somatic location of the substratum corresponding to the para-orbes cerebri et medullae linked with the renal orb (o. renalis). Also it sports the outward manifestation of the renal orb, the hair of the head, which in turn furnishes information about the orthopathic strength of the xue (i.e. of individually specific structive energies).

1) Inspecting the Shape and Movement of the Head (Inspectio motus somatisque capitis)

With infants, a depressed fontanel points to a deficiency of the paraorbes cerebri et meduallae; inversely, a protruding fontanel indicates a pathological change in the same orbs.

If the fontanels do not close properly, or if the head of the baby droops sidewise, this is a sign of congenital deficiency of energies in the renal orb.

Continual uncontrolled shaking or twitching of the head, with infants or adults alike, points to ventus internus[159].

2) Inspection of the Hair of the Head (Inspectio crinis)

A full head of even-coloured[160] hair is a sign of powerful energy in the renal orb, hence of a strong constitution.

Bleached hair may indicate a deficiency of the xue, the individually specific structive energy.

---

[159] On this term of pathology cf. p. 58 and p. 67 above.

[160] Chinese texts here always have "black".

Alopecia (the loss of hair) may be a symptom of an enfeebled energy of the renal orb (qi renale dilabens). (By contrast, the time at which hair becomes grey, no matter whether this happens at middle age or at an advanced age, in the opinion of the Chinese, is essentially a matter of constitution, and hence only of slight diagnostic value.)

Very often alopecia is a consequence of calor xue ("a heat lesion to individually specific structive energy"), hence of a depletion of the fluids. If alopecia sets in after prolonged illness, this indicates that the structive potential (jing) has been exhausted (inanitas jing).

Stiff, dry, brittle hair is a symptom of reduced or depleted active energies.

With infants, unclean looking, clinging hair indicates a disturbance of the oo. intestinorum, often from premature or incorrect weaning.

INSPECTION OF THE FACE AND COMPLEXION (inspectio vultus)

During every diagnosis, a close look should be taken at the face of the patient, because by this simple procedure a number of fairly subtle facts can be obtained. (Concerning the precautions to be taken, in particular as far as lighting is concerned, cf. what has been said above about inspection of the colour of the tongue.)

1) Correspondences and Sites of the Face

The most significant correspondences between the different sites of the face may be taken from Fig. 7.

Thus, according to widely accepted traditions, the items in the left-hand column correspond to those in the right-hand column.

Upper forehead	Complexion as a whole
Middle forehead	Pharynx and trachea
Space between the brows	o. pulmonalis
Bridge of the nose	o. cardialis
Middle section of the nose	o. hepaticus
Tip of the nose	o. lienalis
Nostrils	o. stomachi

INSPECTIO, THE DIAGNOSIS BY INSPECTION 157

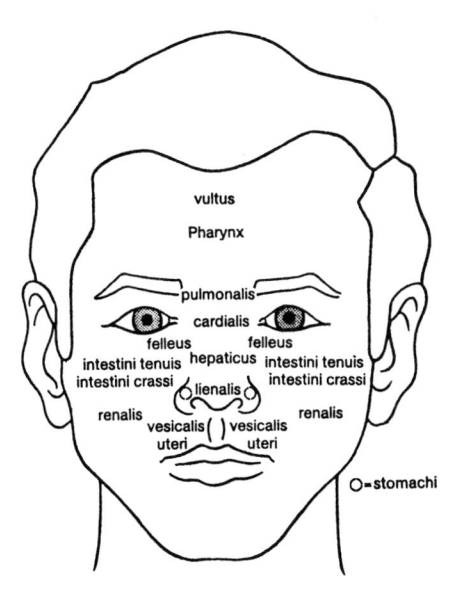

Fig. 7.

In addition, on the upper lip flanking the philtrum, symmetric sites are assigned to the urinary bladder orb (o. vesicalis) and to the para-orb of the uterus (paraorbis uteri). Symmetric sites also correspond to the oo. renalis, intestini crassi et tenuis, felleus (renal, large and small intestine, gall bladder orbs), these aligned on two lines, originating at the centre of the cheeks and converging at the root of the nose.

For the sake of completeness, mention is made here of a "classical"[161] but otherwise quite secondary correspondence between sites of the face and the orbs:

The	Corresponds to
Left cheek	o. hepaticus
Right cheek	o. pulmonalis
Forehead	o. cardialis
Chin	o. renalis
Nose	o. lienalis.

---

[161] Because first mentioned in the Inner Classic of the Yellow Sovereign, Chapter 32.

158   THE ESSENTIALS OF CHINESE DIAGNOSTICS

Of course, all aulic orbs (yang orbs, orbes aulici) indirectly partake of the correspondence of the horreal orbs. As in other diagnostic procedures, practice alone will permit us to decide which of these correspondences must be given preference.

Inspection of the Colour of the Face, Diagnosis of the Complexion (Inspectio coloris vultus)

a) A green or blue-green tint in the complexion is a symptom either of ventus, algor, dolor or ventus pavoris ("wind", "cold", pain, (infantile spasms due to disturbances of the hepatic orb). And, by the qualification of the E.P., where the green or blue-green colour corresponds to the E.P. Wood, this tinge also establishes a direct connection with the hepatic orb and its conduit, the sinarteria yin flectentis and its symptoms[162].

The appearance of a greenish tint as a frequent corollary of pain is due to the fact that very often pain is the sequel of a block of energetic conduits, hence of the congestion of active or structive energies.

The disturbance called ventus pavoris ("wind due to fright"), like any kind of fright symptom, is ultimately[163] promoted by any instability of the hepatic and gall bladder orbs (oo. hepaticus et felleus).

If a dark green (hence a mixture of green and black) tinge appears, this points to pain from an algor-block (dolor algoris). By contrast, if a light green tint is observed, this is a sign of ventus developing on the basis of exhaustion (ventus inanitatis).

A complexion showing green and red portions, indicates ardor orbis hepatici ("glare in the hepatic orb"); if from this mixture of green and red, a dirty looking complexion results, we may deduce an extreme congestion from ardor.

If the greenish or blue-green tint is not limited to the face but also extends to the lips, an extreme preponderance of yin must be inferred.

A greenish complexion during affections of the lienal orb (o. lienalis) indicates that the energies of the hepatic orb encroach upon those of the lienal orb - resulting in a very hard to treat disturbance.

b) A red or scarlet complexion is a sign of calor ("heat"). Within the conventions of the evolutive phases, the red colour corresponds to summer, the heat of summer

---

[162] I.e. of the conduits of the hepatic orb.

[163] Pavor, jing, "fright", is primarily related to the renal orb, but may also affect the cardial and the hepatic orbs.

(aestus), the cardial orb, and its conduit of yin minor of the hand.

Moderate redness of the face indicates calor inanitatis ("heat resulting from exhaustion"); an intensive red colour points to calor repletionis ("heat resulting from repletion"). The first possibility should be taken into consideration after prolonged illness, when after noon the cheeks of the patient acquire a red tint, thus indicating ardor brought on by deficiency of the structive energies (ardor structivus) and flare-up from the hepatic and renal orbs.

A complexion looking as if makeup has been applied, that is, a pink face with a whitish lustre, and showing quick changes in the intensity of the redness, corresponds to a yang-cap-syndrome[164].

If redness occurs with disturbances of the pulmonary orb, this is a symptom of encroachment difficult to treat.

c) A yellow complexion is a sign of humor ("humidity"). In conformity with the conventions of the evolutive phases, any yellow tinge points to the o. lienalis and its conduit, the sinartery of yin maior of the foot.

A resplendent, lemon yellow complexion indicates that there is relatively little "humidity" (humor) present, against a great quantity of calor ("heat"); a complexion yellow like smoked crab indicates that there is much humor and little calor. Also, if a yellow complexion is accompanied by emaciation, these symptoms indicate that there is calor ("heat") in the oo. lienalis et stomachi.

A pale yellow tint indicates exhaustion of the energies (inanitas) in the orbs just mentioned. A sallow looking yellow complexion is a symptom of humor algidus ("a cold heteropathy resulting from humdidity") in these very orbs.

A yellow complexion, with a faint tinge of bluish red or purple, points to stagnating xue. A pale yellow complexion with red spots, streaks or blotches must be taken as a symptom of exhaustion of the energies in the lienal orb (inanitas o. lienalis), and concomitant congestion of individually specific structive energy (xue) in the o. hepaticus, especially if the centre of the body is bloated.

If the nose, in particular its tip, shows a vigorous yellow tinge, this indicates that the energies of the o. stomachi are being re-established, and consequently indicates recovery. If, on the contrary, the tip of the nose shows a murky, vague colour as if parched, one must deduce the extreme depletion of these energies and an illness

---

[164] This has already been discussed on p. 111 above.

difficult to treat.

d) A white complexion is a symptom of inanitas or of algor ("exhaustion" or "cold") or, more generally, of deficient active and structive fluids or active and structive energies in general.

Within the context of the evolutive phase qualifications, the white colour corresponds to the o. pulmonalis and its conduits of yin maior of the hand, also to dryness (ariditas) and to autumn. Since, as it will be recalled, the pulmonary orb controls the rhythm of all orbs, the appearance of a white tinge reveals pathological changes which may be understood as disturbances of the rhythmic distribution of energies.

A white face with a faint tinge of red indicates that energy in the splendor yang-conduits[165] flows in harmony. By contrast, if a deficiency in these very conduits occurs, the red tinge disappears.

If a white complexion accompanies disturbances of the hepatic orb, this is a sign that the energies of the hepatic orb overpower the pulmonal orb - hence a situation difficult to treat.

e) A dark, blackish complexion is a symptom either of algor, dolor or aqua ("cold" heteropathy, affection of the renal orb, or of pain).

Within the context of the evolutive phases conventions, black corresponds to winter, to cold, to water, to the renal orb and its conduits of yin minor of the foot.

If algor ("cold") impedes or blocks the flow of energy, pains ensues.

If a darkish complexion shows a pink glimmer, healthy tonus and subdued lustre, these are signs of good health[166]. If, by contrast, the darkish complexion looks lustreless and sallow, these are signs of calor in the renal orb; if, in addition, emaciation and decayed teeth are present, a chronic calor-heteropathy and the concomitant lesions of structive energies must be inferred.

Aside from these correlations, any darkening of the complexion indicates the predominance of yin or an insufficient deployment of active energy - hence, serious disease.

With disturbances of the cardial orb, a darkening of the forehead is a contravective sign: aqua vincit ignis ("an indication of the energy flowing contrary to optimum

---

[165] The conduits corresponding to the o. lienalis and the o. intestini crassi; cf. p. 105 above.

[166] Yet with a functional dominance of the renal orb.

INSPECTIO, THE DIAGNOSIS BY INSPECTION

function, the energies of the renal orb overpowering those of the cardial orb").

If dark tinges appear in the surroundings of the mouth, a complete loss of the energies of the renal orb may be implied.

Diagnosing Modal Changes of Complexion (Inspectio modi coloris vultus)

The basic tints of the complexion just discussed are constantly undergoing modal inflections - whose significance in Chinese inspection diagnosis, is not second to that of the former. Five couples of inflections, i.e. ten such modes, may be distinguished, viz.

a) Superficial and deep colour: A tint which looks like a fleeting shimmer on the complexion is called "superficial", indicating that the corresponding disturbance affects only the species or the aulic orbs.

A colour which apparently impregnates the skin of the face in depth, is called "deep" colour. It implies that the disturbance affects the intima, hence the horreal orbs.

Changes of direction of a heteropathy from outside toward the intima or vice versa, are reflected in a change of the modes.

b) Limpid and murky (muddy) coloration: A limpid, lucid colour implies that the disturbance essentially affects the yang; a murky or muddy coloration points to a disturbance essentially in the yin.

c) Weak and intensive colour: From a weak coloration, we may infer that the orthopathy is exhausted (inanis); an intensive coloration implies a repletion (repletio) of heteropathy.

d) Diffuse and concentrated coloration: A diffuse coloration is the symptom of light or recent illness; concentrated coloration indicates prolonged or serious illness.

e) Lustrous or dull (lustreless) complexion: A lustrous complexion indicates that the disease takes a favourable course; a dull complexion utterly deprived of lustre suggests an unfavourable evolution of the disease.

Inspection of the Shape of the Face (Inspectio formae vultus)

a) A puffed, swollen face often accompanies dropsy. Chinese medicine distinguishes an active and a structive form of dropsy. In the case of active (yang) dropsy, puffiness develops quite rapidly, and becomes apparent more quickly on the face and the upper extremities than on the abdomen and the lower extremities; with structive (yin) dropsy, puffiness sets in slowly, and affects the lower extremities and the abdomen more quickly and intensely than the upper extremities and the face.

A sudden swelling of the lateral parts of the throat [parotitis]: If it occurs with a swelling of the pharynx, a red face with or without a sore throat, and sometimes with hardness of hearing, it is a symptom of a morbus temperatus infection.

c) Asymmetrical movement or paralysis of the face, the eyelids or the mouth indicate vento percussio [apoplexy].

INSPECTION OF THE EYE (Inspectio oculi)

In traditional Chinese medicine, diagnostic inspection diagnosis of the eye is exclusively limited to the macroscopic examination of those parts of the eye, including the lids, which can be clearly distinguished without the aid of instruments. No methodological or practical parallels with the microscopic viewing of the iris or with the inspection of the retina, used in modern Western medicine and ophthalmology, exist.

Sites of the Eye and Their Correspondences

The well defined sites of the eye and their functional correspondences with the basic horreal orbs are as follows (cf. Fig. 8):

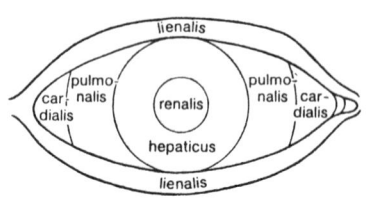

Fig. 8.

1 - Those parts of the scleras clearly showing fine veins, hence close to the canthi, correspond to the cardial orb (o. cardialis) and its specific unfoldment (perfectio), the conduits (sinarteriae).

2 - Those parts of the scleras bordering on the pupil of the eye correspond to the pulmonal orb and its specific unfoldment, the skin.

3 - The bulges of the upper and lower lids correspond to the lienal orb and its specific unfoldment, the flesh.

INSPECTIO, THE DIAGNOSIS BY INSPECTION

4 - The iris corresponds to the hepatic orb and its specific unfoldments, the <u>nervus</u>, i.e. the muscles and sinews representing the motive parts of the locomotive apparatus.

5 - The pupil corresponds to the renal orb and its specific unfoldment, the "bones".

Manifestation of Configurative Force in the Eye (<u>shen oculi</u>)

On a healthy individual, the eye has a limpid and shining appearance, its scleras and pupils are distinctly delineated, and there is a steady gaze. If such signs are present, yet disturbances arise, the latter are of light nature.

If the pupils look muddy, if the scleras show shadows or red, bulging veins, if the gaze is tired, or if the eyes have an unusual glimmer, the configurative force has either been affected by serious disease or been lost.

Significance of Changes in the Appearance of the Eye

a) Redness of the canthi points to <u>ardor</u> ("glare") or <u>calor</u> ("heat") in the cardial orb; redness of the scleras is a symptom of <u>ardor</u> or <u>calor</u> in the pulmonal orb.

b) Yellow scleras indicate the powerful development of a "humid heat heteropathy in the <u>intima</u>" (<u>vigor caloris humidi</u>).

c) An outcurving iris is a sign of <u>ardor</u> in the hepatic orb.

d) Inflamed or sore eyelids indicate <u>ardor</u> or <u>calor</u> in the lienal orb.

e) If the entire eye looks red and swollen, these are symptoms of <u>calor venti</u> in the conduits of the hepatic orb.

f) Strikingly limpid and white scleras are a symptom of <u>algor</u> ("cold"); muddy or murky scleras or a shaded iris indicate <u>calor</u>.

g) Pale canthi imply a deficiency of <u>xue</u> (of individually specific structive energy).

h) Strikingly shining eyelids are symptoms of <u>pituita</u>.

i) Dark-coloured lids, as a rule, indicate exhaustion of the renal orb (<u>inanitas orbis renalis</u>).

j) A slight swelling of the orbita, entailing a barely perceptible protrusion of the eye and a shining complexion, is a precursory sign of dropsy.

j¹) Swelling of the eyelids, accompanied by redness appearing suddenly, indicates calor in the lienal orb.

j²) If the swelling of the eyelids develops slowly and is accompanied by weakness, these are symptoms of inanitas orbis lienalis.

j³) A swollen lower eyelid on elderly individuals points to a weakening of the active energies in the renal orb (qi renale dilabens).

k) A sunken orbit is a symptom of decrepitude of the structive potential (jing) in all orbs. If the symptom is only slightly visible, a favourable prognosis is possible; if it occurs with striking intensity and is accompanied by mental confusion and utterly disharmonious pulses, these are symptoms of imminent death.

l) Napping with half-open eyelids indicates extreme exhaustion of the lienal and stomach orbs (inanitas orbium lienalis et stomachi).

m) Widely dilated pupils and blurred vision indicate a deficiency of the energies in the renal orb.

n) Exophthalmus (widely protruding eyeballs), accompanied by panting and laboured breathing, is a symptom of a bloating of the pulmonal orb (distensio o. pulmonalis).

o) Uncoördinated movements of the eyes or a fixed stare are symptoms accompanying serious disease; squinting, unless present since birth, usually indicates an endogenous ventus hepaticus ("wind heteropathy in the hepatic orb").

p) A slightly fixed stare may indicate a block or obstruction in the intima because of pituita induced by a calor-heteropathy.

Note 1: According to newer findings received into official textbooks[167], inspection of the scleras may aid in rapid diagnosis of inner lesions, in particular of hematoma within the thorax. In the visible triangles of the scleras, such lesions induce dark grey, black or brown spots the size of pinheads, appearing at the end of bluish, purple or red veins (spots not connected with such veins are without diagnostic relevance). Lesions in the thorax close to the back are shown by spots above the horizontal line in the eye, those closer to the chest are shown below this line (Fig. 9). Also, defects in the left side appear in the left eye, lesions in the right side in the right eye.

---

[167] Fujian Zhongyiyao ("Journal of Chinese Medicine and Pharmacology for the Province of Fukien") 1960/8, p. 24, quoted in Zhenduanxue jiangyi pp. 34 - 35.

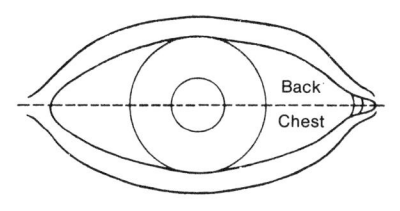

Fig. 9.

Grey, diffuse, cloudy splashes indicate disturbances of active energies, hence functional disturbances), black, sharply defined spots point to lesions of structive energies, hence of somatic changes. The black spots are surrounded by a grey, irregular halo; the lesions are effective in the active as well as in the structive energies. If the veins leading up to the spots are strikingly red, the lesion is accompanied by pain.

Note 2: The presence of ascarids (Ascaris lumbricoides) in about 80% of observed cases, produces similar symptoms on the scleras: blue streaks or spots. In addition, pellucid protuberances on the lower lip, red spots at the tip of the tongue and along the centre line of the tongue, and, in some cases, white spots on the skin of the face, in particular around the cheeks, the size of fingernails have been observed. (The last-mentioned splashes are best seen under diffuse lighting; they tend to disappear under strong direct light.)

DIAGNOSTIC INPECTION OF THE NOSE (Inspectio nasi)

In orbisiconography, the nose corresponds to the opening of the pulmonal orb (o. pulmonalis); by the conduits of sinarteriology, it is linked to the stomach orb.[168]

A puffed or swollen nose indicates the strenght of a heteropathy; a sunken-in, collapsed, shrivelled nose points to an enfeeblement of orthopathy in general and in particular in the orbs mentioned.

Colour Tints of the Nose

A green to blue-green tinge of the nose may accompany pains in the abdomen. A yellow tint is a symptom of calor humidus ("heat on the basis of humidity").

A white tint of the nose indicates the loss of xue (individually specific energy including blood).

From a red tinge of the nose, calor in the conduits of the oo. lienalis et pulmonalis

---

[168] By its paracardinalis, indirectly by its cardinalis.

may be inferred.

A dark, blackish tint of the nose indicates the predominance of the energies of the o. renalis.

A light, lustrous appearance of the nose is indicative either of only light disease, of convalescence or of good health.

Dry nostrils are part of the symptoms of calor affecting the conduits of splendor yang. If the immediate surroundings of the nostrils look as if blackend by soot, this is an indication of extreme glare accompanying a yang heteropathy. However, an identical blackness may also appear around cold and runny nostrils, then indicating extreme algor due to a yin heteropathy.

Discharges from the Nose; Exterior Changes

A thick, murky or yellow nasal discharge indicates exogenous calor venti; thin, fluid, limpid nasal discharge is a symptom of exogenous algor venti.

If the nostrils move with respiration, this symptom during the initial stage of illness indicates that ardor venti or some calor-heteropathy blocks the o. pulmonalis. If the same symptom appears after prolonged illness and is accompanied by perspiration, it points to the imminent depletion of the energies of the pulmonal orb.

DIAGNOSTIC INSPECTION OF THE EAR (Inspectio auris)

In orbisiconography, the ear is related to the o. renalis. Thus the outward appearance of the ear conch may orient us on the state of the constitutive, inborn energies deposited in the o. renalis (qi nativum orbis renalis).

If the ear conch appears to be moderately fleshy and shows a subdued lustre, we may infer a sufficient qi nativum; a puffed ear conch, by contrast, points to the powerful development of a heteropathy; a shrunken, shrivelled ear conch to weakness of the orthopathy.

Pale ear conches are symptoms of algor, bluish to blackish ear conches symptoms of pain.

If, on the back of cold ears red veins appear, this is a precursory sign of measles.

These same veins may also be in evidence with smallpox. A medium-red colour points to a slight infection, purple to an infection of average gravity, whereas bluish or black veins accompany very serious smallpox infections.

INSPECTION DIAGNOSIS OF THE MOUTH AND THE LIPS (Inspectio oris atque labium)

In orbisiconography, the mouth and the lips in particular are correlated to the lienal and stomach orbs.

Colour of the Lips

Medium-red lips indicate good health.

Intensely red (cherry red) lips indicate either repletion or calor.

Pale lips are symptoms of inanitas ("exhaustion") or algor ("cold").

Lips that are at the same time intensely red and dry indicate extreme calor or ardor having affected the structure fluids.

If pale lips look as if covered by a black veil, this is a symptom of extreme algor, a heteropathy which may also manifest itself by bluish or blackish lips.

A green or blue-green tint of the lips is a symptom of pain.

Shape and Movement of the Mouth and the Lips

A gaping mouth, breathing through an open mouth, usually is a sign of exhaustion (inanitas). If in addition the patient appears to exhale only through the mouth, we may infer the imminent depletion of energies in the pulmonal orb.

If a patient gasps for breath through an open mouth like a fish, one may infer the imminent depletion or collapse of the energies of the o. lienalis. If, besides a gaping mouth, the surroundings of the mouth show a bluish tinge, this indicates that the energies of the o. lienalis have been violated, overpowered by ventus hepaticus (a "wind" heteropathy in the hepatic orb).

A puffed philtrum and retracted lips indicate the depletion of active energies in the o. lienalis; a shrivelled, contracted upper lip is a symptom for the imminent exhaustion of structive energies in the o. lienalis.

White spots or white pustules inside the upper lip indicate hemorrhoids.

INSPECTION DIAGNOSIS OF TEETH AND GUMS (inspectio dentium et gingivarum)

The teeth, just as the bones, are part of the "specific unfoldment" (perfectio) of the o. renalis. The jaws are touched by the cardinal conduits of splendor yang of the foot and hand (cardinales splendoris yang pedis et manus), thus indicating a functional relationship with the large intestine and stomach orbs (oo. intestini crassi et stomachi). All these relationships must be kept in mind when, in the context of morbi temperati-diseases, a calor-heteropathy affecting the active energies (calor in the qi and wei) spreads in the splendor yang and endangers the structive reserves of the renal orb (yin renale).

In a healthy individual the teeth and the gums look moist and shiny. If, on the contrary, they seem dry or even parched, we may infer the absence of active and structive fluids, consequently a depletion of structive energies.

If the teeth look as if they were polished or look dry like stones, this is a symptom of calor vigens sinarteriarum splendoris yang (rampant "heat" in the conduits of splendor yang). If, on the contrary, the teeth look dry and dull like dried bone, this same heteropathy has affected the renal orb, leading to the exhaustion of structive energies and hence of all fluids.

If the gums look as white as the teeth, this is a sign of deficient xue.

Bleeding and/or swollen gums indicate - if accompanied by pain - ardor vigens o. stomachi; if there is no pain, this is a symptom of ardor in the renal orb.

Gnashing the teeth usually indicates an endogenous ventus-heteropathy affecting the hepatic orb. The gnashing of teeth during sleep observed in children is a sign of local congestion or block of the energy flow.

INSPECTION DIAGNOSIS OF THE INNER THROAT (Inspectio faucium)

From an inspection of the inner throat, additional diagnostic data on disturbances of the pulmonal, stomach and renal orbs may be obtained.

Pain, redness and puffedness (dolor, rubor, turgor) of the throat usually are symptoms of a calor-heteropathy affecting the pulmonal or stomach orb.

The same diagnosis may be deduced from a putrid membrane that can easily be wiped off from the fauces.

If this membrane cannot be wiped off, and if, instead, intense wiping provokes bleeding, or if this covering is quickly formed anew, this is a sign of diphtheria.

A slight redness of the fauces accompanied by moderate pain is indicative of a deficiency of the energies in the renal orb as a consequence of which the active energies of that orb flare up and outwards (ardor inanitatis).

INSPECTION DIAGNOSIS OF THE MEMBERS (Inspectio membrorum)

General Appearance of Hands and Feet

Swelling or puffiness of the extremities, as a rule, may be taken as a symptom of repletion; atrophy, shrivelling, as a rule, as a sign of exhaustion (inanitas).

With all other symptoms, especially those accompanying arthritic swellings, inflammations, pains and stiffness, conclusions may be drawn only from other diagnostic data.

Wrists and Ankles

A healthy colour and a good tonus of the flesh and the skin covering the wrists and ankles indicates the availability of sufficient supplies of fluids and liquids; dryness and shrivelling of these parts are a symptom of deficiency of the fluids.

Nails on the Fingers and Toes

The nails are the outward manifestation (flos) of the hepatic orb. Their medium-red appearance and dull lustre indicate that active and structive energies are available in sufficient quantity.

Intensely red nail regions point to calor, pale red nail regions to algor or to inanitas; a bluish tinge of these same parts is a symptom of inanitas xue ("exhaustion of the individually specific structive energies"), a yellow tinge comes with an icterus, a dark or black tinge with hematomas and congestions.

INSPECTION OF THE INDEX IN PEDIATRIC DIAGNOSIS (Inspectio indicis infantum)

Since, in pediatrics, quite important methods of Chinese diagnostics such as the inspection of the tongue or the palpation of the pulse can only be applied and relied on to a very limited extent, the diagnostic inspection of the index, on infants and small children up to their 3rd year, partly must make up for this limitation.

1) Topology and Manipulation

The palmar side of the index, starting from the 1st phalanx, is divided into three sites called clusa fortunae, clusa qi, clusa venti (Fig. 10).

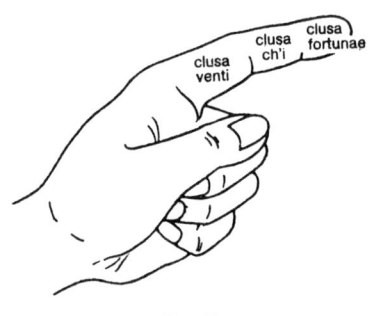

Fig. 10.

The clusa venti ("pass gate of wind", fengguan) is correlated to the system of reticular conduits and hence to quite superficial affections;

the clusa qi ("pass gate of qi", qiguan) is correlated to the cardinal conduits, hence to superficial affections and disturbances;

the clusa fortunae ("pass gate of fate", mingguan) is correlated to the orbs, hence to penetrating and serious disturbances.

In order to make the lines and colours on the sites described stand out well, the physician strokes the palmar side of the passively stretched index of the child several times in proximal direction with his thumb.

2) Appearance

The palmar side of the index, on a healthy child, is pink coloured with a slight yellow tinge. In the presence of pathological changes, persistence of the light tints indicates slight disease, the appearance of intense colours serious disease.

A vivid red indicates an exogenous heteropathy; purple is a symptom of calor.

If the light tints pale out, this points to inanitas; if colour becomes more intense, concentrated, this is a symptom of repletion.

Any green or blue-green tint is a sign either of ventus or of pain; if from this blue-green tint transitions into purple or even black occur, these signs of congestion or stasis on an infant represent an extremely critical condition.

If the lines visible on the different sites (clusae) become more distinct, this indicates penetration, aggravation of disease; by contrast, if the lines become obliterated, disappear, disease rises to the surface and convalescence sets in.

INSPECTIO, THE DIAGNOSIS BY INSPECTION

DIANGOSTIC INSPECTION OF THE SKIN (Inspectio cutis)

In Chinese medicine, inspecting the skin produces only dermatological or infectious diagnoses which neither complement nor improve on those of Western medicine. This is why in a book giving the essentials of Chinese diagnosis, we may completely dispense with those, albeit elaborate, instructions.

THE INSPECTION OF EXCRETIONS (Inspectio excrementorum)

Saliva and Mucus

If saliva and mucus have a limpid, bubbly or foamy appearance, this points to the presence of ventus and is called mucus venti.

If saliva and mucus have a whitish, milky, viscid appearance and are easily ejected, this is called mucus humoris and points to a "humidity" heteropathy.

Clear and thin secretions are symptoms of algor and are called mucus algoris.

Thick, lumped, yellow phlegm is a symptom of calor and is called mucus caloris.

Frequent expectoration indicates algor in the o. stomachi; the continuous secretion of thin saliva is a symptom of algor; the continuous excretion of a thick, sticky discharge indicates calor in the o. lienalis.

Vomitus

The evacuation of a watery, limpid, odourless vomitus (completed by symptoms such as the desire for and the amelioration by hot drinks) indicates an algor-heteropathy.

A clotty, sour-smelling vomitus - and additional symptoms such as the desire for and the amelioration by cold beverages - points to calor.

A slimy, viscid vomitus in the absence of thirst in spite of a dry mouth indicates that there is an accumulation of pituita ("phlegm").

Vomitus including undigested food, of putrid or sour smell, is called an "undigested-evening-meal vomitus".

A purulent, extremely malodorous, bloody vomitus indicates internal ulcers.

The intermittent vomiting of small quantities of undigested food, of slightly foul or sour smell, is a symptom of the congestion of energies in the stomach orb.

Faeces

Stools	Indicate
Yellow, pulpy, malodorous	calor orbium intestinorum
Watery, containing undigested food	algor orbium intestinorum
Liquid and watery, accompanied by symptoms of shuddering, fever, headache	ventus
Watery, accompanied by fatigue and rumbling noise in the abdomen	humor

All other symptoms point to infectious or somatic changes in the intestines, for which, essentially, a diagnosis of Western medicine is competent.

URINATION

Light-coloured, limpid, copious urination indicates algor ("cold"); dark-coloured, murky, sparing urination is a symptom of calor ("heat").

Chapter Two: The Diagnosis by Auscultation and Olfaction
(Auscultatio et Olfactio, Wénzhen)

The Chinese term wén (in the 2nd tone) designates at once acoustic and olfactory perception. Consequently, the diagnostic methods labelled wén include the auscultatory diagnosis of acoustic phenomena just as it does the olfactory assessment of excreta.

AUDITIVE DIAGNOSIS OF VOICE AND SPEECH

On healthy individuals the human voice, independent of personal varieties, sounds distinct, harmonious and coherent; the lack of these qualities indicates pathological disturbances.

The Voice

The loss of one's voice at the very beginning of an illness points as a rule to exogenous "cold"-induced "wind" (algor venti), impeding the deployment of energies of the pulmonal orb. If the voice is lost after prolonged illness, this indicates a lesion of the pulmonal orb.

A hoarse, raucous, jangling voice is, as a rule, a symptom of repletion due to exogenous calor or the powerful development of a calor-heteropathy.

A piping (high pitched, clear yet feeble) voice usually is a symptom of inanitas brought on by algor internus.

The Flow of Speech (sermo)

From particularities of speech, conclusions may be drawn regarding all guiding criteria.

Thus exogenous heteropathies produce a loud, vigorous, at first glib and easy, later on faltering speech.

Endogenous lesions lead to a low, timid, in the beginning halting, later on fluent speech.

Algor manifests itself by the reluctance to speak, and sparing words.
Calor manifests itself by volubility.
Inanitas produces a weak, low, frequently interrupted speech.
Repletion manifests itself in a loud and jangling voice.
Raving, incoherent, confused speech, accompanied by dulled senses, also points to repletion.

A repetitive mutter, accompanied by great nervous prostration, is a symptom of inanitas orbium cardialis sive renalis ("exhaustion of the energies in the cardial or renal orb"), as is a propensity to mutter to oneself, or to say things which are immediately denied.

Respiration

Loud, audible respiration, as a rule, is a repletion symptom; however, noisy respiration may also appear after prolonged illness as a symptom indicating the imminent exhaustion of the energies in the pulmonal and renal orbs.

Barely audible respiration usually is a symptom of inanitas; however, it may also occur with calor affecting the o. pericardialis.

Panting (anhelitus, chuan)[partly congruent with asthma] is present in a patient who breathes with difficulty through his mouth, pulling up his shoulders and who, very often, cannot bear a horizontal position. Such symptoms may either be due to repletion or to exhaustion (inanitas). Panting due to repletion is very loud, accelerated and accompanied by replete pulses and is observed when in a strong constitution a calor-heteropathy has developed in the pulmonal orb or, in the case of an obstruction by pituita ("phlegm").

Panting due to inanitas has a much slower respiratory rhythm and occurs in a patient showing lassitude, speaking with a feeble voice and sighing frequently.

A buzzing or purring respiration (xiao) is defined as respiration accompanied by a buzz or purr at the end of each respiratory movement. This intermittent, hence sometimes latent, yet chronic symptom points to either
1 - "hidden phlegm" (pituita subrepta) tied up at the surface of the flesh by an exogenous algor-heteropathy, and from where it sometimes emerges; or to
2 - an identical heteropathy deversating in the conduits of the pulmonal orb; or, finally, it may be the consequence of
3 - the prolongued stay in cold, moist places or of

THE DIAGNOSIS BY AUSCULTATION AND OLFACTION

4 - an excessive addiction to sour or salty food.

Gasping or puffing (shangqi), symptoms accompanying difficult respiration, are contravective signs (i.e. indicating a flow of energy contrary to the physiological direction) as the consequence of pituita in the respiratory tracts. We may distinguish
1 - a symptom of pituita in the thorax, in which case the patient continuously clears his throat, expectorating opaque phlegm and is unable to bear a horizontal position; or
2 - a symptom of contravective "glare" (ardor) as the consequence of the exhaustion of the yin of the renal orb (inanitas yin orbis renalis), if the patient complains of a sore throat; finally it may be
3 - an indication that a heteropathy fixed in the skin has tied up the energies of the pulmonal orb, thus pushing it back into, and hemming it in within the intima, where it conflicts with the fluids. (Because of the latter mechanism, there very often appears the corollary symptom of puffiness.)

Shortness of breath (duanqi) is defined as a comparatively shallow, accelerated and at the same time nervous and instable respiration which may be, but is not necessarily accompanied by movements of the shoulders. Shortness of breath may be due to
1 - residual thin phlegm in the thorax, if corollary symptoms such as thirst, painful joints and submerged pulses are present;
2 - exhaustion of energies in the pulmonal orb, if, in addition, copious excretion of urine and general weakness are observed; or
3 - repletion of the intima, in particular of the oo. cardialis et intestinorum, if after an algor laedens-disease, a distended and hard abdomen is observed; or
4 - exhaustion of the intima (inanitas intimae) if, as a sequel to an identical disease, the distended abdomen is soft.

Respiratio minor [hypoventilation] (shaoqi) designates a rather regular yet shallow, too slow and too weak (hence inaudible) respiration. This is a symptom of exhaustion (inanitas) and of the collapse of all energies.

The Sound of Coughing (Tussis)

Cough is essentially a symptom of a disease in the o. pulmonalis, which may be due to
  exogenous algor venti, if the cough is loud and raucous and produces clear and white expectoration; also obstructed nasal passages may be observed; or

calor orbis pulmonalis, if coughing produces a muffled noise, yellow and thick expectoration, difficult to eject, and is accompanied by a sore throat, a hot yet open nose; or

algor or humor and/or the massive accumulation of "phlegm" (pituita), if a muffled cough produces great quantities of phlegm; or

inanitas, if the patient feels irritation that produces the desire to cough yet does not to so, and simply draws some deep breaths; or

repletion, if cough has a paroxysmal quality and sometimes is accompanied by hemoptea; or, finally,

"glare" (ardor), if cough never produces any expectoration, but at best some sticky liquid.

Diagnosing the Sounds of Retching and Vomiting

Traditional Chinese medicine distinguishes among vomiting (ou): a noisy process ejecting matter;
spitting (tu): a noiseless process ejecting matter; and
retching (ganou): a noisy act producing nothing.

Each of these anomalies may be due to contravections of energy in the stomach orb.

Vomiting induced either by algor or by inanitas ("cold" or "exhaustion") evacuates matter slowly and is accompanied by moderate noise.

Vomiting induced by calor or repletio is characterized by the sudden loud evacuation of copious matter.

The Sounds of Hiccup and Eructation

Hiccup (eni) and eructation (aiqi) also are due to contravections of energy from the o. stomachi. In a strong and healthy-looking individual, showing no other striking symptoms, hiccup may be due either to

1 - a meteorological contravection;
2 - an affection of algor venti contracted after eating; or
3 - too hasty ingestion of food. In all these cases, the symptom corresponds to a very slight disturbance requiring no treatment at all.

By contrast, hiccup in an exhausted, emaciated individual, and after prolonged illness, represents a very serious symptom and may indicate either

1 - an algor-heteropathy, if it is accompanied by cold extremities, white coating of

the tongue, stale taste in the mouth, slowed-down pulses; or

2 - calor, if the sound of hiccuping is loud and abrupt and accompanied by a dry mouth, thirst, and accelerated pulses; or

3 - inanitas, if hiccuping is only slightly audible and long drawn out, and accompanied by exhausted pulses (pp. inanes) and other symptoms of inanitas; or, finally,

4 - repletion (repletio), if it is clearly audible and accompanied by replete and slippery pulses (pp. repleti et lubrici).

Eructation may be a symptom of

1 - an algor-heteropathy deversating in the o. stomachi;

2 - a momentary disharmony of the energies of the o. stomachi from extreme or even excessive dispulsive applications such as diaphoresis or vomiting (sudatio sive purgatio);

3 - an undigested meal ("undigested-evening-meal syndrome") if foul- or sour-smelling air is also expelled; or

4 - inanitas of energies in old people, if foul-smelling air is expelled.

DIAGNOSIS BY OLFACTION *(olfactio)*

Olfactory diagnosis aims at determining the smell of excretions and evacuations of the body and the smell of the sickroom. Very often olfactory diagnosis acquires critical significance when the relative strength of a disease is to be determined.

Odour from the Mouth (Bad Breath)

Bad breath, except for clearly defined somatic causes such as decayed teeth and stomach ulcers (usually diagnosed and treated by Western medicine) may be due to a calor-heteropathy in the stomach orb.

Smell of Perspiration

If perspiration has a clearly perceptible or even a penetrating strong smell, this is a symptom that a ventus-, calor- or humor-heteropathy[169] has accumulated for some time in the skin, that is, in the specific unfoldment (perfectio) of the pulmonal orb, there vitiating or depleting the fluids.

Odour of Excretions

If excretions such as faeces, urine or menstrual blood have a strong penetrating odour or malodour, this indicates calor or, in the case of urine, also humor; an inoffensive or weak smell, e.g. that of fresh meat, may indicate algor.

Odour of the Sickroom

Independent of the cleanliness of the sickroom, a putrid or dead-body smell is a symptom of very critical lesions to the orbs; an odour of blood usually indicates a depletion of xue (individually specific structure energies, including blood).

---

[169] For the differential diagnosis of these agents, cf. the folding table.

INTERROGATION DIAGNOSIS 179

Chapter Three: Interrogation Diagnosis *(Interrogatio, Wen)*

Questioning of the patient or of his relatives, besides personal data for the file, must produce such information as cannot be obtained by any other methods, e.g. on subjective sensations, emotions, past diseases, their treatment, accidents, living habits and so on. Just as with anamnesis of Western medicine, many questions will be prompted by the course of interrogation. Still, every new patient should be questioned on the following items:

1. Sensations of temperature
2. Perspiration
3. Pains
4. Stools and Micturition
5. Appetite and thirst
6. Breathing
7. Vision and hearing
8. Fatigue and sleep
9. Past diseases and their treatment
10. Menstruation.

SENSATION OF TEMPERATURE

Knowing how a patient experiences temperature, his changing sensations in this regard, constitutes an essential element of any Chinese diagnosis and, consequently, should be ascertained at the very outset. Distinctions should be made between

a^1) Being cold, "shuddering", "shivering": "abhorrence of cold" (wuhan), that is, the generalized subjective sensation of being cold, independent of or even in contrast to, available clothing, surrounding temperature, surface temperature etc.

a^2) Being chilled: "abhorrence of wind" (wufeng), that is, a subjective sensation on the skin, there liable to produce "gooseflesh" as if one were exposed to draughts of air - independent of the objective situation; shuddering, being cold, being chilled may equally be present with "heat" or "cold" (calor- or algor-heteropathies), as well as with inanitas or repletio. Therefore, additional data must be taken into account.

b) Oppressive heat: "abhorrence of heat" (wure), that is, the subjective sensation of oppressive heat, independent of the temperature of the body or its surroundings or of clothing.

b[1]) Fever (fare), i.e. an objective but also subjectively perceived rise in temperature of the entire body beyond the physiological average.

b[2]) Hot flushes, i.e. intermittent or sudden occurrence of the disturbance described under b), oppressive heat.

b[3]) Periodic fevers (chaore), i.e. intermittent rises in temperature occurring by fits or returning periodically, sometimes accompanied by shuddering.

From the patient's sensations of temperature, inferences may be drawn as to the relative strength of the orthopathy or of heteropathies, as to inanitas of yin or yang, concerning exogenous influences or endogenous disturbances.

Symptoms indicating the action of exogenous pathogenic factors are: the sudden onset of symptoms, fever with shuddering, higher temperature of the back of the hand than of the palm, higher temperature of the back of the body than of the abdominal side.

We may deduce an endogenous origin of the disturbance if symptoms develop gradually, if there is an alternation between heat and cold, if the cold the patient feels can be improved by additional covers, if the palm shows a higher temperature than the back of the hand, and the abdominal side a higher temperature than the back of the body.

The relative intensity of shuddering and fever is in direct proportion to the intensity of the heteropathy (or heteropathies) and, as a rule, in inverse proportion to the strength of the orthopathy.

If the aggravation of the symptoms always sets in during the day, this is an indication that the active energies (= yang) are primarily affected; if symptoms always worsen at night, this indicates that structive energies (= yin) are primarily affected.

If, for a prolonged period, temperature always rises in the afternoon, this indicates exhaustion of the yin (inanitas yin). Chilliness, spontaneous perspiration and cold extremities are symptoms of the exhaustion of yang (inanitas yang).

PERSPIRATION

Perspiration is formed in the body by the action of yang (= active energy) on yin (= structive energy, substratum), and surfacing through the pores of the skin. In other words, the appearance of perspiration always indicates that in an individual, a shift in the dynamic balance between active energies and structive potentials has taken place. Thus perspiration appears if activity is increased beyond the measure of the structive potential balancing it; but it also sets in if, in spite of an unchanged level of activity (even if this corresponds only to the maintenance of physiological functions) the available structive energies have been reduced. The first eventuality would correspond to a diagnosis of redundant yang or calor, the second to a case of deficiency or inanitas of yin.

In the wake of exogenous disturbances, perspiration may be present or absent. The absence of perspiration is a symptom of repletio speciei ("repletion of the surface") inducing the tight stopping up of the pores; the presence of perspiration with an exogenous disturbance indicates inanitas speciei ("exhaustion of the surface") completely relaxing and widely opening the pores.

A clear grasp of these correlations permits us to understand why, with an exogenous, light species-affection marked by the absence of perspiration, the therapeutic "unbending" (liberatio) by the administration of mm. liberantia speciei of the repletion of the species, immediately brings on perspiration and not only produces immediate subjective relief but, very often, complete recovery – with normal pulses and disappearance of the unusual coating of the tongue. Of course, in all these cases, the additional information just mentioned must be taken into account if we want to confirm a recovery.

Different from the perspiration appearing with great exertion, the following varieties of perspiration have diagnostic significance:

a) 'Spontaneous perspiration' (zihan), i.e. perspiration appearing without any exertion. This, as a rule, indicates inanitas yang ("exhaustion of active energies").

b) 'Perspiration appearing during sleep' (daohan), literally "predatory perspiration", designates sweating setting in immediately after the patient falls asleep and stopping when he wakes up. Such perspiration usually[170] indicates inanitas yin.

---

[170] To make this diagnostic statement, of course, other data, especially those of the pulse, must be taken into account.

c) 'Perspiration limited to the head': This is accompanied by persistent thirst, yellow coating of the tongue, and superficial and accelerated pulses and indicates ardor ("glare") in the upper calorium (calorium superius).

If this symptom is accompanied by lassitude, fatigue, and a slippery, yellow coating of the tongue, we may infer an accumulation of calor in the wake of "humditiy": calor humidus; accompanied by cold extremities, shuddering, a slippery, white coating of the tongue and submerged pulses, this symptom indicates inanitas yang.

If perspiration is limited to the forehead and accompanied by panting, this is a symptom of the collapse of the active energies.

d) 'Absolute perspiration' (juehan), the profuse and uninterrupted perspiration accompanying extremely critical phases of disease, indicates a total disruption of the interrelationship between yin and yang and, consequently, a "rootless yang", hence active energies dispersing outside.

e) 'Trepidation perspiration' (zhanhan) is the perspiration appearing immediately after a fit of shivering. Its appearance indicates the beginning of the crisis. It must be ascertained from corollary diagnostic data whether this crisis is followed by improvement or if an extremely depleted orthopathy is insufficient to re-establish the normal interaction between all functions. Symptoms indicating the former are: falling temperature immediately after the fit of perspiration, normalizing tendency of the pulses; symptoms indicating the latter are subnormal temperatures after perspiration, and hard, narrow, weak pulses.

PAINS

In Chinese medicine, pain is not a symptom but an integral and essential part[171] of many diseases. This is why the exact qualification and localization of pains has great diagnostic value.

---

[171] This view is very different from that of modern Western medicine, for which, in all cases, pain is an empirical accident to somatic modifications. In Chinese medicine primarily oriented toward the actual, positive perception of function, hence of present movement, present sense experiences, feelings..., pain is a very dramatic and important modification of ordinary feeling, hence cannot be treated independently from other functional disorders determined by diagnosis. Cf. pp. 14 f. above.

INTERROGATION DIAGNOSIS

Pains in the Head ("Headache").

An acute headache usually is brought on by repletion or by an exogenous heteropathy; by contrast, the chronic disposition of intermittent or fitful headaches is due to endogenous factors, in particular to inanitas of the constitutional energy reserves (qi primum). Still, there are many exceptions to these rules, as a more detailed diagnosis will often show.

Headache accompanying menstruation usually points to a deficiency of the yin hepaticum, which indirectly lets the active energies of the hepatic orb rise upward (into the head), there inducing a local repletion.

Particular attention should be given the precise correlations between the sites of a headache, its other modes and the conduits; thus,

headache tending to radiate into the neck and back points to the major yang conduits;

headache developing in the forehead or above the orbits points to the splendor yang conduits;

headache in the temples (very often felt like a drill near the foramen clusa superior, (foramen 3 on the cardinalis fellea) points to the yang minor conduits;

headache accompanied by heavy limbs, a tense, hard abdomen, and spontaneous perspiration points to the conduits of major yin;

headache felt deep within the head, radiating into the teeth and accompanied by cyanosis of the nails is related to the conduits of minor yin; and

headache affecting the top of the head and radiating into the temples, sometimes accompanied by eructations and nausea, points to the yielding yin conduits (sinarteriae yin flectentis).

Dizziness

Like other symptoms, dizziness, whether acute or chronic, may be induced either by repletion or by inanitas ("exhaustion").

Sudden, intense dizziness is a symptom of repletion, either because of ardor flaring up from the hepatic orb, or because of pituita which has not yet precipitated.

Chronic dizziness is a symptom either of deficiency, in particular in the renal orb, or of accumulated humor or pituita impeding the deployment of active energies.

Pains in the Body

Diffuse pains throughout the body occur with exogenous algor venti ("wind"-induced "cold"), here indicating a superficial (species) affection.

Intense pain at an advanced stage of phthisis indicate an already extreme exhaustion of structive energies which, for this reason, no longer suffice to maintain the functions of the nervus and bones (the specific unfoldments - perfectiones - of the hepatic and renal orbs).

A woman's abdominal pains after birth, as a rule, are due to exhaustion of xue (inanitas xue) to the loss of blood or, on the contrary, to congested xue in the conduits.

Pains in the joints (bi) may be due to ventus-, algor- or humor-heteropathies, viz.
1 - if pain remains firmly localized and is accompanied by heavy limbs and lassitude, this is called "sticking pains of the joints" (zhaobi), essentially induced by a humor-heteropathy.
2 - If these pains wander about, affecting one joint and then another, they are called "wandering pains of the joints" (xingbi), essentially ascribable to ventus.
3 - If the pains in the joints are intense and piercing, they are called "intense pains of the joints" (tongbi), essentially induced by algor.

Pains in the loins [ischiatic pains] preponderantly are due to affections of the renal orb, viz.
a - If one feels weakness of the loins, if the pains are persistent yet difficult to localize and to qualify, if they are accompanied by copious, clear urination and diarrhea, and by a sensation of cold in the loins, this is a sign of inanitas yang renalis ("exhaustion of the active aspects of energy of the renal orb").
b - If pains as described are accompanied by constipation, limited, dark-coloured urination, and repeated active congestions in the head and upper thorax (induced by ardor flaring up, and by inanitas) this is a symptom of inanitas yin renalis ("exhaustion of the structive aspects of the energies of the renal orb").
c - Pains in the loins accompanied by the sensation of "sitting in water" or of "carrying a heavy burden tied around the midriff", accompanied by heavy limbs, and aggravated during overcast or humid weather and when sitting down, constitute a symptom of a humor-heteropathy.

Pains in the back, which may radiate into the shoulders and the neck, point to disturbances in the major yang conduits. If these pains persist for some time, an

INTERROGATION DIAGNOSIS

inanitas orbis renalis or a humor-heteropathy from ventus - humor venti - may have induced the symptom - which must be cleard up by additional diagnostic investigation.

DEFECATION AND MICTURITION

To the extent that the circumstances of defecation and micturition escape inspection and olfactory diagnosis, they must be ascertained by questioning.

Stools

Constipation, that is, the suspension of defecation up to several days, may, as a rule, be due to a deficiency of fluids in the oo. intestinorum, or it may be the symptom of the repletion of the active energies in these orbs.

Repletion constipation from a deficiency of fluids brought on by calor, is accompanied by symptoms such as periodic fever, thirst, dry tongue with yellow coating, and hard, tense abdomen.

Inanitas-constipation, likewise due to deficient fluids, occurs in old age or in women after birth, when the xue has been depleted.

Constipation accompanied by a greenish pale complexion, the desire to have hot beverages and the appearance of submerged or slowed-down pulses (pp. mersi atque tardi) is due to algor.

Diarrhea, if accompanied by the sensation of burning heat in the anus during defecation, and by very malodorous faeces, is a symptom of a congestion of calor.

Diarrhea accompanied by abdominal pains, cold extremities, white tongue and stale taste, points to an algor-heteropathy in the orbs: "algor intimae".

Stools, at first hard, then diarrheic, are symptoms of inanitas in the lienal orb because of a humor-heteropathy.

Matutinal diarrhea before sunrise is a symptom of inanitas yang renalis (an exhaustion of the active energies of the renal orb).

Micturition

a) A strikingly increased excretion of urine indicates a deficiency of active energies.

If this increased excretion, however, is accompanied by continuous, intense thirst and increased absorption of liquids, this is part of the sitis diffundens [diabetes] syndrome, not discussed here.

a^1) Increased quantities of urine in the absence of thirst, are a symptom of inanitas orbis renalis.

b) A clearly reduced excretion of urine is a symptom of fluid imbalance from calor (The fluids, in this case, may have been depleted either by excessive diaphoresis or by purging).

c) The frequent excretion of small quantities of dark-coloured urine indicates calor humidus in the lower calorium ("a heat heteropathy induced by humidity in the lower heated space").

c^1) The frequent excretion of limpid urine points to algor inanitatis calorii inferius ("a cold heteropathy due to the exhaustion of energies in the lower heated space").

c^2) The frequent excretion of minute quantities of urine ("urine trickle") is a symptom of calor intimae (calor-heteropathy affecting the orbs) having exhausted structive energies there.

d) Difficult micturition usually is a symptom of calor.

e) Incontinence, i.e. the inability to check the flow of urine, also enuresis nocturna in adults, very often is due to algor inanitatis calorii inferius ("an exhaustion induced cold heteropathy in the lower heated space") or, in the wake of serious disease, is due to a lesion of the qi primum (i.e. of the inborn constitutive energies of the renal orb).

f) A complete retention of urine, unless there are definite somatic obstacles, is due to a more or less extreme deficiency of active energies in the o. vesicalis.

APPETITE AND THE INTAKE OF FOOD

Information available on the appetite and the intake of food, facilitate the evaluation of the functions of the central orbs, oo. lienalis et stomachi. Also, information on food idiosyncrasies may give hints as to existing weaknesses or overactive functions in certain orbs.

Thirst

a) Continuous intense thirst, as a rule, points to calor.

b) The desire for drinks, which, however, cannot be swallowed, and a stale taste,

INTERROGATION DIAGNOSIS

point to algor.

c) Massive thirst, raving speech and constipation indicate calor repletionis ("heat" brought on by repletion).

d) The persistent desire for drinks, only a mouthful of which can be swallowed at a time, is either a symptom of inanitas or of calor humidus ("exhaustion" or "heat" brought on by "humidity").

e) The desire for hot beverages may be due either to
a potent humor-heteropathy: humor vigens, or
algor inanitatis (a "cold" heteropathy brought on by the exhaustion of energies); or finally,
an accumulation of pituita in the middle calorium.

f) Thirst after vomiting is a consequence of a perceptible depletion of fluids.

Hunger, Appetite, Eating

With most diseases, the decrease or increase of appetite is indicative not only of the strength of the qi stomachi, hence of the energies in the stomach orb, but also indirectly of the strength of the orthopathy altogether, and hence very often can reveal the gravity of an illness.

Reduced appetite indicates that the active energies in the oo. lienalis et stomachi have been reduced; increase of appetite is an indication of renewed vigour of these energies.

If eating makes the patient feel better, this indicates general inanitas; if eating makes the patient feel worse, this is a symptom of local repletion.

a) Reduced appetite accompanying exogenous affections indicates an active congestion in the oo. lienalis et stomachi.

b) Reduced appetite accompanying endogenous disturbances is a symptom of inanitas oo. lienalis et stomachi.

c) Total loss of appetite at the beginning of a disease or during a light disease points to a lesion of the qi stomachi (the active energies in the stomach orb), requiring particular attention.

d) Hunger and/or leanness in spite of copious eating point to ardor vigens o. stomachi ("intense glare" in the stomach orb) which, of necessity, entails a lesion of the structive energies of the orb. Finally,

e) hunger, yet no appetite, is a symptom of the lesion of the structive energies of the o. lienalis.

Taste

a) A bitter taste is a symptom of overflowing energies from the o. felleus.

b) A sour taste indicates calor o. hepatici.

c) A pungent taste indicates calor in the pulmonal orb.

d) A salty taste points to calor in the o. renalis.

e) A sweet or sweetish taste indicates that murky energies coming from the o. lienalis are pushed upward and overflow there. Finally,

f) a stale taste in the mouth indicates a humor-heteropathy in the stomach orb (humor o. stomachi) leading to an insufficient assimilation of the qi aquaticum (i.e. the influences exercised by the o. renalis). During convalescence, a stale taste may occur, indicating inanitas o. stomachi, and having the same consequences.

Sapors[172]

In diagnosis, the correlations between sapors and orbs (given in orbisiconography) may be used as complementary orientations; they must under no circumstances be used schematically and without due respect to other diagnostic data.

HEARING

Hearing is a sensory faculty primarily dependent upon the function of the renal orb. The following disturbances of hearing have diagnostic relevance:

Deafness

A comparatively sudden onset of acute deafness is due either to algor laedens of minor yang[173]; or to a calor-heteropathy (morbi temperati). In both cases, the degree of deafness and the gravity of disease are direclty correlated.

Deafness may also supervene because of

a - inanitas orbis cardialis,

b - a depleted structive potential (jing), especially in advanced age;

---

[172] Cf. note 16 on p. 21 above.

[173] Cf. pp. 106 f. above.

INTERROGATION DIAGNOSIS

c - inanitas yang renalis ("exhaustion of the active energies of the renal orb").

Hardness of Hearing

Hardness of hearing, as a rule, is brought on by a ventus-heteropathy or by calor in the conduits of the renal orb.

It may also occur with inanitas yin orbis renalis and resulting repletio yang in the head (exhaustion of structive energies in the renal orb and the resulting repletion in the head).

Tinnitus (Ringing of the Ears)

The sudden and powerful onset of tinnitus which seems to be re-enforced by covering the ear with the hand, is a symptom of repletion. A gradually developing, relatively weak tinnitus, which diminishes if the ear is covered with the hand, is a symptom of inanitas.

EYES AND VISION

Vision is a sensory perception directly and primarily depending upon the functions of the hepatic orb.

Pains in the Eye and Its Surroundings

Piercing, racking pains in the eye, often accompanied by headache and vertigo, are symptoms of a calor-heteropathy in the o. cardialis.

Excessive sensitivity to light, redness, pains in the eyes and eyelids, together with a puffy face, preponderantly occur in summer and either point to
calor venti ("wind-induced heat"), if it is accompanied by chills; or
calor humidus ("humidity induced heat"), if the eyes are watery and inflamed.

If an oversensitivity to light occurs without pain or inflammations, this indicates inanitas xue (exhaustion of the individually specific structive energies).

Reduced Acuity of Vision

Reduced acuity of vision always is due to energetic deficiency, brought on either by prolonged exhausting disease, by excessive crying or by emotional stress.

Blindness at Night

Blindness at night is always a symptom of inanitas orbis hepatici.

SLEEP AND THE DESIRE TO SLEEP

Insomnia

Insomnia, if it is the consequence of exaggerated reflection (cogitatio), may be taken as a symptom of deficiency of the xue orbis cardialis.

If insomnia is accompanied by an oppressive feeling in the region of the heart, by difficult micturition, panting, or irregular breathing, it may be adduced to a disturbance of the functions of the o. lienalis and hence to congested fluids in the centre.

Insomnia accompanied by palpitations, a dry mouth and minute or accelerated pulses is a symptom of deficiency of the structive energies.

In advanced old age, insomnia, as a rule, is due to general inanitas and, consequently, to insufficient coördination between the energies of the different orbs (ultimately an exhaustion of the energies of the o. cardialis, controlling this coördination).

Somnolence

If active energies are exhausted (inanes) and structive energies very powerful (vigentes), this usually brings on somnolence.

If somnolence is accompanied by heavy limbs, pp. languidi, we may infer that there is a preponderance or excess of humor.

MENSTRUATION

Advanced Menstruation

If the onset of menstruation is advanced, if the menses are of red, purple or blackish colour, if these symptoms are accompanied by a dry mouth, accelerated pulses or pains in the abdomen, this indicates calor affecting the xue.

INTERROGATION DIAGNOSIS

If advanced menstruation occurs during the first half of the cycle, if it is of light colour, if there is normal moisture in the mouth, slowed-down pulses and a painful abdomen, these symptoms indicate inanitas xue.

If menstruation is preceded by pains in a hard and tense abdomen, this indicates a congestion or stasis of active and structive energies.

If menstruation is followed by pains in the abdomen without any other symptoms, we may infer an endogenous algor-heteropathy due to inanitas xue.

Absence of Menstruation

If pregnancy has been ruled out, the absence of menstruation may be due to an exhaustion or a congestion of the xue, to extreme stress or to congestions of energy in the oo. hepaticus et lienalis.

Faltering Menstruation

Menstruation which starts but then stops may have been affected either by ira ("wrath") or any other extreme emotion, or by algore percussio (i.e. a sudden algor-heteropathy).

If a disease with fever is present, it is conceivable that calor has affected the xue.

Fluor albus

Fluor albus, as a rule, indicates

algor inanitatis (i.e. a "cold" heteropathy brought on by exhaustion), if it is thin,

calor humidus (a "heat" heteropathy brought on by "humidity"), if it is yellow and malodorous.

In the context of menstruation, questions bearing on somatic data, and those relating to the topology of organs, also questions asked to determine certain epidemiological and gynecological diseases associated with somatic disturbances may be left out here since their diagnosis and treatment is better achieved by Western medicine.

Chapter Four: Palpation Diagnosis *(Palpatio; Qiezhen, Anzhen)*

At first sight, Chinese medicine seems not to be different from any other traditional medical system in that it assigns considerable significance to palpation, i.e. the palpatory examination of the body and the pulses.

However, to properly use and understand the techniques of Chinese palpation, we must keep in mind that, true to its basic rationale and by contradistinction say to traditional Galenic (Western) medicine, Chinese palpatory diagnosis is <u>not</u> primarily and exclusively aimed at ascertaining the sensitivity to pain, the tension, temperature, tumescence of muscles or inner organs; <u>its foremost objective is to obtain authentic and highly discrete data on the actual situation of all vital functions of an individual</u>. Hence, the palpatory exploration of certain critical foramina, and hence the outstanding role of pulse diagnosis.

PALPATION OF THE PULSES *(qiemo,* "pulse diagnosis"*)*

IMPORTANT PRELIMINARY CONSIDERATIONS: PREREQUISITES FOR MASTERING PULSE DIAGNOSIS

Practical experience in pulse diagnosis in East Asia and in Europe, and almost a decade of teaching it to Western physicians, have thoroughly convinced me that what prevents many gifted persons from mastering Chinese pulse diagnosis is factors quite different from what the layman would imagine.

Indeed, three kinds of obstacles to mastering pulse diagnosis must be considered, viz.

1. An inadequate endowment,
2. A wrong intellectual perspective, and
3. An inapt pedagogical approach.

The first "obstacle" is mentioned just for the sake of completeness and may be dismissed for good and all. In fact, during all these years, I never saw anyone practicing medicine professionally with at least average abilities who was not amply provided with the physical endowments (sensitivity of fingers, capability of concentration) and intellectual gifts (the ability to distinguish, coördinate and synthezise observed data) for perfect mastery of pulse diagnosis.

The second "obstacle" must be discussed explicitly at somewhat greater length because it constitutes a real impediment to the study of pulse diagnosis (and sometimes of Chinese medicine altogether). To the layman and, worse still, to the misinformed pseudo-expert on Chinese medicine, pulse diagnosis offers at the same time aspects of crudeness and of widely speculative oversophistication - neither of which proves to be true after one has mastered the method.

The impression that pulse diagnosis must be a crude method results from the educational background of practically all Western physicians. During their years at medical college, they have been more or less thoroughly inculcated with very subtle and sensitive diagnostic techniques which, however, achieve their extraordinary precision and reliability only by inserting highly complicated apparatus between the patient and the doctor registering the patient's symptoms. Worse still, in many countries even the most elementary kind of pulse diagnosis has been eliminated from the curricula of medical colleges - thus leaving future doctors to experiment on their own or to completely drop palpation, in particular palpation of the pulse, as completely irrelevant to a scientific medical diagnosis. - There is some justification in the attitude if, as we pointed out in the first lines of this chapter, the only or the primary aim of diagnosis is to ascertain somatic disturbances; it is an absurd and preposterous limitation if, on the contrary, our interest is in the subtle and positive determination of functional phenomena.

The contrary aspect of diagnosis appears if somebody tries to approach this technique not, as should be the rule, with a good deal of basic medical knowledge and clinical experience but, instead, through the narrative of perhaps highly imaginative but otherwise little-qualified authors who enumerate countless and incoherent details of pulse diagnosis as an oriental storyteller would enumerate the multifarious electronic gadgets in a modern intercontinental plane. What I am driving at is that what to the uninformed glance of someone utterly unfamiliar with the coherent theories of function-oriented Chinese medicine, sometimes unfamiliar also with most elementary medical theory and clinical experience, appears to be a wilful array or a chaotic accumulation of incoherent rules and data, immediately falls into place when the requirements just mentioned are met - then forming an extremely elastic, reliable and

PALPATION DIAGNOSIS

precise tool for determining data which cannot be positively defined with such precision and dispatch by any other method thus far known to mankind and to medical science.

In other words, people often refuse to look at Chinese pulse diagnosis or at Chinese medicine simply because they are utterly oblivious of the intrinsic limitations of their own methodology, hence oblivious also of the complementary nature - and consequently of the complementary methodology required to understand, learn and apply it. Consequently, they attempt to assess and describe the statements of Chinese medicine by using the yardstick of Western methodology - thus obliterating the very facts which they strive to discuss.[174]

The "wrong intellectual perspective" is an obstacle that must be taken seriously by all those who want to teach and to communicate about Chinese medicine in general, and pulse diagnosis in particular. It plays a role in the "no man's land" between Western and Chinese medicine. Still, according to my experience, it does not constitute the most difficult and forbidding obstacle to the mastery of Chinese pulse diagnosis.

Indeed, this qualification is reserved for the last-mentioned impediment, termed "an inapt pedagocial approach".

Most of the failures in mastering pulse diagnosis - I should say at least 80 percent - are due to ignorance of this formidable obstacle, or to approaching it too lightly. What does it consist of?

Chinese pulse diagnosis is a skill. There are artistic skills and scientific, i.e. intellectual, skills. Playing the violin is an artistic skill. Pulse diagnosis is essentially an <u>intellectual skill</u>, just as is the diagnosis by means of an EEG or EKG. Now the acquisition of a skill requires training. And in such training the right balance must be struck between physical and intellectual input. As any teacher knows, at infancy, the physical input precedes or at least has greater importance than the intellectual input; with adoclescence and definitely in adulthood, the situation is reversed. Then in the acquisition of any skill, intellectual information must <u>precede</u> physical training. This precedence must be observed in a twofold manner: The intellectual data must be presented before physical instruction is given; and the intellectual data actually constitute the indispensable premise for the effective acquisition, assimilation and integration of physical experience.

---

[174] It may be worthwhile to read my article <u>The Quandary of Chinese Medicine</u>, published in EASTERN HORIZON, Hongkong, December 1977.

Let me explain. Whereas the infant constantly assimilates new impressions without as yet having an adequate vocabulary to class and to reproduce these, the adult is extremely refractory towards new impressions unless he has such a vocabulary enabling him to link up what his much more sophisticated senses can perceive. Applied to the training and mastery of pulse diagnosis, consequently, the problem is not that the students cannot feel what must be felt, but that they usually are at a loss to describe, hence to assimilate, to permanently learn and keep what they have physically perceived - unless. . . This, precisely, is the critical issue: There is no point in attempting practical training in pulse diagnosis <u>unless all pertinent theory and, more important, the complete iconography of the pulse has previously been absorbed intellectually</u>. In other words, no student of pulse diagnosis should attempt practical training unless he has not only memorized, but understood by frequent rehearsal, every single term and technical relationship instrumental to Chinese pulse diagnosis. (This terminology, as will become evident, has not been wilfully invented but is the result of almost 2000 years of clinical experience and heuristic maturing.) Only on this condition will he be able to immediately describe and express with precision and stringency what he feels when actually putting his fingers on the pulses of a patient's arms. And only on this premise will he be able to recall, reflect upon and communicate to his colleagues what he feels.

If this essential condition has been met, practical mastery of pulse diagnosis in normal medical practice is - at worst - a question of several months; with proper guidance it should take only weeks to gauge, correct and refine one's sensitivity so that the error rate drops to insignificance within one month. If, on the contrary, this warning is ignored, even with the best intentions, a student may not master quite basic notions even with years trying. He proceeds like someone attempting to interpret an EKG without the slightest notion of physics or modern physiology, just by comparing the outward inspection of the patient with the erratic curve traced by the EKG machine. Trying to make sense of the subtle differences felt at the pulse sites without the most strict reference and conscientious attention to the intellectual tools prepared <u>for this very purpose</u> in the course of almost 2000 years is like attempting to interpret an EKG while spurning all knowledge of what is taught about this technique in medical colleges by physics, physiology and clinical medicine.

PALPATION DIAGNOSIS

HISTORICAL AND THEORETICAL BACKGROUND OF PULSE DIAGNOSIS

In China, the palpation of the pulse, since the inception of scientific medicine there - i.e. since the compilation of the Inner Classic of the Yellow Sovereign (Huangdi Neijing Suwen) during the 3rd century before our era - constitutes an integral part of the healing arts.

The first monography devoted to the subject, the so-called "Pulse Classic" (Mojing) was compiled by Wang Shuhe living approximately from 265 to 316. Between the appearance of this work and the last general scientific treatment of this subject to appear thus far, the "Sphygmology ('pulse studies') of Li Shizhen"[175], a continuous refinement of theory and method thanks to the efforts of famous and less famous physicians took place.

Pulse diagnosis, without any doubt, constitutes the foundation and the backbone of any Chinese diagnosis properly and completely carried out. For the data obtained from the palpation of the pulse not only may be used to confirm or to correct the different results obtained by other diagnostic procedures such as inspection, auscultation, olfaction and interrogation; more important still, and strange as it may sound to laymen and beginners, pulse diagnosis is less open to error or manipulation, and at the same time affords a more direct, a more subtle and more objective access to the situation than any other procedure used in Chinese diagnosis.

Chinese pulse diagnosis does not presuppose any exceptional, little known, paranormal endowment or ability in the person applying it. All that is required is a solid grounding in its coherent theory and a trained and well kept hand.

Strange to say, it is the latter requirement of a trained and of a well kept hand which, even in East Asia, in spite of all lip service to the idea and acceptance of pulse diagnosis, in former times and, to some extent even today, keeps down the number of persons having really mastered this method. It should be recalled that in former times and even today - just think of the barefoot doctors digging in the earth, mixing mortar or operating heavy machinery - traditional medicine is exercised as a kind of side activity, the side activity of farmers, craftsmen, businessmen, administrators, apothecaries. And, in spite of their adaptability, certain manual

---

[175] Binhu moxue - The precision of some and the definition of not a few of the iconograms of the pulse used today are due to Li Shizhen's work. However, this amazing scholar, whose life extended from 1518 to 1593, has earned even greater fame by the compilation of the monumental "Systematic Pharmacopoeia" (Bencaogangmu), elaborately describing some 1800 drugs and assembling almost 10.000 prescriptions.

activities really do affect the sensitivity of the palpating fingers.

We have already touched upon another obstacle, a wrong intellectual perspective. Today, not a few physicians, thoroughly trained in Western medicine, yet with no comparable knowledge or even utterly ignorant of the epistemological and methodological foundations of Chinese medicine, argue that it is simply against logic and reason that all the information which Chinese medicine pretends can be gained from the palpation of the pulse, positively can be obtained in this way.

We have repeatedly alluded to the wilful and illegitimate confusion and inversion of Western and Chinese methods and modes of cognizance; we also have mentioned the consequences of the pseudo-scientific and wilful attitude which pretends that in order to arrive at a rationally stringent statement in Chinese medicine, we must start out from a premise of anatomical and physiological data identical with those postulated by Western medicine[176]. In this practical presentation of the subject, we cannot go into the details of arguments developed at length elsewhere. However, a reminder should be given that, for more than two generations, scientific physiology - that is, physiology of Western medicine - has abandoned the mechanistical hypothesis that the circulation of blood and humors is exclusively effected by the pumping effort of the heart. If this hypothesis were true, man would have to have a pumping organ many times the size actually present in order to overcome the enormous resistance to the circulation in the capillary part of the circuit[177]. In other words, the physiological circulation of blood and humors is the result of the synergy exactly controlled by nervous impulses between the rhythmic impulses of the heart in the large arteries, and the active propulsion of liquids in the capillaries.

Moreover, to produce the "pulse iconogram" at a definite site of an artery such as the ostium pollicare (at the processus styloides radii), a wealth of additional factors and influences must be taken into account, each of which may be known separately, but whose in vivo interaction within a certain individual at a given moment, it is impossible to analyze completely, let alone to measure. For besides the arterial pressure and the frequency of the heartbeat there are the thickness and flexibility of

---

[176] We have very often dealt with this problem, e.g. in Porkert, The Dilemma of Present-Day Interpretations of Chinese Medicine, published in MEDICINE IN CHINESE CULTURES, Comparative Studies of Health Care, Dept. of Health, Education and Welfare, Washington D.C., 1975, pp. 61 - 70.

[177] Any modern textbook of medical physiology will describe these relationships, including the so-called Law of Poiseuille (Jean-Marie Poiseuille, 1799 - 1869), as well as the vasomotor effect of the capillaries. - Cf. e.g. Arthur C. Guyton, Textbook of Medical Physiology, Philadelphia 1971, pp. 230 ff.

PALPATION DIAGNOSIS

the walls of the artery, the tonus of the wall of the artery, the thickness and turgor of tissue between the bone and the artery and between the artery and the surface of the skin, the length of the artery running through elastic tissue and so on. At any rate it is not mere conjecture but a well known law of physics that overtones forming in a vibrating medium or body are very much influenced by the configuration and hardness of this oscillating body and its support. From the viewpoint of physics, consequently, an identical wave of the pulse passing over three consecutive sites of manifestly different anatomical configuration, e.g. the sites pollex, clusa and pes of the ostium pollicare, must manifest themselves by three different modulations.

It is quite a different matter to define how these qualitatively discrete pulse data are correlated to other data of a comprehensive system. But here again, the reply can be given with ease and precision: Palpation of the pulse and pulse iconography are organic parts, hence essential and perfectly integrated constituents of China's system of medical science. By contrast, these very data are in no way related - or, if they appear to be, only in a very approximate and indirect way - to the scientific postulates of Western anatomy and physiology. Or, put differently, to suppose that Chinese pulses are correlated to "organs" is a gratuitous invention of amateurish modern literature on acupuncture - and has no foundation whatsoever in the authentic insights and theories of specifically Chinese medical science.

TECHNIQUE OF PULSE DIAGNOSIS I: PRACTICAL REQUIREMENTS AND PRECAUTIONS

Fundamentals

Palpation of the pulse, according to the classical rules of Chinese diagnosis, is done by applying (the index, middle and ring fingers of) one hand first to the pulse sites of one, and after this, of the other arm of the patient. This implies that a right-handed diagnostician as a rule will only train his right hand and execute palpation with this hand only, and a left-handed person will proceed inversely.

It is, however, conceivable that a tennis pro, reluctant to abandon his sports hobby, in order to do Chinese pulse diagnosis may train his left hand for taking the pulse.

Incidentally, I have never seen Chinese pulse diagnosis as described executed in Japan, not

even by the stars of today's kampo-medicine and acupuncture[178]. Japanese traditional doctors usually take the pulse simultaneously with both hands, which they apply only for the fraction of a minute – thus precluding that anything resembling the elaborateness of Chinese pulse diagnosis is obtained.

Prospective diagnosticians should also be warned against the idea that during the working day of a physician, a complete pulse diagnosis can be done on any number of patients. If it is true that an experienced diagnostician will be able to arrive at a perfectly stringent and precise diagnosis within five to ten minutes, if average conditions[179] prevail, intricate and very difficult cases may take up to thirty minutes of palpation. Consequently, such diagnosis, in addition to demanding great concentration, may also – in particular when feeling the pedal sites – put physical strain on the diagnostician. Therefore a responsible and conscientious diagnostician will avoid doing more than twelve complete and detailed diagnoses, spread over the day.

Still, as has already been said, the Chinese method of taking the pulse requires no exceptional endowment but only a trained and well kept hand. Thus proper pulse diagnosis may become impossible for days or even weeks if the palpating fingers have been brought into contact with strong alkaline solutions, with mortar, acids or sometimes only with powerful detergents. The sensitivity of the fingers is also impaired by professional piano playing, by playing plugged string instruments, by rope climbing, mountaineering etc. As can be deduced from these examples, all kinds of activities and sports which either affect the skin on the finger tips and/or produce an excessive thickening of the tissues between the skin and the bones, e.g. rowing and tennis, may impair the quality of pulse diagnosis.

Finally, an influence not to be taken lightly is the cold of winter. A hand warming up after having been thoroughly chilled may have its sensitivity impaired at least during palpation of the first one or two patients.

Timing of Pulse Diagnosis

It is true that the palpation of the pulse may have to be effected during any hour of the day or of the night. Still, for the obtention of particularly critical diagnoses, an

---

[178] The literal meaning of the Japanese word kampo is "Chinese prescriptions", a designation given since the 8th century of our era to that branch of Japanese medicine, developing from the imported Chinese medical tradition.

[179] Cf. the next two pages.

effort should be made to see the patient just after he has awakened from sleep and before taking his breakfast. Second-best alternatives are the hours between the times of the usual main meals, in which cases, for optimum results, diagnosis should take place two hours after the preceding and one hour before the following big meal.

The ingestion of an ordinary lunch even on a perfectly healthy person without any digestive symptoms, will temporarily push the clusal pulses in the direction of "overflowing" (pp. exundantes)[180]. But the digestive process, depending upon the quality and quantity of food and drink absorbed, may indeed affect all pulses.

When establishing a first comprehensive diagnosis on a patient, late afternoons and nights should be avoided for pulse diagnosis at least with the critically ill, since on these, functions then tend to drift off significantly from the diurnal average.

Accidental Influences to be Reckoned with or Avoided

As a rule, all influences and factors momentarily affecting the patient - in addition to constitutional ones, those of meteorology, emotions and social setting - enter into the iconogram of the pulse obtained.

It is likewise true that the effect of brief, ephemeral stimuli and momentary regulative adaptation can and should be kept out of the pulse iconogram, such as driving a car, climbing stairs, passing from the winter cold into the overheated surroundings of a doctor's study, etc. In other words, an attempt should be made to determine what may be called an average or "typical" pulse of the patient at rest - a pulse which reflects all the continuous and typical stresses to which the patient is subjected anyway, but which excludes the untypical, accidental and momentary ones. Thus on outpatients, pulse diagnosis should be attempted not sooner than a quarter of an hour after their arrival.

Of course, any kind of medication will affect the pulse. Thus any comprehensive pulse diagnosis must be preceded by a detailed interrogation clearing up these factors. If the patient states that he takes powerful stimulants or sedatives, a final diagnosis may need to be postponed.

---

[180] The iconogram of the flooding pulse will be found on p. 214. The general influences of meals on the pulse are discussed on p. 246.

Constitution of the Diagnostician

With the diagnostician in perfect health and in full command of his bodily resources, all momentary influences resulting from a change of weather, from the moderate intake of food or even permanent slight hypertension[181], do not affect the precision and subtlety of pulse diagnosis.

By contrast, this precision is impaired by all unusual strains such as momentary stress due to driving a car, exhaustion as the consequence of disease or of excessive exertion, emotional shocks, the use of strong stimulants or medicines[182], and so on. For, indeed, these factors may produce either a significant repletion or, inversely, a significant exhaustion (inanitas) in the palpating finger, thus temporarily disturbing the individual standards.

Thus, e.g. an extremely irritated or excited diagnostician may feel a replete pulse of the patient as a normal pulse or a superficial pulse as an exhausted (inanis) pulse, a pulse showing just a mere tendency towards inanitas as a latent pulse, etc.

Indeed, there is agreement among all authors of former times and among present practitioners of Chinese pulse diagnosis that a diagnostician should take the pulse only if he himself is perfectly relaxed, at ease and hence capable of concentration.

We should mention here that even under seemingly ideal conditions, a diagnostician should not take his own pulse: The complicated mixture of subjective and objective impressions as well as an impossible-to-gauge re-enforcement of impulses which, in being synchronous, have different modulations in the fingers and at the pulse sites, prevent good results. At best, after having acquired a certain routine, he may try to take his own pulse by the so-called emergency method described below.

TOPOLOGY AND SIGNIFICANCE OF THE GENERAL BODY PULSES

It is true that in Chinese diagnostics, palpation of the radial pulses taken at the so-called ostium pollicare, as far as sophistication of method and practical usefulness is concerned, clearly takes precedence over the palpation of any other pulse sites.

---

[181] The Western diagnosis of hypertension may, under no circumstances, be equated to the Chinese qualification of repletion!

[182] The effects of smoking and liquor must be assessed individually, depending upon the constitution of the individual and the quantity taken.

PALPATION DIAGNOSIS 203

Still, if viewed in historical perspective[183], and as a bridge to the postulates of Western medicine oriented toward somatic sites described by anatomy, the description of general pulses of the body precedes that method of pulse diagnosis which is limited to taking the radial pulses only. As with some other major diagnostic procedures, the interpretation of the body pulses is approached on two seperate levels, viz.

by comparision of 3 x 3 pulse sites on the head, the hands and the feet, and

the palpation of respectively one representative pulse on the head, hand and foot.

The 3 x 3 Pulses of the Body

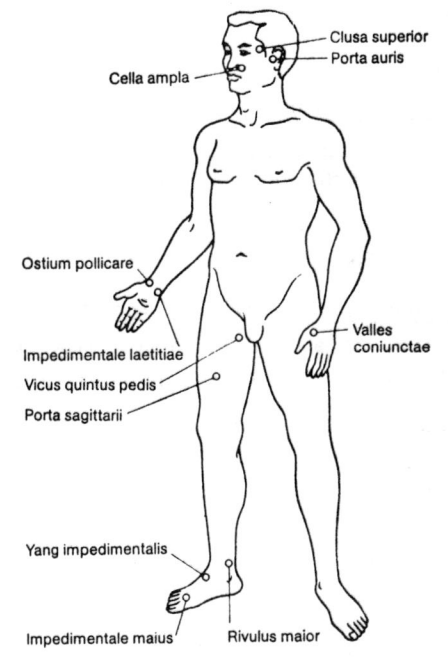

Fig. 11.

Upper Pulses (Pulses of the Head): Of these

(1) the temple pulse - corresponding to the foramen <u>yang maioris</u> = <u>clusa superior</u> (foramen 3 on the "gall-bladder conduit") - permits an assessment of energy in the

---

[183] Chapter 20 of the Inner Classic of the Yellow Sovereign.

sides of the head;

(2) the pulse of the ear - corresponding to the foramen porta auris (foramen 21 on the tricalorium conduit) - gives indications of the energy in the ears and eyes; and

(3) the nasolabial pulse - corresponding to the foramen cella ampla (foramen 3 of the "stomach conduit") - permits assessment of the energy in the mouth and teeth.

Central Pulses (Pulses of the Hand). Of these

(1) the pulsus yin maioris manus - corresponding to the ostium pollicare - gives information on the energy in the pulmonal orb;

(2) the pulsus yin minoris manus - corresponding to the foramen impedimentale laetitiae (foramen originalis and inductorium, no. 7 on the cardial conduit) - gives information on the energy in the cardial orb; and

(3) the pulsus splendoris yang manus - corresponding to the foramen valles coniunctae (foramen inductorium quinque inductoriorum, no. 3 or 4 on the "large intestine conduit") permits assessment of the energies in the chest.

Lower Pulses (Pulses of the Foot). Of these

(1) the pulsus yin flectentis pedis - corresponding to the foramen vicus quintus pedis ("hepatic conduit" for. no. 10), and to the foramen impedimentale maius (id. no. 3, originalis, inductorium) - permits assessment of the energy in the hepatic orb;

(2) the pulsus yin maioris pedis - corresponding to the foramina porta sagittarii (cL11) and yang impedimentalis (O - cS42) - permits assessment of the energies in the stomach and lienal orbs; and

(3) the pulsus yin minoris - corresponding to the foramen rivulus maior (i - cR3) - gives information on the energy in the renal orb.

Representative Pulses on the Head, Hand and Foot

The representative pulses are as follows:

(a) on the head, the pulse felt in the foramen accipiens hominum (cS9) approximately corresponding to the carotis-pulse of Western medicine - for gauging the energy of the stomach orb (qi stomachi);

(b) on the hand, the ostium pollicare corresponding to the site of the arteria radialis passing the processus styloideus radii, to assess the energies of the 12 cardinal conduits; and

(c) on the foot, the foramen yang impedimentalis (O - cS42), corresponding to the arteria dorsalis pedis, likewise informing us about the qi stomachi.

At the sites of the body pulses as well as in those of the representative pulses, only general qualities of the pulse[184] such as repletion or inanitas, acceleration or slowness, superficial or deep quality are defined - and considered to have diagnostic relevance. These representative pulses have first been described in the Shanghanlun.

Palpation of the sites accipiens hominum, yang impedimentalis and rivulus maior is done in emergency cases, when it is difficult or impossible to feel the pulse at the ostium pollicare, and it is nevertheless imperative to determine whether energy still is available in the oo. lienalis et renalis, the respective depositories of acquired and congenital energies (qi ascitum, qi nativum).

TOPOLOGY AND CORRELATION OF THE PULSES IN THE ostium pollicare (cunkou), I.E. OF THE "RADIAL PULSES"

General Remarks, History, Terminology

The designation of the site ostium pollicare (cunkou), hence literally "inch opening", results from the fact that the site so designated is situated one inch (in Chinese: cun, in Latin: pollex) proximally of the linea piscis ("limit resembling [the belly] of a fish) (yuji) - as the thenar is called in traditional Chinese medicine because of this line defining its limit.

The term cunkou, as has been explained in a preceding section, although first used in the Inner Classic, does not acquire all its implications and diagnostic associations except in the Classic of Objections (Nanjing)[185]; and the essential theory concerning the cunkou almost reaches maturity in the Pulse Classic[186].

In the terminology of sinarteriology the site so defined corresponds to the foramen vorago maior (O-i for. 9 of the pulmonal cond.), which is considered to represent a point in which all 12 cardinal conduits convene (conventus 12 cardinalium). But

---

[184] For more details cf. page 209 below.

[185] Probably compiled during the 4th century of our era.

[186] A text already mentioned above on p. 197.

different from such a foramen, which by definition always corresponds to a punctual site with a circular perimeter, the site called <u>ostium pollicare</u> extending in proximal direction comprises two additional pulse sites called <u>clusa</u> and <u>pes</u>.

The designation "foot", in Chinese <u>chi</u>, in Latin <u>pes</u>, is explained by the fact that starting from the foramen <u>lacus ulnaris</u> (= <u>lacus pedalis</u> - c -cP 5) situated in the bend of the elbow, it takes one biometric foot to reach the site called 'foot' (<u>pes</u>) in distal direction.

On the adult wrist the sites called <u>pollex</u> (inch) and <u>pes</u> (foot) are separated by a small space designated as <u>cl(a)usa</u>, a Latin term expressing, as the Chinese word <u>guan</u> does, a "natural defile" as well as a "fortification" or "fort". Therefore <u>clusa</u> (<u>guan</u>), from the etymology of the term as well as by the ontogenetic development of the site, is not a site of palpation with measurable extension but, instead, the postulated line of separation or delimitation between the sites <u>pollex</u> and <u>pes</u>. It is only when these two sites gradually move away from each other on the adult, that the <u>clusa</u> can be defined as a third pulse.

The pulses to be felt at these three sites are defined by their names as "pollicar pulse", "clusal pulse" and "pedal pulse" (Fig. 12).

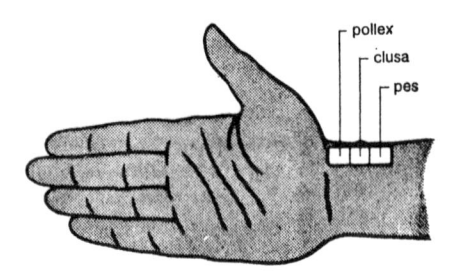

Fig. 12.

Regions of the Body and Radial Pulses

As was the case with the tongue and with certain body pulses, the radial pulses have correlations on two different levels, viz. with the orbs and with general regions of the body. These alternative interpretations are of considerable usefulness since, depending on how far diagnosis has advanced, two different patterns may be discerned, a general and rough one for determining the general site of the disturbance by referring to the correlation between radial pulses and body regions, and a much finer functional

PALPATION DIAGNOSIS

pattern resulting from the correlations between orbs and radial pulses. Very often the first pattern may be used in the beginning, or if other diagnostic methods did not or could not yet furnish any data (e.g. on an unconscious patient); and it will be the sole mode of correlation if we are interested in topologically localizing a somatic lesion.

To illustrate the latter possibility, we might adduce the case of a 30 year old woman who 17 years earlier, when jumping into a too shallow swimming pool, had struck the bottom with her head. Since this accident, she had suffered continuously from exasperating headaches which could be controlled only by extremely strong doses of analgetics. X-ray and neurology did not produce any conclusive diagnoses. The patient had undergone treatment twice for abuse of analgetics, had tried out most physiotherapeutic methods such as massage, underwater massage and acupuncture. Now, painstaking diagnosis of the pulses during an acute seizure of pain produced just a shade of tense pulses (pp. intenti)[187] solely at the clusal sites. When, based on this, the paravertebral sites of the back were explored by palpation, two extremely replete foramina between the vertebrae of the thorax were evident. Acupuncture of these sites immediately brought complete disappearance of pain and relaxation.

The correlations valid for both hands are that
  the pollicar pulses correspond to the region from the head to the chest (mamillary line);
  the clusal pulses correspond to the region between the mamillary line and the navel line; and
  the pedal pulses correspond to the region from the navel to the feet.

Of course, these indications imply a certain overlap between the corresponding regions. A disturbance which according to the concepts of Western medicine is situated in the upper thorax region - e.g. a serious bronchitis - may produce significant changes either in the pollicar or in the clusal pulses - probably in both and, sure enough, these correspondences already imply an approximation to the more subtle correspondences between orbs and radial pulses.

---

[187] Cf. p. 216 below.

Orbs and Radial Pulses

Approximately since the 1st century of our era[188], each radial pulse is correlated to one specific orb, or to a small number of specific orbs. Also, in this way, the horreal orbs are directly, and the aulic indirectly, correlated to one particular pulse site. Still, as was to be expected, the theorectical pattern prescribed by the existence of six individual pulse sites on the adult could not be parallelled by perfectly symmetrical empirical or clinical data. Today, almost 2000 years later, the following correlations may be taken to have stood up under prolonged clinical experience as best conforming to the requirements of a flexible yet very stringent diagnosis[189]:

manus sinistrae		pulsus	manus dextrae	
Mediate	Direct		Direct	Mediate
[*o. intestini tenuis*]	*o. cardialis*	*pollicaris*	*o. pulmonalis*	[*o. intestini crassi*]
o. felleus	*o. hepaticus*	*clusalis*	*o. lienalis*	*o. stomachi*
o. vesicalis	*o. renalis* (*oo. intestinorum, paraorbis uteri*)	*pedalis*	*renalis* (*oo. intestinorum, paraorbis uteri*)	[*o. tricalorii*] (*o. vesicalis*)

The orbs given in [ ] must be taken into consideration only if other diagnostic data indicate a significant disturbance of their functions; consequently, as a rule and in other cases, they need not be considered when feeling this site.

The orbs or para-orbs given in ( ) at all times affect the changes manifesting themselves at the given site; their functions must, however, be distinguished from those of the other orbs mentionend by differential diagnosis.

---

[188] When the terminology found in the Inner Classic was applied to clinical practice. This early development drew to a temporary close with the compilation of the Mojing, already mentioned on p. 197 above.

[189] By this cautious wording we already imply that, in Chinese medical literature, different correspondences for some of the pulse sites have been proposed; yet also that such differences, at all times, stayed within narrow limits, linked as they were to clinical experience. This is why in a textbook written for practical purposes, such historical discussions may be omitted.

PALPATION DIAGNOSIS

SPECIFIC ICONOGRAPHY OF THE RADIAL PULSES: THE PULSE ICONOGRAMS (moxiang)

General Characteristics of the Pulses to Be Felt at the ostium pollicare

Each pulse that can be felt under an exploring finger at the ostium pollicare is defined by its length, width and depth.

By length of the pulse, the palpable extension of the pulse at one site, consequently under one exploring finger is defined in the direction of the artery.

Width of the pulse defines its extension at one site parallel to the skin, yet at right angle to the direction of the artery.

Depth of the pulse defines the apparent position of a pulse felt at one site relative to its support and relative to the surface of the skin.

Accordingly, a distinction is made between
superficial pulses (pp. superficiales), pulsating "on the flesh yet below the skin";
submerged pulses (pp. mersi) pulsating "under the flesh, yet on the bone"; and
middle pulses (pp. mediani) pulsating between the superficial and the submerged pulses (Figs. 13 and 14).

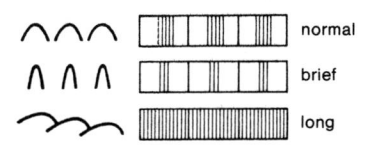

Figs. 13/14.

The depth of a pulse must be determined by varying the pressure of the exploring finger (cf. below); the width and length of a pulse, by contrast, may vary under different pressures, but do not necessarily do so.

Already here attention should be drawn to the fact that normal pedal pulses are situated half a step, or one step deeper than the normal pollicar and clusal pulses (Fig. 19). Consequently, the palpation of the pedal pulses normally requires greater pressure than that of the other two sites.

ICONOGRAPHY OF THE PULSES: THE CONVENTIONAL ICONOGRAMS

Each of the pulse iconograms may be found at one single site, at several sites or at all six sites of a patient.

(1) The Superficial Pulse (pulsus superficialis, fumo) 浮 脉

Iconography: The pulse beats at the surface and can already be felt under slight pressure; under increasing pressure it gets weaker; as pressure is released, the pulse regains its full strength.[190]

Diagnosis: A species-symptom; if the pulse is strong, we may infer repletion of the species, if it is weak, inanitas of the species.

Explanation: An exogenous heteropathy has developed in the species, i.e. in the skin and in flesh, and is combatted there by the defensive energy (wei). In this case a strong superficial pulse indicates repletion in the species. But even if the active individually specific energy (qi) is already exhausted (inanis), a certain amount of defensive energy may still flow into the species - then producing a weak superficial pulse.

Important note: It must be clearly understood that a superficial pulse as defined, is not automatically an exhausted pulse (p. inanis)! Although a superficial pulse gets weaker under increased finger pressure, it will not completely disappear - unless, in addition, there is inanitas. If this symptom prevails (the combination of this superficial pulse with an exhausted one, hence inanitas speciei), the therapeutic accent must be on correcting the exhaustion.

(2) The Submerged Pulse (pulsus mersus, chenmo) 沈 脉

Iconography: The pulse moves "below the flesh", hence with slight or moderate pressure of the exploring finger cannot be perceived at all; it requires strong pressure.

Diagnosis: A disturbance in the intima. If the pulse is strong, we may infer repletion in the intima, if it is weak, inanitas in the intima.

Explanation: This pulse may be due to two different factors: A heteropathy may have condensed in the intima, hence in an orb, impeding the flow of active and structive energies. The consequence will be a replete submerged pulse. Or the active energy of

---

[190] This is the classical description of the iconogram. It should be underscored, however, that a superficial pulse can be determined correctly only under released pressure! Cf. page 237 below.

PALPATION DIAGNOSIS

the affected orb is <u>inanis</u> and is no longer deployed sufficiently. This produces an exhausted submerged pulse (<u>p. mersus inanis</u>).

(3) The Slowed-Down Pulse (<u>pulsus tardus, chimo</u>) 遲 脈

<u>Iconography</u>: A slowed-down pulse with less than four beats per breath (in the adult)[191].

<u>Diagnosis</u>: A symptom of <u>algor</u> ("cold"), either of <u>algor inanitatis</u> (the pulse is weak and slowed down), from an <u>algor</u>-heteropathy as the consequence of exhaustion; or from massive attack of a climatic excess: <u>algor,</u> thus producing <u>algor repletionis</u>.

<u>Explanation</u>: <u>Algor</u> ("cold") slows down movement, hence reduces activity (yang); this is why all active energy including the defensive energy (<u>wei</u>) appears to be impeded and dampened - a fact also manifest by the slowing down of the pulse.

However, a slowed-down pulse may also appear as the consequence of a heteropathic accumulation of <u>calor</u> extensively slowing down the flow of energy in the conduits; in this case, however, the slowed-down pulse <u>always</u> shows repletion. This latter eventuality must, of course, be clearly distinguished from the former by the different corollary symptoms[192]. Usually they may be defined as a <u>splendor yang</u>-syndrome of <u>algor laedens</u>[193].

(4) The Accelerated Pulse (<u>pulsus celer, shumo</u>) 數 脈

<u>Iconography</u>: An accelerated pulse with the frequency of more than five beats per breath (on the adult).

<u>Diagnosis</u>: A symptom of <u>calor</u> ("heat"). If this pulse is strong, we may infer repletion, if it is weak, <u>inanitas</u>.

<u>Explanation</u>: The acceleration of the pulse is an indication that yang, active energy, is copiously deployed (<u>yang vigens</u>), or that it is driven by a <u>calor</u>-heteropathy - in this case producing a replete accelerated pulse.

An accelerated pulse may also appear after prolonged disease, when the structive

---

[191] For all the details on how the frequency of the pulse is assessed in Chinese pulse diagnosis, cf. the paragraphs on p. 238 below.

[192] E.g. the colour of the body of the tongue, the presence or absence of thirst, and so on.

[193] Cf. pp. 105 ff. above.

energies have become depleted and exhausted (inanes), thus depriving active energy of a sufficient foundation - in which case an exhausted accelerated pulse (p. celer inanis) will be observed.

A particular variety is an exhausted superficial accelerated pulse (p. celer inanis superficialis), indicating that the remnants of an exhausted yang are pushed into the species. This pulse, felt under the slightest pressure, abruptly collapses if the pressure is increased and can no longer be felt.

(5) The Exhausted (Depleted) Pulse (pulsus inanis, xumo) 虚 脉

Iconography: A weak pulse which can be made out only in one of the three levels[194] by very careful palpation. It disappears, is lost immediately and completely if the pressure of the finger is decreased or increased.

Diagnosis: Inanitas of the orthopathy.

Explanation: The active energies are not sufficient to keep the structive energies moving: this produces a weak exhausted pulse. Or the structive energies are insufficient to maintain the active energies, thus producing a hollow, easily collapsing pulse.

(6) The Replete Pulse (pulsus repletus, shimo) 实 脉

Iconography: A strong pulse manifesting itself on any of the three levels. Usually it can already be detected under slight pressure, and even heavy pressure will not make it disappear. Still, the pulse shows its greatest strength and deployment on one particular level, "its specific level".

Diagnosis: Repletion of a heteropathy.

Explanation: When a heteropathy clashes with the orthopathy, active energy is mobilized massively, thus producing a jam in the conduits.

(7) The Slippery Pulse (pulsus lubricus, huamo) 滑 脉

Iconography: The pulse comes and leaves easily, gliding along, and feels like a round, slippery object, e.g. a ball in a polished bowl.

Diagnosis: It may indicate one of three disturbances, viz.: 1. pituita ("phlegm"), 2. an

---

[194] Cf. Fig. 14 and the text on p. 209 above.

PALPATION DIAGNOSIS   213

active indigestion (shi) in infants; 3. calor ("heat") as the consequence of repletion (calor repletionis).

Explanation: The slippery pulse (p. lubricus) is classed as a yang-pulse, for active energy is replete, making the xue gush up - with ensuing slipperiness. This repletion of active energy may be due either to an accumulation of pituita, to a momentary block of the digestion in an infant or to a calor-heteropathy affecting constructive and defensive energies.

In women, if absolutely no pathological symptoms obtain, the slippery pulse may indicate pregnancy[195].

(8) The Grating Pulse (pulsus asper, semo) 涩 脉

Iconography: The pulse comes and recedes gratingly, chafingly or scrapingly - as if there were friction - producing a sensation of bamboo being scraped with a light knife.

Diagnosis: This pulse indicates a variety of factors: 1. stagnant active energy; 2. an impaired structure potential (jing) or deficiency of the individually specific structure energies (xue); 3. in some cases it appears when pituita affecting the stomach orb in infants produces a block of digestion.

If this pulse is strong there is repletion, if it is weak, inanitas.

Explanation: If the individually specific structure energy (xue) is reduced, if consequently the fluids are depleted, a grating, rasping pulse results. The same iconogram may ensue from inveterate, hardened pituita, stases, hematomas, concretiones (i.e. structive, hence somatic, material neoplasms), keloids.

(9) The Long Pulse (pulsus longus, changmo) 长 脉

Iconography: The long pulse "has a strait head and tail"[196], hence exceeds its site.

Diagnosis: Redundancy of energy.

Explanation: A long pulse, no matter at which site it appears, if showing a shade of harmonious languidity, is an indication of a plentiful qi medium[197], hence of strong

---

[195] Details on the pulses of pregnancy are found on p. 247 below.

[196] Illustration 13 and the text on p. 209 above.

[197] In other words, it indicates that considerable reserves of energy are present in the buffering reservoirs of the oo. lienalis (et stomachi).

214   THE ESSENTIALS OF CHINESE DIAGNOSTICS

and healthy energy.

Long pulses may also occur when the yang hepaticum (active energies of the hepatic orb) are redundant, or if there is plentiful yang and calor in a horreal orb (intima) - in all these cases with a tendency toward stringiness.

For these reasons, if a long pulse appears, additional qualities and tendencies of the pulses are of particular relevance.

(10) The Brief Pulse (pulsus brevis, duanmo) 短 脉

Iconography: "A pulse with a shortened head and tail", thus unable to completely fill its site[198].

Diagnosis: If a brief pulse is strong, it indicates an agglutination, congestion of the qi, i.e. of active individually specific energies; if it is weak, it points to a lesion or depletion of this energy.

Explanation: Qi, the active individually specific energy, is insufficient to move or to bring to the surface the xue, the individually specific structive energy. In addition to such a deficiency of active energy, a brief pulse may also be due to stagnant xue, agglutinated qi, hence any kind of congestion brought on by factors such as pituita, undigested food etc. Care should also be taken to distinguish between a strong and a weak brief pulse[199].

(11) The Flooding Pulse (pulsus exundans[200], hongmo) 洪 脉

Iconography: The pulse feels like a tidal wave: it arrives with great power and only recedes slowly and gradually; it is a wide and flooding pulse.

Diagnosis: Calor vigens ("profuse heat").

Explanation: Internal "heat" (calor intimae) spreads profusely in all directions and is

---

[198] Cf. Fig. 13 and the text on p. 209 above.

[199] Cf. the text on p. 236 as well as Fig. 17 there.

[200] Readers of our Theoretical Foundations..., whose original text was written as early as 1968, will note some variance from the pulse iconography used there. These modifications are due to our intensive practical experience taking the pulse, before writing the present textbook of diagnostics. Thus the terms exundans (in the place of redundans), fixus (in the place of firmus), minutus (in the place of subtilis), mobilis (in the place of movens), agitatus (in the place of turbulentus), concitatus (in the place of rapidus) constitute modifications of certain normative terms in order to establish an even closer agreement with sense experience.

PALPATION DIAGNOSIS   215

drawn off insufficiently.

A flooding pulse may also be brought on by <u>inanitas</u> of the yin in the <u>intima</u>, as a consequence of which <u>calor</u> from an uncontrolled yang smashes into the <u>species</u>.

If a flooding pulse - and consequently the disturbances just mentioned - persists for some time, a dissociation of active and structive energies is to be feared. Consequently, if during convalescence a patient with chronic <u>inanitas</u>, with phthisis, after severe losses of blood or fluids, or with severe diarrhea, shows a flooding pulse, this is a serious symptom indicating grave danger.

(12) The Large Pulse (<u>pulsus magnus, damo</u>) 大 脉

In the majority of Chinese texts on pulse diagnosis, the large pulse is usually taken as a synonym for the flooding pulse, hence receives no separate treatment. Clinical experience, however, shows that it can and must indeed be distinguished from the flooding pulse.

<u>Iconography:</u> A pulse that is wider and longer than the ordinary pulse, yet does not well up.

<u>Diagnosis:</u> A large pulse is a symptom of either 1. a rampant heteropathy (<u>vigor heteropathiae</u>), 2. a spreading, rapidly increasing heteropathy, 3. under some circumstances even, <u>inanitas intimae</u> (hence, a symptom of the exhaustion of the energies in a horreal orb).

<u>Explanation:</u> When evaluating this pulse, particular care must be taken to distinguish whether it is strong or weak, hence to determine whether it expresses repletion or exhaustion.

(13) The Evanescent Pulse (<u>pulsus evanescens, weimo</u>) 微 脉

<u>Iconography:</u> Independent of the level at which it can be felt, this pulse is extremely weak, extremely frail, like a shadow - so that the exploring finger may sometimes feel it, sometimes lose it.

<u>Diagnosis:</u> The collapse or extreme deficiency of active energies (<u>yang dilabens</u>). Under certain conditions it may indicate <u>inanitas</u> of all forms of energy.

<u>Explanation:</u> If active energies collapse, and/or structive energies have been exhausted (<u>inanes</u>), the pulse no longer can be clearly felt, hence becomes vague, like a shadow. Now if the criteria used for evaluating pulses at the different levels - from

a superficial to a submerged pulse - are applied, we may conclude that an evanescent pulse disappearing under the slightest pressure indicates the ruin of active energies, whereas an evanescent pulse disppearing under increased pressure would point to the exhaustion of structive energies.

If an evanescent pulse appears after prolonged disease, this is a symptom of the imminent collapse of the orthopathy. If such a pulse, however, occurs after recent and not too profound affections, a favourable prognosis is quite possible.

My repeated experience with a number of remarkable cases has shown that it may be prudent to qualify as "evanescent", pulses at sites where momentarily no pulse can be felt at all. As explained below, the total absence of certain pulses, in particular at the pedal sites, is a sure sign of imminent death. On the other hand, as explained in the section on the "Varieties of the Normal Pulse" below, all six sites of an individual in fair health may show evanescent pulses.

In this connection I remember a rare case shown to me in Bombay: On a boy of twelve, absolutely no pulses could be felt. He was considered a curiosity to the extent that the American heart surgeon C. - the boy had repeatedly been operated on because of complications with his ductus Botalli - considered that he must have utterly atypical arteries. Also my friend in Bombay, a cardiologist, thought this hypothesis was worth considering. When I first tried to take the boy's pulses, I too was utterly unable to detect any. On the other hand I had to admit that the boy was of fairly normal complexion, that the warmth and humidity of his hands were quite normal too, etc. Now while I was still puzzling how to reconcile these observations, my friend the cardiologist had put two needles into the arm of the patient and stimulated these by electricity. I had kept palpating the arm of the patient, and to our amazement, after about a quarter of an hour of stimulation, all pulses at the six sites appeared, with a tendency to minuteness, hence with a slight weakness, but perfectly clear and well defined. This experience has brought home to me the extreme limits which we must allow for an evanescent pulse.

(14) The Tense Pulse (pulsus intentus, jinmo) 緊脈

Iconography: This pulse feels tense and vibrating like a twisted rope.

Diagnosis: The tense pulse is the classic symptom for the chronic disposition to, or the presence of, pain. (Any prolonged pain, regardless whether it results from endogenous or exogenous, even mechanical factors, produces a tense pulse.) By

PALPATION DIAGNOSIS

contrast brief, recent and momentary pain, such as that experienced when one accidentally bumps one's leg against an obstacle or sprains an ankle, does not necessarily entail a tense pulse. The tense pulse may also indicate an algor-heteropathy or a momentary block of digestion.

Explanation: If, in the presence of a tense pulse, there is preponderance of yin, this indicates that a structive heteropathy has accumulated either because an algor-heteropathy at the surface (algor speciei) ties up the defensive energy; or because algor intimae holds down active energies there.

A similar explanation - algor - holds good for other symptoms accompanying the tense pulse: pain or undigested food blocking the stomach. In all these cases, algor impedes the deployment of warm, harmonizing activity.

The tense pulse has particular significance when Chinese diagnosis is used as a complement to Western diagnosis. With cases of chronic pain, sometimes persisting for years without any practicable and treatable specific diagnosis, the precise location of the tense pulse (cf. the correlations between the pulse sites and the body regions, above) produces these conclusive indications needed for initiating specific and directed therapy.

(15) The Languid Pulse (pulsus languidus, huanmo) 緩 脉

Iconography: Although this pulse shows a normal frequency of four beats per breath (on the adult), it comes and recedes languidly, gradually.

Diagnosis: Humor ("humidity").

Explanation: Humor is the quality of climate corresponding to the E.P. Earth, and to the o. lienalis. If this quality occurs in excess, it impedes activity.

Still, an even, balanced languid pulse, showing configurative force (shen), on certain individuals, may be an indication of excellent health.

Also, during convalescence, a harmonious languid pulse indicates the recovery of the orthopathy.

(16) The Stringy Pulse (pulsus chordalis, xianmo) 弦 脉

Iconography: The stringy pulse is felt as "sharp and taut, like the string of a lute", in other words, this pulse is exceedingly narrow ("sharp","keen"), at the same time strikingly long and taut, independent of the level at which it is felt.

Diagnosis: The stringy pulse may indicate 1. all lesions and affections from ventus ("wind") striking the o. hepaticus; 2. may indicate pain accompanying the aforementioned disturbances. 3. It can be a symptom of a congestion produced by pituita. 4. It may accompany malaria.

Explanation: The stringy pulse is the specific pulse of the E.P. Wood; consequently it accompanies all kinds of heteropathies induced by ventus, and all affections of the o. hepaticus, including the concomitant other symptoms, in particular pain.

The stringy inflection of the pulse is due to a violation of functions qualified by the E.P. Earth by energetically redundant functions corresponding to the E.P. Wood. Under these circumstances humor is blocked or reduced, the conduits are depleted of moisture, and the corresponding sharp, incisive, keen pulse results.

If such a pulse accompanies a phthisic disease, it indicates the loss of the qi stomachi, consequently a critical stage.

(17) The Onion-Stalk Pulse (pulsus cepacaulicus, houmo) 芤 脉

Iconography: This is a large, superficial pulse, hollow within, comparable to an onion-stalk. In other words, this is a wide and long superficial pulse which readily collapses under the exploring finger and disappears, only to reappear in depth upon increased pressure of palpation.

Diagnosis: The onion-stalk pulse reveals a deficiency of structive energies from either the loss of xue (also the loss of blood), or a lesion of other structive forms of energy such as constructive energy, structive potential (jing) or fluids.

Explanation: Excessively reduced structive energy offers only an insufficient basis for active energy; consequently active energy disperses at the surface, as evidenced by the wide superficial pulse with an empty centre.

If in the complete pulse iconogram containing one or several onion-stalk pulses, a stringy pulse or a grating pulse should also be in evidence, it may be inferred that a stasis, an inner congestion of structive energy is present. Great care must be taken to determine such a repletive factor amid a majority of otherwise inanitas-symptoms.

(18) The Tympanic Pulse (pulsus tympanicus, gemo) 革 脉

Iconography: A superficial and very taut pulse, hollow within, feeling like the leather of a drum.

PALPATION DIAGNOSIS   219

Diagnosis: The interrelated factors producing a tympanic pulse are 1. a deficiency of xue ("individually specific structive energies, including blood"); 2. the loss of structive potential (jing); 3. serious hemorrhages after birth, miscarriage.

Explanation: The tympanic pulse showing outward strength with inward depletion indicates that extremely exhausted resources of structive energies fail to control active energy, a situation corresponding to a vicious circle which pushes active energy to the surface, permitting it to disperse completely.

(19) The Fixed Pulse (pulsus fixus, laomo)[201] 牢 脉

Iconography: A deep, replete and long pulse which feels as if it sticks to the bone.

Diagnosis: Endogenous algor affecting the structive energies, inducing repletion; painful blocks in the abdomen, e.g [ileus].

Explanation: Strictly speaking and taken isolatedly, a fixed pulse always indicates structive concentrations (induced by algor), blocks, concretiones - and never inanitas. It is the typical repletion pulse occurring with disturbances of structive, indirectly sometimes also of active energies. If a fixed pulse and the repletion to which it points occurs as part of a general "exhaustion" (inanitas) diagnosis, there is immediate danger of death.

(20) The Frail Pulse (pulsus lenis, rumo) 濡 脉

Iconography: The frail pulse is a superficial, small, yielding and weak pulse.

Diagnosis: The frail pulse indicates either inanitas or humor.

Explanation: A frail pulse combining the qualities of a minute and a soft pulse, as a rule points to deficiency of active as well as of structive energies. A frail pulse to be qualified as soft, superficial and small, may, however, also occur with humor impeding the flow of energy, and without the presence of inanitas.

(21) The Soft Pulse (pulsus mollis, ruanmo) 软 脉

Most authors consider the soft pulse to be identical with the frail pulse. As the subsequent iconogram indicates, a distinction of the two pulses appears justified.

---

[201] Cf. note 200 on p. 214.

220   THE ESSENTIALS OF CHINESE DIAGNOSTICS

Iconography: A soft, yielding, superficial and weak pulse which, however, shows normal width and length.

Diagnosis: Inanitas.

Explanation: Because of deficiency essentially of active, to some extent also of structive energies, the energies available in the conduits - corresponding to the species - are reduced in quantity.

(22) The Infirm Pulse (pulsus invalidus, ruomo) 弱 脉

Iconography: A yielding, thin (minute), at the same time deep pulse.

Diagnosis: Weakness from inanitas of active and structive energies.

Explanation: This pulse must be distinguished from the preceding two pulses not only by its particular iconography - it is a deep (!) pulse - but also by the fact that it has considerable significance during convalescence: It indicates that the orthopathy is still exhausted - a situation perfectly normal after prolonged, exhausting illness. However, if the infirm pulse appears with recent diseases and in the company of symptoms of repletion, we may infer a contravective, atypical and very often critical course of disease.

(23) The Dispersed Pulse (pulsus diffundens, sanmo) 散 脉

Iconography: A superficial, dispersed or dispersing pulse without root. When the pressure of the palpating finger is gradually reduced, this weak pulse can only be felt after some time and vaguely; if pressure is increased again, it disappears completely.

Diagnosis: The qi primum, i.e. the structive part of the qi nativum (the resources of energy acquired at birth and stored in the renal orb) has dispersed, has become diffuse.

Explanation: If the contours of a pulse do not appear despite cautious and complete application of the palpating finger, this indicates that the energy of all orbs is about to be depleted.

(24) The Minute Pulse (pulsus minutus[201], ximo) 细 脉

Iconography: The minute pulse is thin and tenuous like a silk thread yet, independent of the level at which it appears, it can be felt clearly and distinctly.

PALPATION DIAGNOSIS   221

Diagnosis: The minute pulse may indicate either 1. inanitas of active and structive energies; 2. states of weakness and exhaustion because of excessive efforts; 3. humor ("humidity") affecting and impeding the circulation of energy.

Explanation: If a minute pulse occurs in an individual of good health on the whole, it usually indicates a lesion of the qi merum orbis renalis (of the active aspect of constitutional energy resources stored in the renal orb), brought on by excessive speculation or anxiety (cogitatio or sollicitudo). Hence, if a minute pulse appears on individuals apparently in good health and complaining only about some shortness of breath, or if it accompanies diseases with fever, together with dazedness and reduced acuity of the senses, this must be taken as a serious symptom.

(25) The Small Pulse (pulsus parvus, xiaomo) 小 脉

Usually the small pulse is taken to be entirely synonymous with the minute pulse; the actual distinction between these two pulses, however, quite often has significance.

Iconography: A narrow and short pulse which can be felt clearly, independently of its level.

Diagnosis: Inanitas.

Explanation: Depending upon the level at which this small pulse occurs, we may conclude that inanitas of the active, of the active and structive, or primarily of the structive energies is present.

(26) The Recondite Pulse (pulsus subreptus, fumo) 伏 脉

Iconography: A pulse hidden away in the depth. It can only be detected weakly upon the application of extreme pressure against the bone or the sinews, and even then is easily lost again.

Diagnosis: The recondite pulse may indicate the presence of either 1. energies that have been completely hemmed in, confined by a heteropathy; 2. flexus ; or 3. intense, excruciating pain induced by repletion.

Explanation: The recondite pulse points to a constriction, hemming in, confinement of energy and to repletion resulting from this. Flexus (the retreat, yielding of energy) and intense pain may also be consequences of this situation.

If the pulses on the sites of both hands show reconditeness, if in addition the pulses in the foramina yang impedimentalis and rivulus maior[202] can no longer be felt, this indicates imminent death.

(27) The Mobile Pulse (pulsus mobilis[201], dongmo) 動 脉

Iconography: The mobile pulse is at once slippery, accelerated and strong, and feels like a bean moving back and forth on its stem.

Diagnosis: A mobile pulse, within the context of classical Chinese medicine has been interpreted as a sign of pain (dolor) or of anguish and fright (pavor). However, under conditions where Chinese diagnostics is applied as a complement to Western diagnostics, the significance and value of this iconogram is much wider: The mobile pulse reflects the incompatibility of outward stimuli with the constitutional or momentary disposition of an individual. Thus, any excessive or, in whatever way, inappropriate medication, in particular the excessive use of tonics or of antiphlogistic drugs, also very often the use of cortisone, induces a mobile pulse, thereby indicating that the individual cannot integrate the therapeutic influence.

If we are faced with the decision to maintain, reduce or completely stop a previous medication, if we have doubts about the sincerity of the patient who says that he is taking no medication whatsoever, the presence or absence of the mobile pulse is a principal clue to guide us.

Explanation: Dissonance, disharmony, a clash between active and structive energies.

(28) The Agitated Pulse (pulsus agitatus[201], cumo) 促 脉

Iconography: An agitated, excited, raging pulse, stopping at irregular intervals.

Diagnosis: An agitated pulse may indicate 1. a profusion of active energy (yang vigens); 2. repletion because of calor; 3. very powerful congestion of energy, induced by pituita or undigested food; or 4. painful swellings.

Explanation: If an agitated pulse is strong and large, it may indicate an excess of active energies; if it is weak and small, we may conclude, on the contrary, that structive energies are present in excessive quantity or intensity; or we may infer inanitas algoris ("cold induced by a depletion of active energy").

---

[202] Cf. Fig. 11 on p. 203 above.

PALPATION DIAGNOSIS

The pulse stops intermittently because from the preponderance either of yang or of yin, the harmonious rapport between the two forms of energy is frequently disrupted.

(29) The Adherent Pulse (pulsus haesitans, jiemo) 结 脉

Iconography: A pulse beating languidly, lazily, stopping at irregular intervals.

Diagnosis: An adherent pulse may be due to an excess of yin, leading to agglutinations or blocks, concretiones et congelationes[203], also producing obstructions induced by pituita [blocks in the intestines].

Explanation: Because of the excessive strength of structive energies, the active energies are thrown out of kilter and, at the same time, cannot deploy as they should.

(30) The Intermittent Pulse (pulsus intermittens, daimo) 代 脉

Iconography: A pulse stopping at regular yet strikingly long intervals.

Diagnosis: An intermittent pulse may indicate 1. that the energy of an orb has become enfeebled or evanescent; or 2. that a ventus-heteropathy is present, accompanied by pain; or it may indicate 3. the consequences of either intense emotions or of mechanical lesions and wounds.

Explanation: An intermittent pulse may, if no other symptoms contradict this, point to an imminent collapse of energies in the intima, in particular in the lienal and stomach orbs.

It also occurs on pregnant women. It then may indicate a momentary and transitory collapse of the function of a single orb, and hence does not in all cases warrant a sombre prognosis.

(31) The Racing Pulse (pulsus concitatus, jimo) 疾 脉

Iconography: An extremely excited and accelerated pulse attaining 7 to 8 beats per respiration in the adult.

Diagnosis: After a collapse of the yin, the yang, having lost its foundation, is

---

[203] These terms indicate palpable indurations, neoplasias. More precisely, concretiones are yin indurations, clearly localized and, as a rule, not painful; congelationes are yang indurations, often changing the site, without clear somatic modifications, yet very painful.

mobilized in the extreme: A symptom of the imminent collapse of the qi primum[204].

Explanation: The racing pulse indicates that the yin merum, the structive energies representing the constitutional resources and reserves present since birth and stored in the renal orb, have been depleted and that, consequently, yang, active energies, disperse uncontrolled. At the same time, it is a symptom that this yang, this active energy has already been greatly depleted or is about to be depleted. If a racing pulse accompanies extremely high fever with algor laedens or morbi temperati-diseases, or if it occurs during the terminal stage of phthisis, it must be considered a very serious symptom.

It is possible, when diagnosing a racing pulse, to distinguish between the preponderance of active or of structive energies: If, when increasing pressure of the finger, the racing pulse offers increased resistance (hardness), we may infer an utterly uncontrolled and unleashed yang; if, by contrast, it yields under increased pressure of the palpating finger, we infer an uncontrolled yin. In the first case, the patient will also show symptoms of extreme excitation, in the second case lassitude. Under all circumstances, if a racing pulse occurs, the overall harmony of the pulses has been disrupted: "Loss of qi stomachi". Nevertheless, provided the racing pulse still shows average strength and size, i.e. that it is neither too large (magnus) nor too small (parvus), there is still hope left for the patient.

Remarks on Reduced Iconographies of the Pulse

Because of the absence of competent instruction and teaching aids, acupuncturists in and outside China have, at all times, put up with a simplified, reduced iconography, distinguishing at best inanitas and repletio, calor and algor, superficial and submerged pulses.

Moreover, as I explicitly witnessed during my visit to most of the Academies of Traditional Chinese Medicine in the Chinese People's Republic in 1978, till the seventies, and partly from the pernicious influence on science and academic research of the Great Revolution of Proletarian Culture, these Academies, too, have drastically reduced the scale of iconograms of the pulse, usually to 8.

There is no denying that such simplified iconography may have some justification if

---

[204] Cf. the note 58 on p. 47 above.

used by medical aides ("barefoot doctors") not pretending to any definite and final diagnostic statement on intricate and complicated disturbances.

However, this very simplification, if made the rule and guideline for the teaching and application of Chinese diagnosis, not only will represent a pseudo-scientific and detrimental intermission; it will in fact render completely worthless and inane the use of Chinese diagnosis as a scientific complement to the methods of modern Western diagnostics.

Let me illustrate by one example: According to the simplified iconography (comprising only 8 iconograms instead of 30 or 32) there is no 'mobile' pulse. What constitutes a mobile pulse is subsumed under the "slippery" pulse. Now if we refer to the corresponding iconograms above, we see that the mobile pulse has paramount significance for a physician who must decide whether a certain medication administered thus far, has helped or harmed the patient, consequently whether the medication should be maintained, stopped or replaced. The slippery pulse, in turn, is a very clear indication of a precise pathological factor: humor ("humidity") and its sequels. To confuse the mobile pulse with the slippery pulse would put an additional, very often excessive strain on the information to be derived from other sources of (Chinese!) diagnostics. Usually it will overstrain these other methods, thus diminishing the stringency of diagnosis or completely obliterating it.

Hence, for the consistent application, verification and rational development of the diagnostic methods evolved in China through more than two millennia, the maintenance of the complete iconography as here described is utterly essential.

Comparison of Iconograms of the Pulse

The iconograms of the pulses just described are the outcome of 18 to 20 centuries of maturation, and they represent an ideal foundation for every precise, univocal and lucid diagnosis of function, provided that the diagnostician has completely mastered them in all details and is able to reproduce them at will. In view of this aim, it may be useful to compare those of the iconograms resembling others, and those directly opposed to certain other iconograms.

Similar Iconograms of the Pulse

The slowed-down pulse and the languid pulse.

In the adult, the slowed-down pulse corresponds to approximately 3 beats per breath and appears to be somewhat reduced in size and strength (tendency to a small and weak pulse). By contrast, the languid pulse showing 4 beats per breath on the adult, appears to be large, with a tendency to redundancy.

The submerged pulse and the recondite pulse.

A submerged pulse is imperceptible under slight pressure, yet it can be clearly felt with increased pressure. - The recondite pulse, even when strong pressure is applied, can still not be felt clearly; it only makes its appearance when extreme pressure against the support (sinew or bone) is exerted.

The accelerated pulse, the tense pulse, and the slippery pulse.

The accelerated pulse appears, as the name implies, accelerated to 6 beats per breath on the adult. The tense pulse, under the palpating finger, feels like a twisted rope. The slippery pulse tends to slip away or to slip back and forth under the palpating finger, comparable to a pearl in a polished bowl.

The superficial pulse, the exhausted pulse, and the onion-stalk pulse.

The superficial pulse, under slight pressure gives the impression of redundancy and fullness, under increased pressure the impression of deficiency and weakness. The exhausted pulse (p. inanis) often gives the impression of being large yet weak, quite independent of the level at which it occurs. The onion-stalk pulse (p. cepacaulicus) can be felt as well at the surface (under slight pressure of the finger) as in depth (under strong pressure of the finger); it cannot be felt in the intermediate level (i.e. when average pressure is applied with the finger).

The infirm pulse, the frail pulse, and the soft pulse.

The infirm pulse (p. invalidus) is thin and yielding and can only be felt with increased pressure of the finger (in depth).

The frail pulse (p. lenis) is superficial, at the same time small, i.e. narrow, short and soft.

The soft pulse (p. mollis) has normal or increased length and width, is superficial and soft.

The evanescent pulse, the minute pulse, and the exhausted pulse.

The evanescent pulse is like a shadow which can only be felt vaguely and indefinitely, comparable to the sensation of a pulsating cobweb.

The minute pulse, although very tenuous and tender, always can be clearly perceived.

The exhausted pulse (p. inanis) often appears rather enlarged to the touch, at the

PALPATION DIAGNOSIS

same time is weak, yet clearly perceptible at its level.

The stringy pulse and the long pulse.

The stringy pulse is narrow and long and, most important, taut like the string of a lute: Very often the individual pulsebeat cannot be perceived because of this extreme tautness.

The long pulse exceeds its site like a bamboo stick - which again makes it difficult to distinguish individual pulse waves.

The brief pulse and the mobile pulse.

The brief pulse (p. brevis) is a yin pulse, in the sense that it is not only much shorter than normal but often somewhat slowed down, slow in coming and going.

The mobile pulse is a yang pulse; although as short as the brief pulse, it is, by contrast, accelerated, even and strong.

The flooding pulse and the replete pulse.

The flooding pulse (p. exundans) gives the impression of a tidal wave: it is wide and full, but loses this character under increasing palpatory pressure.

The replete pulse always is felt as taut and hard, irrespective of the pressure applied.

The fixed pulse and the tympanic pulse.

The fixed pulse is a deep pulse, with a tendency to stringiness, hence to increased length and tautness; yet it sticks to the bone and does not move.

The tympanic pulse is a superficial pulse; in addition it is very taut and large.

The agitated pulse, the adherent pulse, the grating pulse, and the intermittent pulse.

The agitated pulse (p. agitatus) is a very excited pulse, stopping at irregular intervals.

The adherent pulse (p. haesitans) moves slowly and sluggishly, slowing down to a full stop at irregular intervals.

The grating pulse (p. asper) is slowed down, brief, and at the same time may scrape and have irregularities.

The intermittent pulse (p. intermittens) stops a long while at regular intervals.

Complementary Iconograms of the Pulse

The superficial pulse and the submerged (deep) pulse.

The surfacing or submersion of the pulses gives a clue as to whether yang or yin, species or intima is accentuated. The superficial pulse indicates that the activating, dynamizing, light, loose and limpid aspects are dominant, the submerged pulse indicates the preponderance of the structive, materializing, consolidating, heavy and murky qualities and tendencies.

The slowed-down pulse and the accelerated pulse.

In the adult[205], 4 to 5 beats per respiration constitute a normal or harmonious pulse rate. A slower frequency is considered a slowed-down pulse, a higher frequency an accelerated pulse.

The exhausted pulse and the replete pulse.

Excessive hardness or resilience is indicative, respectively, of redundancy or deficiency, of the repletion of a heteropathy or of the exhaustion (inanitas) of the orthopathy.

The slippery pulse and the grating pulse.

By these qualities, the mobility of the pulse is defined. A slippery pulse (p. lubricus) indicates that there is much xue and little qi, a grating pulse (p. asper), inversely, that there is much qi and little xue.

The flooding pulse and the evanescent pulse.

These qualities deal with the power of the pulse: A flooding pulse (p. exundans) occurs when there is abundance of xue or when there is repletion in the presence of calor. The evanescent pulse usually is accompanied by algor or inanitas of the qi and is a symptom of deficiency.

The tense pulse and the languid pulse.

These are terms qualifying the tension of the pulse. A pulse is tense and taut when algor has impaired the structive energies (xue and constructive energy: ying). Inversely, it is relaxed, sluggish, without tension if ventus has affected the defensive energy (wei) so that structive energies are not dynamized sufficiently.

QUALITATIVE AND SYSTEMATIC CATEGORIES OF THE PULSES

In order to achieve precision and stringency in pulse diagnosis, the integration of the individual pulses into a system is at least as important as the descriptive comparison

---

[205] Cf. pp. 239 f. as well as p. 238 below.

PALPATION DIAGNOSIS

of their qualities. The systematic order of the pulses results from their division into
1. pulses of the orbs,
2. pulses defined by their form,
3. pulses expressing a mode of activity; also
4. the qualification of the pulses by yin and yang, and
5. their grouping under descriptive characteristics.

The Pulses of the Orbs

For practical purposes, this group is of cardinal importance[206]. For the pulse of an orb or, more precisely, the specific quality of the energies characterizing an orb appearing at any site (consequently not only at the site corresponding to that particular orb!) indicates a disturbance, usually redundancy, of the energies of that orb. The following correspondences between pulse qualities and orbs have been established:

	Corresponds to the
The superficial pulse	orbis pulmonalis
the submerged pulse	orbis renalis
the flooding pulse	orbis cardialis
the languid pulse	orbis lienalis
the stringy pulse	orbis hepaticus.

Pulses Defined by their Form

There are 8 pulses defined by their form. This form, besides expressing an affinity with one or several orbs, may indirectly give a hint of the relative level of energy. Thus

A pulse qualified as	Points to	And implies
Long	oo. hepaticus et lienalis	Redundancy
Brief	oo. hepaticus et lienalis	Deficiency of active energy
Fixed	o. renalis	Repletion

---

[206] Cf. the discussion on pp. 248 f. below.

A pulse qualified as	Points to	And implies
Tympanic	oo. renalis, hepaticus, pulmonalis	Extreme deficiency, depletion
Onion-stalk	oo. renalis, hepaticus, pulmonalis	Deficiency of structive energies
Dispersed	oo. renalis et hepaticus	Deficiency
Minute	oo. renalis et lienalis	Deficiency
Recondite		Repletion

The Modal Pulses

There are 15 modal pulses which, as their name indicates, point to the quality, i.e. the direction in which a disturbance tends to "bias", to make the orthopathy deviate.

Thus a(n)	Is a Symptom of
Accelerated pulse	calor,
Slowed-down pulse	algor
Tense pulse	Pain, algor
Slippery pulse	pituita
Replete pulse	Repletion
Exhausted pulse	Exhaustion (inanitas)
Grating pulse	Stasis, congestions; concretiones
Frail pulse	inanitas from humor
Soft pulse	inanitas speciei
Infirm pulse	inanitas during convalescence
Evanescent pulse	Depletion of energy, first of yang, then of yin
Mobile pulse	Effects of inappropriate stimuli; pain, anguish
Adherent pulse	Redundancy of yin, concretiones
Intermittent pulse	ventus, pain, shock
Agitated pulse	Overexcited yang or repletion of calor
Dispersed pulse	Imminent depletion of the qi primum
Racing pulse	Flare-up of active energy during the depletion of the qi primum

PALPATION DIAGNOSIS

The Qualification of the Pulses by Yin and Yang

Within the wider context of Chinese medical theory, the qualification of the pulses by yin and yang may be taken note of.

Yin Pulses	Yang Pulses
Slowed-down (p. tardus)	Accelerated (p. celer)
Submerged (p. mersus)	Superficial (p. superficialis)
Grating (p. asper)	Slippery (p. lubricus)
Exhausted (p. inanis)	Replete (p. repletus)
Brief (p. brevis)	Long (p. longus)
Evanescent (p. evanescens)	Flooding (p. exundans)
Languid (p. languidus)	Tense (p. intentus)
Tympanic (p. tympanicus)	Onion-stalk (p. cepacaulicus)*
Fixed (p. fixus)*	Stringy (p. chordalis)*
Soft (p. mollis)	Mobile (p. mobilis)
Infirm (p. invalidus)	Agitated (p. agitatus)
Dispersed (p. diffundens)	Racing (p. concitatus)
Minute (p. minutus)	Large (p. magnus)
Small (p. parvus)	
Recondite (p. subreptus)	
Intermittent (p. intermittens)	
Adherent (p. haesitans)	

Pulses marked with * are considered to be yang in yin or yin in yang.

The Pulses Grouped under Descriptive Characteristics

(1) Superficial Pulses:
    the superficial pulse,
    the flooding pulse,
    the large pulse,
    the tympanic pulse,
    the frail pulse,

the soft pulse,
the stringy pulse,
the onion-stalk pulse.

(2) Submerged Pulses:

the submerged pulse,
the recondite pulse,
the fixed pulse.

(3) Slowed-down Pulses:

the slowed down pulse,
the languid pulse,
the grating pulse,
the adherent pulse,
the intermittent pulse.

(4) Accelerated Pulses:

the accelerated pulse,
the agitated pulse,
the mobile pulse,
the tense pulse,
the racing pulse.

(5) Exhausted Pulses:

the exhausted pulse,
the dispersed pulse,
the minute pulse,
the brief pulse,
the infirm pulse,
the evanescent pulse.

(6) Replete Pulses:

the replete pulse,
the long pulse,
the slippery pulse.

PALPATION DIAGNOSIS

THE TECHNIQUE OF PULSE DIAGNOSIS II

Position and Support of the Patient's Arm

During palpation of the pulses situated at the processus styloides radii, special care should be taken with the adequate position and support of the patient's arm. If this arm is stretched, if there is tension in the muscles, if the patient wears close-fitting garments, certain exhausted pulses may be influenced or disappear altogether; other pulses, with the exception of the replete ones, may be changed in their quality, thus impairing the diagnosis.

For these reasons, the forearm on which the pulse is to be examined, should be supported from the hand at least to the middle of the ulnar bone by a specially prepared "cushion for pulse diagnosis", resting upon a support of appropriate height in such a manner that the patient may extend his hand during the required time for palpation without the slightest tension or undue movement. For this purpose, a small table to be adjusted in height should be ideal; but otherwise, other pieces of furniture adjusted with care should do.

Palpation of the pulse on a patient in bed will require at least as much consideration. Indeed, as will be apparent from what follows, correct palpation, according to the rules of Chinese pulse diagnosis, on a patient unable to move, who can be approached only from one side of the bed, is a next to impossible undertaking.

Needless to say, no proper pulse diagnosis can be done with both patient and diagnostician - or for that matter only one of the two - standing up.

Application of the Fingers

As already stated, the 2 x 3 sites of the ostium pollicare of the adult, are palpated by applying the index, middle finger and ring finger of the hand trained for palpation, i.e. of the "palpation hand" of the diagnostician. This is done by first advancing the tactile bulb of the middle finger to find the prominence of the processus styloides radii in order to get a general bearing - thus defining the site called "clusa" (Fig. 15).

Fig. 15.

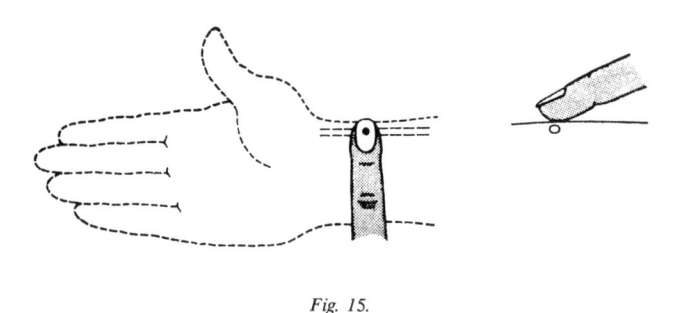

Then, while keeping the tactile bulb of the middle finger on this spot, those respectively of the index and the ring finger are brought up to contact the sites of the pollicar and of the pedal pulse. With some practice, the diagnostician should be able to locate these three sites on the average patient within seconds.

Atypical configurations of the arteria radialis do occur. If absolutely no trace of a pulse can be detected at the usual sites, these should be looked for by completely checking laterally from the normal sites, and even on the back of the wrist.

The bifurcation of the arteria radialis immediately beyond the clusa is the rule. Yet even then, more often than not, only one pulse at the pollex will be felt: that of the main branch of the artery, before diving away below the sinews of the wrist.

Still, one may be confused by the frequent appearance of the lateral branch, in other words, of two pollicar pulses. Of these, the correct one is on line with the clusa and the pes. The other, a "secondary pollex", is situated closer to the median axis of the wrist and usually produces an iconogram of a more distinct yet rather thin ("minute", "tense") pulse. The temptation to accept this secondary pulse as the pollex, of course, is the greater, the more difficult it may appear to assess the correct pollex. If the correct pollex shows an inanis pulse or if, because of the shortness of the wrist – frequent on female patients – distinguishing it from the clusa requires special care, it seems convenient to simply grasp what one can get. One must not give in to this temptation unless 1. even after the most careful and cautious palpation, absolutely no pulse could be determined at the usual site; and 2. the qualitiy of this secondary pollex is not in striking disharmony with the rest of the diagnostic data. Such a decision, to be sure, requires some experience, but it is in fact only a very slight problem to someone with an average amount of experience in the palpation of the pulse.

PALPATION DIAGNOSIS

The three palpating fingers - index, middle finger and ring finger - should be applied to the "spine" of their corresponding pulses so as to produce an even and horizontal contact between the bulbs of the fingers and the sites of the wrist. (For evident reasons, this evenness of contact must always be an approximation because of the different lengths of the three fingers applied simultaneously. Since the tips of all three fingers must be aligned on the artery, the middle finger will have to be slightly retracted, hence applied to its site at a slightly different angle from that of the index and ring finger.)

The centre of the tip of one particular or of all three fingers may be advanced beyond the spine of the pulse in order to achieve even fuller contact between the finger and the site. (Fig. 16)

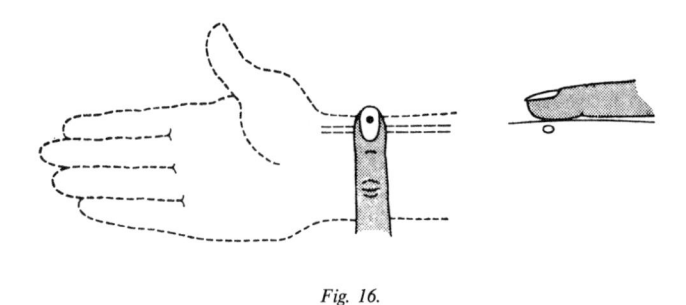

Fig. 16.

With some diagnosticians and under certain conditions, this positioning may produce an even better definition of the pulse. However, it may also produce the contrary effect, because the pulsation in the finger artery of the diagnostician may seriously blur the sensation sought for.

Applying and Slackening Pressure: Tilting and Sliding the Fingers

After all three palpating fingers have been applied to the corresponding sites as described, even pressure is applied on all three fingers and then slowly released. By this manipulation, an overall impression of the pulse, in particular as regards its strength, depth, length and width, is sought. Subsequently, this general impression must be filled in with supplementary details, by separately pressing down each of the three fingers.

During this palpation of the individual site, all attention is concentrated on one site or on the finger palpating it; the other two fingers barely touch their sites in order to ensure proper alignment.

The individual and specific palpation of a single site now must produce with utmost precision the iconogram of the corresponding pulse, including eventual modulations or tendencies[207]. This is why for this part of the diagnosis, most of the time and concentration should be reserved.

Although the application of the fingers as described in Fig. 15, and with varying pressures, will be perfectly adequate to define most iconograms, certain qualities can be registered with greater certainty if particular movements of the fingers are executed.

To gauge the length of the pulse precisely, tilting or rolling the palpating fingers sidewise (Fig. 17) is a useful and proven method.

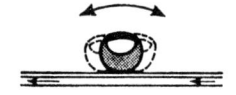

Fig. 17.

To distinguish a flooding pulse from a large pulse or from superficial pulses in general, proceeding as has been recommended in Fig. 16, should be tried.

To gain greater assurance when defining slippery, fixed, mobile or onion-stalk pulses, a lever-like movement of the palpating finger, as described in Fig. 18 is recommended.

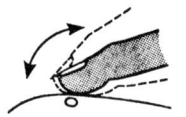

Fig. 18.

---

[207] What is meant by "modulations" or "tendencies" can be seen on p. 242 below.

With the exception of the submerged pulses, the precise depth (level) of all other pulses must be determined by slackening pressure! In other words, even if the diagnostician believes that he has clearly defined a superficial pulse when putting down his finger(s), and applying pressure, he must further increase pressure to the extent that all the other levels, including a pulse present at the deepest level will have been perfectly perceived[208], and then slowly release pressure to find his superficial pulse confirmed. This procedure must be the standard method because only by reviewing all three levels can he, so to speak, perceive the complete extension in depth also of a superficial pulse, and state with assurance that nothing has escaped his attention - quite aside from the greater clarity which even a superficial pulse gains, when perceived under released pressure.

At this juncture, it should be recalled that all pedal pulses under normal conditions, that is, "physiologically", are situated barely one level deeper than the corresponding pollicar and clusal pulses (Fig. 19), and this standard, of course, must also be applied to the submerged pulses.

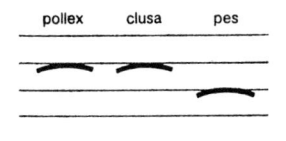

Fig. 19.

Consequently, for the palpation of a pedal pulse, higher pressure is required than for the palpation of the pulse at any other site; a pedal pulse situated on the same medium level of a clusal pulse, already must be defined as a "superficial" pulse; also, a pedal pulse situated on the same level as a submerged clusal pulse, may be defined as a medium pulse.

The high pressure required for the palpation of the pedal pulses, which, in spite of this, must be sensed and defined with quite the same care and precision as the other pulses, is one of the reasons why even persons with some experience should not feel a large number of pulses without interruption. For, of course, this difficulty must not be avoided or circumvented by changing fingers, e.g. applying the middle finger to the pedal site.

---

[208] A recondite pulse, however, will still require additional attention. Cf. its iconogram on p. 221 above.

To ensure absolutely even and comparable results in the palpation of the pulses, it is imperative that identical fingers be applied to identical sites. Consequently, not only must the diagnostician always use the same hand for palpating the pulses on both wrists of the patient; the patient must also change position when the other hand is examined.

Determining and Assessing the Frequency of the Pulse

Although the Chinese are a very time-conscious people, in Chinese pulse diagnosis, the absolute frequency of the pulse - representing today perhaps the only characteristic still registered by Western medicine - plays no role, and the relative frequency plays only a secondary one.

The relative frequency of the pulse is usually determined with reference to the breaths of the patient. One breath corresponds to the time elapsing between the beginning of an exhalation to the end of a following inhalation. In the adult, i.e. beginning approximately with the 15th year, 4 to 5 beats per breath may be considered a healthy average.

The corresponding standards for children and adolescents are:

up to the 3rd year:	8 beats per breath;
during the 4th year:	approximately 7 beats per breath;
between the 5th and 12th years:	approximately 6 beats per breath.

Time Taken for Pulse Diagnosis

There is no fixed and set rule prescribing the duration of pulse diagnosis. However, the time required for the continuous observation of a site during 50 beats of the pulse[209] constitutes the absolute minimum. Usually, when first seeing a patient, considerably more time should be taken if one hopes to arrive at reassuring and practicable conclusions. Thus an expert with long experience will normally still devote 5 minutes to define an exceedingly clear iconogram of the pulses; pulse iconograms of average difficulty will usually require 10 to 15 minutes of concentrated attention. And if under anatomically difficult conditions, a very intricate and complex pulse, corresponding to a critical and difficult situation of the patient, is to be defined with

---

[209] If less time is taken, it will be impossible to define precisely an adherent or an intermittent pulse.

PALPATION DIAGNOSIS

ultimate precision, half an hour must not be considered a waste of time. The inexperienced diagnostician should consider taking twice as long.

Quick, Summary and Emergency Diagnoses

Under exceptional conditions and in emergencies, the requirements for an appropriate and comprehensive diagnosis of the pulse cannot be met even approximately. Therefore, the diagnosing physician should not waste time in the attempt to obtain a fragmentary yet highly doubtful partial diagnosis. It is much preferable then to execute a "one-site" diagnosis by applying the bulb of the thumb (not the whole thumb!). Applying the bulb of the thumb to the ostium pollicare, he concentrates on the perception of the precise level at which the pulse beat is most distinct - and will, as a side product, also gain information about the relative firmness ("repletion/inanitas") of the pulse. Using this method, the following correspondences should be noted:

Correspond	On the Left Hand to	On the Right Hand to
Superficial pulses	orbis cardialis	orbis pulmonalis
Medium pulses	orbis hepaticus et felleus	orbis lienalis et stomachi
Submerged pulses	orbis renalis	orbis renalis

This kind of summary diagnosis is useful in emergency cases, on critically ill patients and after deliveries. It would be incorrect procedure to use it on all patients.

Palpation of the Pulses of Infants and Adolescents

The ostium pollicare does not attain the length required for cleary distinguishing the three sites until around the age of 15. Before that age, for anatomical reasons, it is difficult or absolutely impossible to distinguish them. Therefore, for palpation diagnosis of young patients, Chinese medicine has established that

up to the 6th year of age, only one pulse may be felt and defined at the ostium pollicare: the pollicar pulse. (Such palpation of the pollicar site must not be confused with the emergency method just described in the preceding section! And, of course, it must be executed and interpreted according to the rules applying to the pollex pulses[210].)

Palpation diagnosis of a fairly lively infant of less than a year should be avoided if possible. But even beyond that age, and up to the 4th year, the data obtained from such palpation should only be used as corollary orientations: Some diagnosticians are wont to underestimate the disturbing effects on the precision of diagnosis produced by the restlessness of the child, by the efforts of the mother to calm it, and by the efforts of the diagnostician to compensate for these factors through increased concentration <u>and a firmer grasp</u>.

Approximately after the 6th year, next to the <u>pollex</u> site, a pedal site may also be palpated (with the ring finger!) and interpreted in consequence.

Approximately at the 12th year, it will become practicable and justified to distinguish all three sites. If, at first, on short wrists, there is not sufficient room for all three palpating fingers, after having located the <u>processus styloides radii,</u> only the index and ring finger are applied, and the pollicar and pedal pulses are taken first. During a second course of diagnosis, the middle finger is applied to the pulse at the <u>processus.</u> (This same method, very often, is warranted when the short wrists of female patients offer the same difficulty.)

Different Sensations When Palpating with One or with More than One Finger; Halos

During palpation of the <u>ostium pollicare,</u> it is not a rare occurrence that simultaneous pressure applied to all three fingers will produce the sensation of a fairly strong pulse, whereas when pressure is applied with only one finger, a weak pulse appears; but the opposite case may also be met with, viz. that where combined pressure of three fingers produces a weak pulse, pressing down one finger only produces the sensation of a strong pulse. Part of this paradox is due to the effect of the so-called "halo on the pulse" (<u>yun</u>).

A Pulse Slipping out from under the Finger: If simultaneous pressure of three fingers produces a strong pulse, pressure applied with one finger only, a weak pulse, this pulse surely must be qualified as a stringy and at the same time a slippery pulse - with a fairly good level of energy. If this extremely narrow and at the same time slippery pulse is touched in one single spot only, it literally slips out from under the finger.

---

[210] In heeding the instructions and the advice given above on p. 237.

PALPATION DIAGNOSIS

When applying three fingers at once, the slipping away is prevented so that, consequently, the energy flow really concentrated into only one narrow yet slippery strip will be felt as a strong pulse.

Error Induced by a Distinct yet Weak Pulse: If a pulse, when felt with one finger only, appears to be strong, whereas pressure applied with three fingers produces a weak sensation, we must infer a basically weak pulse. If attention is concentrated on the sensations in one single finger only, perhaps on the particularly sensitive index, even a fairly weak pulse, by showing distinct shape, may give the impression of relative strength. If, however, attention is distributed evenly on all three fingers, this sensation disappears completely.

A Halo Surrounding a Weak Pulse: When palpation by all three fingers produces the impression of a large pulse and palpation by only one finger that of a minute pulse, we must infer a minute or stringy pulse surrounded by a halo. This halo, when pressure is applied simultaneously to all fingers, produces the impression of a wide and strong pulse.

A Large Halo Surrounding a Narrow Pulse: If palpation of a pulse with all fingers produces the sensation of a minute pulse and, by contrast, palpation with one finger only gives the impression of a large pulse, we may definitely infer an exhausted pulse surrounded by a rather large halo. When attention is focused on one finger only, this halo produces the impression that a large pulse is present; the wider focus and the more vague impression achieved when simultaneously palpating with all three fingers, definitely prevent such deceptive perception.

A Halo Surrounding a Submerged Pulse: A fairly rare case, likewise due to the presence of a halo is a pulse felt at the surface, when palpated with one finger only, yet in depth, if all fingers are applied. It is the halo which produces the erroneous impression of a superficial pulse.

Note: Not in every case where the pulse at one moment appears to be small and weak, at another large and strong, is it surrounded by a halo! Very often such vacillation may be attributed to wrong application of the fingers[211], to the neglect of basic precautions or to insufficient experience of palpation.

---

[211] If there are doubts, the reader is referred to pp. 234 f. above and the figures 15 and 16.

Recording the Pulse Data

When recording pulse data in the patients' files, no strict and narrow rules need be observed. Still, a warning should be given against undue simplification or undue definition. It is bad, incorrect practice to record a pulse as a "lung pulse", pulsus pulmonalis, when actually referring to the pollex-site of the right hand; or as a "liver pulse" ("pulsus hepaticus") when designating the clusal pulse of the left hand. This habit, used by some apparently experienced practitioners, introduces unnecessary restrictions into the highly precise, yet at the same time flexible statements of Chinese pulse diagnosis; and, of course, it may impede a thorough re-evaluation of former diagnoses in the light of newer diagnoses of the same patient.

Consequently, when recording pulses, it should be a rule
1. to qualify them exclusively by their site, never by whatever correlation may exist between this site and certain orbs.
2. To adduce, wherever possible and significant, in addition to the basic quality of the pulse, all modulations and tendencies of the pulse at each individual site.

Consequently, good examples of how complete iconograms of pulses may be recorded are the following:

	Left Hand	Right Hand
Pollicar pulse	Mobile > exhausted	Accelerated > minute
Clusal pulse	Mobile	Accelerated > minute
Pedal pulse	∅ superficial	∅ minute

or

	Left Hand	Right Hand
Pollicar pulse	Exhausted > submerged	Flooding > exhausted
Clusal pulse	Flooding/	Flooding > mobile
Pedal pulse	Flooding/	Flooding/

PALPATION DIAGNOSIS   243

The sign ∅ indicates that at this site no significant deviation of the pulse could be detected. An isolated stroke indicates that no modulation has been determined.

EVALUATION OF THE PULSE DATA

The Normal Pulse

To evaluate any pulse iconogram, we must have a clear idea what a normal pulse looks like. Such a normal pulse meets three requirements, viz. it has

        1. qi stomachi,
        2. configurative force (shen), and
        3. roots (stirps).

Qi stomachi: It is already stated in the Inner Classic of the Yellow Sovereign[212] that a pulse must show weiqi, i.e. the harmony resulting from a strong central orb: "If [the energy of the] stomach orb is present, there is life, if [the energy of the stomach orb] is absent, there is death".

As will be recalled, the stomach orb in orbisiconography corresponds to the orb actively organizing and maintaining the harmonious balance of the energy flow between all other orbs. It is this force of the active and spontaneous maintenance of a harmonious balance, and of the distribution of all strains, stresses and disturbances, that is meant if the term "qi stomachi" is used with reference to the pulses, not the concrete orbis stomachi, the functions of which may be confined to one single site only.

In other words the expression "having qi stomachi" or "there is qi stomachi" is a synthetic judgement describing the complete concert of all orbs.

How is this qi stomachi perceived in diagnosis? - Firstly by the fact that if the average depth of all pulses is taken into consideration, this will correspond to medium-level pulses. Thus, if at one site, a submerged pulse is present, this submerged pulse will be compensated by a superficial pulse at another site; also, acceleration or slowing down will never be extreme but just manifest as a tendency. Secondly, that all pulses, in spite of individual deviations, are characterized by an even and identical

---

[212] In the Inner Classic of the Yellow Sovereign, viz. in Chapter 18 of the Suwen, respectively Chapter 9 of the Lingshu.

basic rhythm[213].

To repeat, the term <u>qi stomachi</u> describes the general impression of a coherent, internally balanced and clearly defined iconogram of the pulse. The presence of <u>qi stomachi</u>, or conversely its absence, decrease or return, is a necessary, albeit often implicit factor in every diagnosis of the pulse.

The ideal position of the pulses, their relation to the three levels, has already been mentioned with reference to Fig. 19[214]. Accordingly, the pollicar and clusal pulses should be felt strongest in the center of the 2nd level, and the pedal pulses in medium depth, i.e. at the top of the 3rd (i.e. deep) level.

Configurative Force (<u>shen</u>): The configurative force of the pulse is that indispensable flexibility and resilience required to compensate for any pathological deviation by immediate regulative countermeasures in the opposite direction.

Hence, even an evanescent pulse, if it has configurative force, will not be utterly deprived of contours and definition. By appropriate measures[215], it may indeed momentarily become quite clear and distinct. Also, a stringy pulse showing configurative force (hence a certain flexibility) will not resemble the iron tautness of a piano string but still give the impression of living pulsation.

Roots (<u>stirps</u>): The root or roots in the iconogram of the pulse correspond to the pedal pulses. If these may be distinctly felt, the pulse is not deprived of roots. (As will be recalled, the pedal pulses correspond to the energy situation in the <u>o. renalis</u>, the repository of constitutional energy resources (<u>qi nativum</u>). The complete depletion or collapse of this energy, resulting in the total disappearance of the pedal pulses, if confirmed by repeated palpation, is - utterly independent of available medical resources - a sure sign of imminent death.

Varieties of the Normal Pulse

Every diagnostician must be familiar with the varieties and inflections produced upon the pulse by weather, climate, profession, constitution, age, and sex. For such inflections may be due to physiological factors, and then do not constitute pathological symptoms.

---

[213] This certainly cannot be the case if some pulses only are evanescent or recondite, or if racing pulses occur.

[214] On p. 237 above.

[215] Cf. p. 216 above.

Climate and Season

In moderate climates, the regular change of the seasons and their typical weather produces slight inflections of the pulse on healthy individuals which may be described

> in spring as an inflection in the direction of a stringy pulse,
> in summer as an inflection in the direction of a flooding pulse,
> in autumn as an inflection toward a superficial pulse and
> in winter as an inflection toward submerged pulses.

Long-term residence in hot climates enlarges and softens the pulses (large pulses, soft pulses); long residence in very cold climates deepens the pulses (submerged pulses); continuous residence in a very dry climate lifts the pulses to the surface and makes them narrow (superficial or minute pulses); life under very humid conditions produces languid pulses. Yet none of these inflections, taken isolatedly, may be interpreted as a symptom of disease.

Constitution, Constitutional Factors

Healthy, husky individuals show a clear inflection toward submerged pulses. Healthy, slender individuals show a clear inflection toward superficial pulses.

If on a very active individual all six sites uniformly show flooding or uniformly show large pulses - and, after very careful diagnosis, the total absence of any other pathological symptoms - such pulses must be considered to be normal pulses for this individual. Similar conclusions obtain for sanguine or phlegmatic types, if on such individuals <u>at all sites of the pulse</u> languid or minute pulses can be determined.

Age

During infancy, as Chinese medical theory has it, an individual is "entirely made up of yang". Hence, at this age, good health is usually accompanied by rather superficial or accelerated pulses[216], compared with those of the adult.

A consequence of this statement is that the appearance of true adult pulses in an infant or, worse still, the manifestation of true yin pulses such as a submerged or a slowed-down pulse, indicate a more critical situation than would be the case in an adult.

During old age, all pulses, in particular those at the pedal sites, show a tendency toward infirmity (infirm pulses), i.e. yielding, narrow and submerged pulses.

---

[216] Cf. p. 211 above.

Differences of Sex

In the races of East Asia, pulses of the female have a distinct quality of frailty, softness, infirmity, in other words they possess less tension, less force than those of males. This is because in those races female tissue stores more fat and humidity than that of the males. Consequently, palpation on female patients requires increased care and experience.

On Indo-European races, this extreme sex-related difference in the tissues of the wrist is not observed. Except for rare cases, the pulses of women may be palpated by the same technique as that used on men.

Mode of Life, Sexual Activity

Prolonged sedentary life and professional activity influence the iconography in particular of the pollicar pulses in the direction of infirmity (infirm pulses) (i.e. not genuinely exhausted pulses which would constitute a pathological symptom). Inversely, constant bodily activity or great indulgence in sports may produce accelerated or large pulses.

Prolonged sexual continence clearly moves the pedal pulses in the direction of infirm pulses. (In China this kind of iconogram is called a "true monk's pulse" because in this manner a real monk could be distinguished from other inmates of a monastery indulging in sexual relations.) Inversely, excessive sexual activity pushes the pedal pulses to the surface (superficial pulses) or, eventually, produces minute or exhausted pulses at the pedal sites - the latter already constituting pathological symptoms.

Meals, Elementary Poisons

The clusal pulses, after a short fast, tend to show infirmity (infirm pulses); prolonged fasting or starvation will produce exhausted and superficial clusal pulses.

The intake of food may momentarily move the iconography of the clusal pulses in the direction of flooding or languid pulses.

The use of alcohol or coffee momentarily affects the pollicar pulses, there normally accelerating and widening the pulse (accelerated pulses or large pulses). The habitual use of these poisons may produce further pathological changes at the clusal pulses, which must be determined by individual diagnosis.

PALPATION DIAGNOSIS

Pulses in Gynecology and Obstetrics

Menstruation

If the clusal and pedal pulses of the left hand show a distinctly stronger tendency towards flooding and largeness (flooding pulses, large pulses) than those at the corresponding sites of the right hand, if the woman complains neither of bitter taste nor of fever nor of a distended abdomen, menstruation is imminent.

Irregular Menstruation, Disturbances of Menstruation

These in pulse iconography affect the pedal pulses, which usually are weaker in comparison to the harmonious pollicar and clusal pulses.

Blocked menstruation, amenorrhea, may be due either to repletion or to exhaustion (inanitas). The former usually produces slippery pedal pulses, the latter grating pedal pulses.

Pregnancy

Pregnancy is expressed in the pulses by accelerated and slippery pulses in an otherwise well balanced and harmonious iconogram, provided that complementary signs such as the absence of menstruation, unusual appetites such as the desire to have very sour or very salty food etc. also are present.

Changes in the pulse iconography with normal and uncomplicated pregnancies are limited to the pedal pulses (acceleration, slipperiness) and to the pollicar pulse of the left hand (corresponding to the site of the cardial orb[217]): mobile or accelerated pulses.

Healthy pregnancy is characterized by the absence of stringy, onion-stalk, grating, fixed or recondite pulses. The latter pulses, by contrast, are characteristic of pathological events such as abdominal tumors of the female, likewise accompanied by irregular menstruation and sometimes also tense, submerged or adherent pulses.

If irregular menstruation is due to extreme exhaustion, accelerated pulses, if they occur, show a tendency toward grating pulses, whereas pregnancy always produces a tendency toward slippery pulses.

If a grating pulse occurs during pregnancy, this is a symptom that the foetus is in danger or has died.

---

[217] It should be recalled that the cardial orb, within the system of orbisiconography, links up with the paraorb of the uterus. - Cf. Porkert, Theoretical Foundations... p. 163 f.

Twitching, especially in the pedal pulses, is one of several other signs indicating that labour has set in.

CLASSIFICATION OF SYMPTOMS; PRIORITIES

More than on any other method of Chinese diagnostics, we may and must rely upon the palpation of the pulse for obtaining precise and reliable data for defining a disturbance and its quality - and thus furnish exact data for an effective and rational therapy. To achieve these aims, the diagnostician must be able to correctly assess the relative weight of competing information. Thus, above all, he must be able to assess
  1. the correlation with an orb,
  2. the correlation with a site, and
  3. the correlation with the depth level of the pulses observed.

The Significance of the Pulses of the Orbs[218]

If pulse qualities, iconograms corresponding to a particular orb appear, they are a symptom of redundancy of the energies of the corresponding orb - <u>independent of the site at which these qualities are percieved</u>. In other words, if it is true that certain energies are required for the healthy function of a particular orb, such energies, nevertheless, must not directly be identified with that orb, especially not with its structive, material aspect. A preponderancy of energies, consequently, practically always implies a pathological increase of the energy level, increased stress upon the affected orb - without demonstrable somatic changes of its substratum, or even indications of the same.

Thus, if a certain pulse corresponding to an orb appears at one or several sites not corresponding to that orb, the clear and unequivocal implication is that the orb whose quality is expressed by this pulse, modulates, overlays, violates, accroaches by its energies those orbs at whose sites this particular pulse is observed.

To illustrate, stringy pulses are observed at the pedal sites of both hands. The consequence is that the energies of the hepatic orb – the stringy pulse represents the pulse expressing the quality of the hepatic orb! – modulates the renal orb. In order to decide upon a therapy, it must be checked whether this modulation is due to true redundancy or, on the contrary, due to

---

[218] All "pulses of the orbs" are enumerated above on p. 229.

inanitas yin o. hepatici ("exhaustion of the structive energes of the hepatic orb"). Additional clues for deciding the question must therefore be found by examining the clusal pulse of the left hand (corresponding to the site of the hepatic orb). If at this site repletion is present, the direct dispersion of energy from the orb and conduits of the o. hepaticus may be justified; if, by contrast, inanitas, exhaustion, is manifest or even only an indifferent energetic situation, the pollicar site of the left hand, and other tendencies of the pedal pulses must be taken into account.

Another example would be flooding pulses in all sites, with the exception of the pollex of the left hand. At this site, the pollicar site of the left hand, an exhausted pulse is observed. (I clearly remember this striking iconogram because I found it with great similarity in East Asia and in Europe, each time on a teacher). Conclusion: The structive energies of the cardial orb are weakened, unable to support adequately the active energies of the cardial orb. The latter, consequently, is dispersed, thus modulating the energies of all other orbs. Therapy: Suppletio ("completing") the structive energies of the cardial orb.

The Significance of the Site of the Pulse

In the adult, each site at the right and left ostium pollicare corresponds directly to a certain horreal orb, and more or less also to its functional correlate. Consequently, each form pulse or modal pulse observed in this site directly gives information on the functional situation in this orb and, indirectly and approximately also on the substrative or functional endogenous or exogenous factors inducing the observed deformation of the orbic function - hence of the pulses. Stated differently, the fact that a particular iconogram of the pulse appears at a specific site directly indicates that the functions corresponding to that site are disturbed - and indirectly implies that pathological changes have taken place in a substratum corresponding to that site.

For example, a grating pulse at the pollicar site of the right hand indicates serious difficulties of respiration, congestions of structive energies in the o. pulmonalis; at the same time this symptom favours the hypothesis that the organ supporting these functions, in other words the lung, is materially affected or changed: emphysema, hyperemia.

A second illustration would be the following: Minute pulses at the pedal sites point to a function of the renal orb yielding under stress. At the same time they imply that this weakness is due to constitutional weakness of the specific substratum of the renal orb - in the words of Western medicine, to a neurological instability.

The Significance of the Levels of the Pulses (Depth)

Independent of the correlations existing between orbs, sites and the modal qualities of certain pulses, there is a fundamental correlation between the depth (level) of the pulses and the phylogenetic age of the corresponding biological functions and their substratum, thus

superficial pulses correspond to rapid functions, to an accelerated metabolism, to phylogenetically young tissues - essentially represented by the oo. pulmonalis, cardialis, pericardialis, intestinorum;

medium pulses correspond to functions of medium speed, to tissues of medium phylogenetic age - represented by the oo. lienalis et stomachi, tricalorii, hepaticus, felleus [mesenchyme, flesh, glandular tissues]; and

submerged pulses correspond to the slow functions, to extremely slow metabolism, to phylogenetically old tissues - represented by the o. renalis and its correlates: [nerves, bones, teeth].

The correlations just described not only form the premise of the summary or emergency diagnoses described above[219]; more important still, the fact that they have been and are constantly experienced in practice furnishes the real foundation and justification for yoking together e.g. the o. cardialis and the o. intestini tenuis, the o. pulmonalis and the o. intestini crassi and their corresponding specific unfoldments (perfectiones), outward manifestations (flores)[220]. Thus the seeming paradox finds an explanation, viz. that the renal orb on the one hand shares the site of the pedal pulses with the oo. intestinorum, vesicalis, et tricalorii; yet that, on the other hand, the submerged pulses may under no circumstance be correlated to any other orb except the renal orb and its specific unfoldment, bones.

For example, a tense pulse observed at the pedal site of the right hand, by itself permits no conclusion as to which orb or system is affected. If, however, an onion-stalk pulse has been observed at the pollicar site of the same hand, the conclusion is very likely that the patient suffers from pains in the abdomen because of an inner lesion, accompanied by internal hemorrhages.

Another example: The pulses at all sites are superficial yet strong. We may infer a

---

[219] Cf. p. 239 above.

[220] Cf. p. 29 above.

PALPATION DIAGNOSIS

species-affection against which are marshalled actively the energies of the oo. pulmonalis, cardialis, pericardialis and their specific unfoldments: skin and conduits. But indirectly also the oo. intestinorum et vesicalis are involved, because they are – momentarily – deprived of energy needed and mobilized to fight off the exogenous heteropathy.

Summary of the Practical Implications

The multifarious and complex varieties and combinations of pulse iconograms observed during palpation of the ostium pollicare on adult individuals may be interpreted and understood as fitting into one of three patterns:

First, pathological symptoms are found in one site only; the other five sites all show normal pulses.
Diagnosis: The orb(s) corresponding to the site is (are) affected. Therapy may be solely directed to correcting the anomalies in these functions.

Second, at several or all sites of the pulse a single pathological variety of the pulse is observed.
Diagnosis: A clearly circumscribed disturbance of one or several energies. Therapy: Medication directed at the "seat" of the disturbed energy[221].

Third, at different sites of the pulse different pathological varieties of pulse iconograms are observed.
Diagnosis: A disturbance of orbic functions and energies. Therapy: Harmonization of the energy balance by bolstering or dispersing energy in the orbs whose affections are indicated through the site of the disturbance in the pulse.

Simple and Complex Iconograms of the Pulse

For the sake of completeness, a technical definition should be mentioned which is given in all pertinent Chinese texts on pulse diagnosis, namely that for defining certain pulses, more than one qualitative statement, hence, the combination of several standard iconograms may be required. The result is so-called "complex iconograms" of the pulse, for example when

a superficial and at the same time a tense pulse occurs: a double pulse (p. duplex), or
a submerged, small and exhausted pulse is observed: threefold pulse (p. triplex), or even
a pulse must be qualified as superficial, accelerated, slippery and replete: a fourfold

---

[221] I.e. the respective orb, as evident from the correlation between an orb pulse (p. 229) and other diagnostic data, must be treated either by propping up (suppletio) or by dispelling (dispulsio) its energies.

pulse (p. quadruplex).

As should be evident from what has been said above, there are no theoretical or technical difficulties for the expression or interpretation of these combinations. Care should only be taken to really incorporate all the data determined by the palpation of the pulse into the patient's files.

Critical Symptoms in the Pulse

(1) A pulse resembling a kettle boiling over, that is, a superficial and to an extreme degree accelerated pulse, hollow within, without root, indicates extreme calor or the three yang and the absence of structive energy.

(2) A pulse resembling a fish moved by water, i.e. fixed at the head, and moving the tail: surfacing, which now can be perceived, now cannot, indicates extreme algor in the three yin conduits and total depletion of the yang.

(3) A pulse like a knocking stone, i.e. a submerged pulse which deep down knocks against the finger like a stone, is an indication of the collapse of the energies in the renal orb.

(4) A pulse resembling an untwisted rope, i.e. superficial, loose and vague, expresses a total loss of the energies in the renal orb.

(5) A pulse like a dripping gutter, that is, a pulse in the middle level, of which now and then a beat can be perceived, and which is weak and dampened: this pulse indicates that constructive and defensive energies are exhausted and the qi stomachi has disappeared.

(6) A pulse like a swimming crab, that is, a superficial pulse with vague contours, erratically surfacing. It indicates extreme deficiency of the structive energies.

(7) A pulse resembling the pecking of a sparrow, i.e. a very intense and accelerated medium pulse, stopping now and then and continuing as before: collapse of the energies in the lienal orb.

(8) A pulse like the edge of a knife, i.e. on slight pressure the pulse appears to be small and accelerated; under increased pressure it feels as if it were hard, large and racing: total collapse of the energies in the hepatic orb.

(9) A pulse resembling a pea which is tossed about points to the collapse of the energies in the cardial orb.

(10) A pulse resembling sesame seeds swept around by wind, i.e. an evanescent or extremely minute pulse, indicates the exhaustion of defensive energy.

PALPATION DIAGNOSIS

All iconograms just described indicate very serious and critical disturbances which, if not treated immediately and effectively, will end in death.

PALPATION IN GENERAL

Besides the pulses, a number of other regions or sites of the body may be palpated. Here, as with other methods of Chinese diagnosis, the sensory perceptions of qualities at these sites must be interpreted with reference to the Eight Guiding Criteria in order to produce precise and univocal diagnostic data.

PALPATION OF THE INNER SIDE OF THE FOREARM (palpatio cutis pedalis)

In Chinese diagnosis the term cutis pedalis, chifu designates the skin (cutis, fu) at the inner side of the forearm, consequently covering this member between the bend of the elbow (corresponding to the foramen lacus pedalis = lacus ulnaris) and the site named 'pes' at the wrist[222]. Changes of diagnostic relevance that may be observed in this region have already been treated in a special chapter of the Inner Classic of the Yellow Sovereign[223]. There we learn that

a plump and somewhat slippery cutis pedalis indicates ventus;

a rough cutis pedalis is a sign of pains in the joints brought on by a ventus-heteropathy;

a coarse cutis pedalis comparable to the scaly skin of a dry fish indicates redundancy and congestion of juices (stases);

a hot cutis pedalis indicates fever; and

a cold cutis pedalis is a symptom of weakness or exhaustion (inanitas).

PALPATION OF THE SKIN (palpatio speciei carnis): DETERMINING BODY TEMPERATURE, MOISTNESS OF THE SKIN ETC.

Palpation of the skin in Chinese diagnosis is employed to produce data on the warmth and flexibility of the flesh and on the moistness of the skin.

The moistness of the skin is determined by softly stroking the skin with the hand[224].

The body temperature is gauged by palpation, exercising light, intermediate and strong pressure with the fingers.

---

[222] Cf. p. 206 above.

[223] Lingshu, chapter 74.

[224] On the diagnostic significance of perspiration, cf. p. 181 above.

PALPATION DIAGNOSIS

a - If the heat of fever is felt strikingly under low pressure yet seems to be less under the fingers left on the spot for some moments, this is a symptom of calor in the species, i.e. in the pulmonal orb; or it may point to inanitas-fever (fever due to exhaustion of structive energies).

b - Fever felt most strikingly under medium pressure and apparently less under strong pressure indicates that calor in the calorium medium or in the cardial orb is present.

c - Fever felt most strikingly under strong pressure indicates calor affecting the marrow and bones, i.e. fever-induced exhaustion of structive energies (inanitas yin) or fever induced by calor humidus (a "heat-heteropathy brought on by humidity").

Cold extremities, i.e. hands and feet, are symptoms of algor developing in the structive energies, in yin.

If the patient starts if touched with cold hands, this is a symptom of the exhaustion of the active energies (inanitas yang).

If the patient has an exceptionally hot palm, this is a symptom of endogenous disturbances brought on by stress; if the back of his hand is strikingly hot, this indicates algor venti.

THE PALPATION OF ULCERS AT THE SURFACE OF THE BODY (palpatio ulcerum)

Although ulcers, boils and so on clearly constitute bodily, somatic changes to be taken care of by surgery, it may be useful to incorporate the data gained from their palpation into the complete diagnostic picture of an individual. Thus

a) If ulcers show swelling and yield under pressure, this is a symptom of algor.

b) Swollen ulcers felt as hot, point to calor.

c) Ulceration with an extensive yet moderate swelling and a sunken-in, concave centre, is a symptom of inanitas.

d) A fairly small yet strongly protuberant swelling indicates repletion.

e) If the site of disease appears hard, more or less hot and distended, yet if the patient feels no pain when pressure is applied, pus has formed.

f) If the diseased site is very hot, if it appears to be harder on its margins and soft in the centre, and if the patient experiences great pain when pressure is applied, this again points to purulence.

PALPATION IN PEDIATRICS (palpatio infantum)

Since in pediatrics important diagnostic methods like pulse diagnosis and interrogation have only limited uses, other diagnostic procedures applicable to pediatrics must not be neglected.

Palpation of the Members (palpatio membrorum)

a) Hot soles of the feet indicate calor.
b) Cold calves indicate algor.
c) Cold fingertips are a symptom of flexus pavoris i.e. of the retreat, contravection of energies brought on by shock and fright.
d) If only the middle finger of the infant's hand is hot, this points to exogenous algor venti.
e) If only the tip of the middle finger is cold, there is the possibility of a smallpox infection.
f) If the infant has cold palms and continuously opens and closes the hands, this is an unfavourable sign pointing to a total depletion of structive energy.

Palpation of the Forehead (palpatio frontis)

a) If, in the presence of fever, the forehead shows a distinctly higher temperature than the palm, this indicates calor speciei.
b) If during fever the palms clearly have a higher temperature than the forehead, calor inanitatis may be inferred.

PALPATION OF THE FORAMINA (OF ACUPUNCTURE POINTS) (palpatio foraminorum)

Even today, in the presence of quite reliable electrical probes and instruments for locating and diagnosing foramina ("acupuncture points"), the palpation of such foramina still constitutes a significant element of solid acupuncture diagnosis and technique.

Within the wide scale of diagnostic information to be gained from the palpatory examination of foramina, those obtained by feeling the inductoria dorsalia (beishu)[225]

---

[225] Cf. Porkert, Theoretical Foundations... pp. 335 f.

PALPATION DIAGNOSIS

and the foramina originalis (yuanxue)[226] have special significance and usefulness, since they are precisely correlated to the functions of specific orbs.

If, when palpatory pressure is applied with the tip of the finger, one or several of these foramina are sensitive - i.e. the patient experiences pain - this is a symptom of repletion or of congested energy in the corresponding orb.

If, by contrast, the energy in these same orbs is depleted or exhausted (inanis), palpatory pressure applied to the foramen either will be felt as a slight itch or will produce an agreeable sensation.

---

[226] Cf. op. cit. pp. 341 f.

BIBLIOGRAPHY

This bibliography, in its first section, mentions only titles or sources which have actually served for the compilation of the present text.

Chinese Sources and Secondary Texts

1) *Jingyue qüanshu* 景岳全書 ("Collected Writings of Zhang Jingyue = Zhang Jiebin, 張景岳(介賓) 上海科學技術出版社, (1958) 1960

2) *Jinguei yaolue yuyi* 金匱要略語譯 中華人民共和國衛生部 中醫研究院；人民衛生出版社 1959

3) *Zhongyi zhenduanxue jiangyi* 中醫診斷學講義 廣州中醫學院；上海科學技術出版社 (1963) 1964

4) *Zhongyixue gailun* 中醫學概論 (Reprint of the 1st edition of 1958 by 中醫藥衛生出版社, 香港)； 1971 南京中醫學院

5) *Zhongyi neikexue jiangyi* 中醫內科學講義 上海中醫學院 上海科學技術出版社 (1963) 1964

6) *Yixuexinwu* 醫學心悟 compiled by Cheng Guopeng (Zhongling) 程國彭(鍾齡)；人民衛生出版社, 北京 1963

7) *Yibu qüanlu* 醫部全錄 (Medical Chapters of the Encyclopedia 古今圖書集成) reprinted by 人民衛生出版社, 北京 1959

8) *Mojing* 脈經 ("Pulse Classic") by 王叔和 Wang Shuhe 商務印書館, 上海 1956

9) *Neijing jiangyi* 內經講義
北京中醫學院　上海科學技術出版社　(1963) 1964

10) *Pinhu moxue* 瀕湖脈學 and other titles by 李時珍 Li Shizhen
人民衛生出版社, 北京　(1956) 1957

11) *Sanyin ji yibing fangcui (Sanyinfang)*　　　　　　　　　by Chen Wuze
various editions 三因極一病方粹（三因方）　陳無擇

12) *Shanghanlun jizhu*　　　　　editied by Hoang Zhuzhai
傷寒論集註：黃竹齋 ; 人民衛生出版社, 北京　1958

13) *Shanghanlun jiangyi* 傷寒論講義：成都中醫學院 ; 上海科學技術出版社
(1963) 1964

14) *Wenbingxue jiangyi*　溫病學講義：南京中醫學院
上海科學技術出版社　(1963) 1964

Books by the Author

1) The Theoretical Foundations of Chinese Medicine, MIT Press, Cambridge, Mass. 1974, 2nd. ed. 1978

2) Klinische chinesische Pharmakologie, Heidelberg 1976

3) Die chinesische Medizin, Düsseldorf and Vienna, 1982.

ENGLISH GENERAL INDEX

Abhorrence of wind 179
abrupt changes, of temperature 87
abuse of diaphoresis, vomiting 177
abuse of dispulsive applications 177
accidents, mechanical 57
accidents, mechanical 58
accroachment 24, 61, 87
accumulation of phlegm 176
accumulation of pituita in the central calorium 187
action **18**, 34
active aspect 103
active control of fluids and juices 106
active energies 104, 111, 181
active energies exhausted 190
active energies flaring up 168
active energies of the renal orb, exhausted 189
active energies, collapse of 182
active energies, deficiency of 140, 160
active energies, depletion of 150
active energies, dispersing outside 182
active energies, hemmed in 82
active energies, hemmed in by a yin heteropathy 146
active energies, obstruction of 152
active energies, of the hepatic orb, rising upward 183
active energies, of the orbis lienalis, imminent exhaustion of 154
active energies, of the orbis renalis 151
active energies, state of 130
active energies, symptoms of affections of the 180
active energy 211
active energy, impaired, of the pulmonal orb 89
active energy, individually specific 21, **114**
active energy, profusion of 222
active energy, stagnant 213
active fluids, depletion of 149
active impulse 23
active individually specific energies, agglutination of 214
activity 103
activity **18**
activity 22
activity, actual 23
activity, potential 23
activity, sexual, influence on the pulse 246
actual structivity 94
actuality 22
actuality, axis of 111
acu-moxi-therapy 10
acupuncture 10, 100, 11, 200, 49
acupuncture points 29
addiction, excessive, to sour or salty food 175
advantages, heuristic 101
aestus heteropathy 137
aestus excesses 60
affinities with the orbs 50
affinities, of all orbs with the sensorium of the head 132
affinity, olfactory 28
agents 31, 32, 8
agents, exterior (exogenous) 42, 57
agents, inner (endogenous) 42, 57
agents, neutral 57, 58
agents, of disease **56**
agents, pathological 24
age, advanced 156
age, reflected in the tongue 138

aggravation 101
aggressiveness 19
ahorrence of cold 179
alcohol 139
alcoholic excesses 40
alertness 66
algor factor 108
algor heteropathies 180, 184
algor heteropathy 42, 49, 59, 171, 174, 176
algor heteropathy in the large intestine orb 92
algor laedens disease 175
algor laedens pathology 103
algor-symptoms 44, 45
amelioriation 101
analysis, causal 14, 15, 2, 3, 5
anatomy 26
ankles, appearance of 169
antibiotics 138
anxiety 57
62
appearance, lustreless, faded 126
appetite 34
appetite , reduced 127
appetite, good 127
appettitiveness 19
ariditas-heteropathy, exogenous 88
aspects, ambivalent 107
aspects, somatic 2
aspect, outward 39
aspect, perfective 19
assay of drugs 10, 19
assimilation, of energy 129, 80
assimilation, of external influences 62
associations 19
aulic orb 29
aulic orbs 158
aulic orbs 21, 27, 30
auscultation, auditve diagnosis of voice and speech 34, **173**
auto-representation 122
autumn 20, 23, 60
back 21
background, historical, of pulse diagnosis 197
balance of energy 35, 80
balance, dynamic 181
balance, energetic, between all orbs 129
barefoot doctors 197
being chilled 179
belly 21
best time, for pulse diagnosis, 201
biassing 32, 56
black 125
bladder, urinary 27
block of the energies in the pulmonal orb 89
block of the energy flow 168
block of the pulmonal orb, due to calor 166
blocks, inner 145
blocks, obstructions 223
blocks, within the orbs 146
blood 113, 116, 219
blood, odour of 178
bodily shape, inspection of **126**
body 29, 9
body fluids 37
body hair 87
body of the tongue 130, **131**

body of the tongue, colour   130
body of the tongue, shape   130
body of the tongue, specific quality   130
body pulses, general   **203**
body, fat   127
body, lean, and strong appetite   127
body, strong   127
bolstering, energies   77
bone   163, 39
bones   48, 94
bones, largeness of   127
breakdown, total, of an orb   126
breathing, balanced harmony of   123
brightness   20
calor heteropathies   180
calor heteropathy   151, 166, 189, 213
calor heteropathy, affecting the pulmonal or stomach orbs   168
calor humidus heteropathy   149
calor-heteropathies influence cooling of the pulmonal orb   91
calor-symptoms   44
cardial orb   129, 160, 162, 37, 38
cardinal conduit   104
cardinal conduits   103
cardinal conduits, serious disturbances of   170
causes   2, 31, 9
central pulses   **204**
centrifugality   19
certitude   121
changes   19
changes, malignant organic   10
changes, somatic   10
checking sequence   23, 28
check, physiological   28
check, structure   23, 24
circulation of blood   198
circulation of energy, impeded   221
circulation, of energy   115
clash, powerful, between heteropathies   127
cleanliness   178
climate   124, 9
climatic excesses   113, 39, **58**, 81
clinical medicine   100
clinical uses   101
clothing   122
clusal pulse   **206**
clusal pulse, defining the   233
coating of the tongue   130, **131**
coating of the tongue on a healthy individual   142
coating of the tongue, criteria for the description   143
coating of the tongue, diagnostic inspection of   **142**
coating of the tongue, particular structure   130
coating of the tongue, thickness of   134
coating of the tongue, true or false   135
cold medicines   38
cogitation, excessive   75, 97
coherence   74
cohesion, of the personality   73, 74
cold   20, 32, 48, 57, 58, 70, 82
cold drinks, ingestion of   89
cold heteropathy   90
cold remedies   49
cold, extreme   137
cold, heavy   44
collapse of the active energies   182
collapse, imminent, of the functions of the stomach orb   151
collapse, of all energies   175
collusion   23
coloration, concentrated   161

colour   28
colour of the face   **158**
colour of the lips   **167**
colour tinges, correlations with phases, seasons, orbs   125
colour, deversant   125
colour, dominant   124
colour, inspection of   **124**
colour, of early death   126
combinations   33
commandments   15
communication between below and above   106
complementarity, of causal analysis and inductive synthesis   4
complement, functional   28
complete loss of the energies of the renal orb   161
completing energies   77
complexion   125, **158**
complexion, inspection of   **156, 158**
complexion, lustrous   161
complexion, modal changes of   **161**
comprehension, easy   121
concentration of the active energies, of the renal orb   96
concepts, general   31
concepts, synthetic   31
concretion   19
condensation of pituita algoris   90
condensing function, of the pulmonal orb   90
conduit theory   101
conduits   115, 162, 205, 57, 65, 66, 73
conduits, cardinal   103
conduits, depleted of moisture   218
conduits, heteropathies deversating in the - of the pulmonal orb   174
conduits, pathology of   **100**
conduits, reticular   77
conduits, touching the tongue   129
conduit, main   28
configurative force   129, 140, 21, 217, 55, 71, 74, 76
configurative force, as manifest on the tongue   135
configurative force, inspection of   **123**
configurative force, of the eye   163
configurative force, of the pulse   244
confusion, historical   101
congestion   105, 87
congestion of active or structive energies   158
congestion of energies in the oo.hepaticus et lienalis   191
congestion of energy   222
congestion of individually specific structive energy   159
congestion of xue   191
congestions   230, 24
congestions of juices   254
congestion, active, of the oo. lienalis et stomachi   187
congestion, local   168
congestion, of energies in the stomach orb   171
congestion, of the active energies of the hepatic orb   68
conquest sequence   23, 24, 25, 28
conservation, of structive energy   35
considerations, abstract   101
considerations, topological   102
consistency   74
consistency, logical   13
consistency, of reflection   123
constitution   156, 35
constitution, acquired, root of   80
constitution, feeble   96

constitution, inborn, foundation of   94
constitution, influence of, on the pulse   245
constitution, strong   155, 174
constitution, structive   111
constitutive energies of the renal orb   186
constructive energy   103, 113, 115, 21 ,75, 80, 136
contentment   111
contradictions   103
contradictions, basic   103
contravection   126, 62, 52
contravections, of the qi hepaticum   68
contravection, brought on by shock and fright   256
contravection, meteorological   176
contravective energy   52
contravective glare   175
control centre   130
control of calor   103
controls, central   134
convalescence   170, 217, 230
conventional standards   **17**
conventions, normative   17
convention, classical   104
cool ariditas symptoms   61
cool medicines   38
cooling function, of the pulmonal orb   90
cooling off, unwholesome   89
coolness   20
coordination, insufficient, between the cardial and renal orbs   78
coöperation   23
correlations of the pulses with orbs   248
correlations of the pulses with sites   248
correlations of the pulses with the depth levels   248
correspondences   158, 20
correspondences, of the sites of the eye   **162**
correspondences, of the tongue with all orbs   133
correspondence, of radial pulses and orbs   **208**
correspondence, of regions of the body, and radial pulses   206
cortisone   222
coughing, the sound of   **175**
crimson   125
crisis, beginning of   182
crisis, in the course of a disease   143
criteria   121
criteria, eight guiding   **32**, 31, 121 , 5, 49
criteria, polarizing   22, 22
critical excess of yin   38
critical issue, when learning pulse diagnosis   196
critical symptoms, upon inspection of the tongue   **153**
cross   22
crudeness   11
crudeness of pulse diagnosis   194
cue, rhythmic   87
damaging cold   65
danger   62
danger, supposed   63
darkness   20
data, absolute   13
data, empirical   17, 28, 30
data, material   15
data, relative   13
data, sensory   11
data, somatic   15
day   20
decisions, capacity to make   66
decrease, of energy   36
defecation   **185**
defence, outer   74
defense line, foremost   114
defense system   87

defensive energy   103, 113, **114**, 21, 21, 210, 211, 228, 87
defensive faculty, impaired   111
deficiency, extreme, of active energies in the o. vesicalis   186
deficiencies   24
deficiency   54, 75
deficiency of active energies   185
deficiency of energy, in the pulmonal and renal orbs   91
deficiency of individually specific structive energies   219
deficiency, constitutional   94
deficiency, extreme   230
deficiency, extreme of structive energies   141
deficiency, in the renal orb   183
deficiency, of active energies   36
deficiency, of fluids   185
deficiency, of structive energies   230
deficiency, of structive energy   36
deficiency, of the active energies in the central orbs   82
deficiency, of the qi medium   82
deficiency, of the yin hepaticum   70
deficiency, of the yin renale   97
deficient structivity   117
definition   18
deflections   30
deformation   24
depletion   21, 32, 50
depletion, extreme, of the qi stomachi   159
depletion, of active energies of the pulmonal orb   89
depletion, of structive energy   168
depletion, of structive fluids, of the pulmonal orb   88
depletion, of the energy of all orbs   220
deployment, impeded, of active energies   183
depth   130, 20, 39, 42, 59
depth, of the pulse   **209**
desire to sleep   **190**
determination   18
determination, specific, of functional disorders   7
development, rational, of diagnostic methods   225
deversant colour   125
deviation   56
diagnoses, four   **122**
diagnosis, differential   **31**
diagnosis, early   10
diagnosis, economical   14
diagnosis, functional   11, 122
diagnosis, individually specific   8
diagnosis, medical   12
diagnosis, rational   14
diaphoresis, excessive   186
diaphoretics   107, 112
diaphragm   110, 21, 45
diarrhea, control of   92
diet, unwholesome   63
diet, wrong   40
differences, individual   3
differentiation   32
direction   17
direction   32, 28
directionality   31
direction, change of   4
disease   15
diseases of major yang   103
diseases of the liver and gall-bladder orbs   **66**
diseases of the pulmonal and large intestine orbs   87
diseases, constitutional   10
diseases, degenerative   138
diseases, infectious   73
diseases, inner   66

diseases, of the kidney and urinary bladder orbs   94
diseases, of the oo. hepaticus et felleus   **66**
diseases, of the orbes cardialis et intestini tenuis   **73**
diseases, of the renal and vesical orbs   94
diseases, of the stomach and spleen orbs   80
disease, acute   101
disease, chronic   101, 96
disease, exogenous   40
disease, light, recent   101
disease, prolonged   101, 94, 96, 89
disease, recent   39
disease, serious   94, 97
disease, severe   101, 111
disease, somatic   9
disease, superficial   39
disharmony, of the energies of the orbis stomachi   177
disorders, functional   10, 9
dispersion, of blocked energy   79
dispersion, of congested energy   85
disposition, asthmatic   105
disruption of rhythm   87
disruption, total of the interrelationship between yin and yang   182
distension of the pulmonal orb   128
distinction between health and disease   11
distinctness   22
distribution of active and structive energy   109
distribution of heat and cold   109
distribution of structive energy   109
distribution, of energy   129, 80
disturbances, functional   1
disturbances, in the regulation of the quantitative distribution   109
disturbances, of yang minor   107
disturbance, essentially in the yang   161
disturbance, essentially in the yin   161
diuretics   106
dominant colour   124
dosage, correct   52
dosage, of individually specific structive energy   66
dropsy   161
dryness   58
dryness, extreme   **60**
ducts, respiratory and digestive   113
duration   9
dynamization, of the flow of fluids and juices   106

ear conch, colour of   166
ears   204, 94, 20
ear, inspection of   **166**
eating habits   9
eclecticism   11
economy   121
effect   31
effectiveness, diminished   13
effects, dynamic   4
effects, future   9
effects, past   2, 9
effects, present   9
effects, side-   121
efficacy of therapy   10
efforts, excessive   221
electro-dynamics   5
emblems   18
emetics   108, 107
emotion   29
emotional stress, excessive   189
emotions   53, 68
emotions, consequences of intense   223
emotions, directed, deployment of   94
emotions, seven   40, 57

emotions, suppressed   68, 76
emotion, congested   74
emotion, extreme   191
encroachments, of the yang hepaticum   70
endogenous pathogenic factors   180
endowment, exceptional   121
endowment, in pulse diagnosis   193
energetic conduits, block of   158
energetics, medical   65
energies in the 12 cardinal conduits   204
energies in the stomach and lienal orbs   204
energies, active   67
energies, clear   21
energies, constitutive, deposited in the orbis renalis   166
energies, in the chest   204
energies, murky   21
energies, refined   21
energies, unrefined   21
energy exchange, harmony of   106
energy in the renal orb   204
energy level   127
energy of the stomach orb   204
energy supply, balanced   111
energy supply, harmonious   111
energy, blocked   79
energy, constructive   21
energy, defensive   21
energy, in the cardial orb   204
energy, in the pulmonal orb   204
energy, powerful, in the renal orb   155
energy, structive   61
enfeeblement   111
epidemics   64
equipoise   23
errors, of pulse diagnosis   197
error, occasions for   14
evacuation, of sticky mucus   77
evaluation, statistical   3
events, past   4
evening   23
events, actual   4
events, present   4
events, simultaneous   13
events, synchronous   13
event, unique   15
evolutive phases   102
excellent health   217
exertion   181
excess of humor   190
excesses, alcoholic   46
excesses, alcoholic   53
excesses, climatic   57
excesses, sexual   40, 46, 53, 57, 63, 94
excessive purging   186
excessive reflection   57
excess, climatic   57
excretions   103
excretions, inspection of   **171**
exhausted yang   46
exhausted yang, of the renal orb   95
exhausted yin   37
exhaustion   111
exhaustion   127, 221, 254, 61, 81, 87
exhaustion, heat-   88
exhaustion of active energies   141
exhaustion of active energies of the renal orb   185
exhaustion of active energy   50
exhaustion of energy, in the large intestine orb   92
exhaustion of structive energies   97

exhaustion of the energies in the cardial and renal orbs 174
exhaustion of the energies of the orbs 51
exhaustion of the energies of the stomach orb 85
exhaustion of the individually specific structive energy 51
exhaustion of the orthopathy 49
exhaustion of the renal orb 98
exhaustion of the surface 181
exhaustion of the yin of the hepatic orb 183
exhaustion of the yin of the renal orb 175
exhaustion of yang 180
exhaustion of yin 180
exhaustion, bodily, extreme 53
exhaustion, extreme 54
exhaustion, extreme, of structive energy 184
exhaustion, glare of 36
exhaustion, imminent, of structive energy 127
exhaustion, individual standards of the diagnostician 202
exhaustion, of active energies 255
exhaustion, of energies in the pulmonal orb 175
exhaustion, of structive energy 168, 35
exhaustion, of structivity 88
exhaustion, of the active as well as of the structive energies 141
exhaustion, of the active energy of the cardial orb 75
exhaustion, of the energies of the pulmonal and renal orbs 174
exhaustion, of the hepatic orb 158
exhaustion, of the orbis lienalis affects the orbis pulmonalis 91
exhaustion, of the orthopathy 130
exhaustion, of the xue 191
exhaustion, total of active and structive energies 137
exogenous heteropathies 170
exogenous pathogenic factors 180
expansion 18, 19
expansiveness 19
experience, positive 7
expression, firm 123
exterior 20
extremes, cold and heat 87
extroversion 19
eyelids 162
eyes **189**, 204
eye, inspection of **162**
eye, sites of **162**

face, inspection of **156**
face, shape of **161**
face, sites of **156, 157**
factors, constitutional 56
factors, cosmic 56
factors, deviating 49
factors, emotional 56
factors, endogenous 56
factors, exogenous 101, 56
factors, individual 15
factors, social 56
factor, inner 42
faeces, inspection diagnosis **172**
fallacies, major 57
false cold 44, 48
false heat 44
false repletion 53
false symptoms 53
false thirst 48
fear 100, 57, **62**, 63
femaleness 20

fever disease 97
fever diseases, common 100
fever disease, endogenous 42
fire 20
firmness, of the flesh 123
fissures, on the surface of the tongue 139
five E.P.s **22**
five evolutive phases 17
five evolutive phases **22**
flare up of active energies, during depletion 230
flare-up from the hepatic and renal orbs 159
flaring up 38
flaring up, of glare of the hepatic orb 69
flesh 106, 162, 169, 80, 83, 97, 127
flesh, surface of the 174
flexibility 33
flexus-cold 48
fluids 116, 178, 48, 83
fluids and liquids, economy of 94
fluids, active 140, 160, 21
fluids, deficiency of 185
fluids, depletion of 154, 156
fluids, diminishment of 61
fluids, excessively drained 145
fluids, exhaustion of all 168
fluids, impaired 145
fluids, insufficient availability 91
fluids, lesions of 148
fluids, secretion of 151
fluids, serious deficiency of 135
fluids, structive 160, 21
fluids, sufficient supplies 169
food 27, 62
food, energies absorbed from 145
food, hasty ingestion of 176
food, intake of 186
food, separation into clear and murky elements 78
food, transformation of 78
food, undigested 222
foramina 29
forces, external 27
force, configurative 21
forearm, inner side of **254**
forehead 103
forms of energy, active, structive 114
fright 158, 57, **63**
function 4, 56, 9
functions, actual 8
functions, assimilating 132
functions, distributive 132, 82
functions, integrative 82
functions, momentary 8
functions, nervous 94
functions, neurological 94
functions, reproductive 94
functions, simultaneous 17
functions, storing 132
functions, vital 121
function, constitutive 29
function, detached 32
function, dominant 29
function, normal 32
function, pathological 32
function, regulative, of the hepatic orb 109
function, specific 29
function, stability of 15, 4
function, storage 30
fundamentals of technique in palpating the pulse **199**
gall-bladder 27
garments, wet 60

generalization 32
glare 107, 136, 58, **61**, 67, 74
glare spreads uncontrolled 97
glare, extreme 153
glare, in the cardial orb 38
glare, in the upper calorium 182
glare, inner 76
glare, of the hepatic orb 69
good health 221
gradients, extreme, of energy 87
gravity, centre of 22
green 125
guiding criteria, eight **32**
habit 65
habits, eating- 9
hair 39
hair of the head **155**
halo 240
hands and feet, general appearance of **169**
hardness 21
harmful cold 101, 104, 113
harmful cold diseases 100
harmonization 23, 35
harmonization of the energy flow 108
harmonization, of energetic processes 80
harmony, lost, between the orbes lienalis et stomachi 83
head, top of 103
health 11
hearing **188**
heart 198, 27, 59
heat 165, 32, 48, 90
heat congestion 106
heat flares upward 97
heat heteropathy in the large intestine orb 92
heat heteropathy, affecting the stomach orb 85
heat shock 59
heat symptoms 79
heat, extreme 137
heat, false 46
heat, heavy 44
heat, internal 214
heat, oppressive, of summer 57
heat, true 46
heaven 20
hemorrhages serious, after birth 219
hepatic orb 163
hepatic orb 68
hepatic orb, conduits of the 158
hepatic orb, disturbances of the 160
hepatic orb, functions of 189
heteropathies 103
heteropathies, exogenous 173
heteropathies, induced by an exogenous factor 101
heteropathies, intensity of 180
heteropathy **32**, 56, 57, 64
heteropathy, exogenous 152
hidden phlegm 174
homeostasis 32
homogeneity of substratums 15, 3
homogeneity, decreasing 3
horreal orbs 29, 158, 21, 27, 28, 30
hot remedies 49
humdity 105, 221, **60**
humid heat 83
humidity 134, 146, 159, 165, 182, 187, 191, 255, 58, 83
humidity heteropathy 171
humidity, excessive 81,
humidity, transformation of 83
humor heteropathies 184

humor heteropathy 153
humor excesses 60
humor heteropathies 60
iconographies, reduced, of the pulse **224**
iconography, complete, when learning pulse diagnosis **196**
illness, critical state of 116
illness, prolonged 96
imagination 68
imbalance, emotional 9
implements, technical 12
impressions, actual 2
impressions, momentary 2
impressions, present 2
improvement 101, 182
impulse, active 23
inanitas fevers 255
inanitas symptoms 50, 52, 67
inanitas, during convalescence 230
inborn constitution 94
incompatibility, of outward stimuli, with the constitutional disposition 222
increase, of energy 36
index in pediatric diagnosis **169**
indigestion, active 213
indistinction 22
individually specific active energy 113, 210, 50
individually specific structure energies 50, 178
individually specific structure energies, exhausted 189
individually specific structure energies, deficiency of 213
individually specific structure energy 113, 127, 137, 146, 219, 37
individually specific structure energy, at the surface 214
individually specific structure energy, block of 139
individually specific structure energy, congestion of 159
individual, healthy, basic colour of 125
inductive synthesis **4**
indurations, localized 68
infections 166
infection, exogenous 42
infectious disease 137
infectious diseases, initial stage of 148
inflections 30
influences, accidental, on pulse diagnosis 201
influences, exterior 40
influences, of climate and season on the pulse 245
influences, orienting 73
initiative 66
inner orbs 28
inner side 39
innocuousness 121
inner orb 39
inoculation, prophylactic 64
inputs, cosmic 62
inputs, psychic 62
inputs, social 62
insight, clear 73
inspection 33
inspection of the head **155**
inspection of the tongue **129**
inspection, of the bodily shape **126**
instability 28
instability of the active energies, of the orbis renalis 95
instability of the hepatic orb 158
instability, of the orbis lienalis 106

269

integration, of the personality	73	measures, suppletive	52
integration, stringent, rational	7	measures, therapeutic	31

integration, of the personality 73
integration, stringent, rational 7
integrity, functional 49
intensity of the heteropathies 180
interaction 24
interchangeabilty 15
interior 20
internal wind 67
interrogation 34
intestine 26
intima symptoms 40
43
intimacy, sphere of 122
inventiveness 68
inversion 23
iris 163
irregularities, dietetic 58
irregularities, sexual 58
irritation, of the cardial orb 76
juices 127
kampo-medicine 200
kidney 27
large intestine 27
large intestine orb 91
latency 64
layer, deeper, of the individual 114
left side 20
length, of the pulse **209**
lesion in the active energies 108
lesion of the active energies in the stomach orb 187
lesion of the qui stomachi 187
lesions in the thorax 164
lesions, critical of the orbs 178
lesions, endogenous 173
lesions, inner 74
lesions, mechanical 223
lesion, of the pulmonal orb 173
lesion, of the qui primum 186
lesion of the structive energies of the stomach orb 187
levels of correspondence 133
lienal orb 162, 167
life habits, irregular 87
life, manifestations of 8
lining 32, 39
lips, inspection of 167
liquids 127
liver 27
local repletion, in the head 183
location, of radial pulses **206**
locomotive apparatus 163
loss of blood 53
loss of blood, of fluids 215
loss of structive potential 219
loss of the qui stomachi 218
lower pulses **204**
lower side 20

major yang 103
major yin diseases **108**
maleness 20
malfunction 32
malnutrition 81
manifestations, outward 127
manifestation, active, of the personality 111
manifestation, outward 29
marrow 39, 48
marrow and bones 255
materialization 19
matter 17, 2, 9
maxilla 131
meals, influencing the pulse 246

measures, suppletive 52
measures, therapeutic 31
measures, to increase active and structive energies 112
measures, to increase the exchange between above and below 112
measures, dispelling 52
measures, therapeutic 10
medication, effect upon pulse diagnosis 201
medication, inappropriate 222
medicine, empirical 8
medicine, inner 66
melons 60
menstruation **190**
menstruation, disturbances of 247
menstruation, influence on the pulse 247
meteorological contravection 176
methodology 2
methods, empirical 8
metric system 17
micturition **185, 186**
midnight 23
minor yang diseases **106, 110**
misuse of the body 9
mobility 66
mode of life 246
models 26
model, topographical 116
modes of cognizance 2
moist places 174
monk's pulse 246
moon 20
morbi temperati diseases 168
morning 23
motion 18
motions and movements, inspection of **127**
mouth 204, 80
mouth, inspection of **167**
movement 20, 4, 9
movement, contrary 52
movement, erratic 67
movement, erratic, of the yang of the hepatic orb 69
movement, harmonious 103
movement, of xue 113
movement, outward 101
movement, perception of 8
moxibustion 10, 49
mucus, hidden 76
mucus, inspection of **171**
murky energy 103
muscles, and sinews 66
nails on fingers and toes 169
nasolabial pulse 204
nature, thermic, of disease 44
neck 103
negations 19
negative 18, 19
nervous functions 94
nervousness, inanitas-nervus 78
163
neurological functions 94
night 20
noon 23
nose 131, 87
nose, diagnostic inspection of **165**
noxious influence, exogenous 103
numbers, even 21
numbers, odd 21

objective, foremost, of pulse diagnosis 193
objectivity 12, 121
obscurity 20

```
obstruction by pituita      174
obstructions in the intima      164
obstructions, inner      145
obstructions, within the orbs      146
olfaction      34
olfaction, diagnosis by      178
opening, body-      29
orb      101, 26
orbisiconographic paradigm      28
orbisiconography      26, 65, 8
orbs      102, 114, 57
orbs, active      27
orbs, aulic      27
orbs, horreal      27, 28, 30
orbs, inner      28
orbs, outer      28
orbs, transaction-      27
orb, checking      28
orb, complementary      28
organ      26
organ, sensory      29
origin      22
orthopathic yang      108
orthopathy      103, 32, 56
orthopathy, bolstering of the      103
orthopathy, exhaustion of      49
orthopathy, strength of      180
orthopathy, weakness of      166
outer defense      74
outer layer      32
outer orb      39, 28
outward aspect      39
outward manifestation      29
overpowering      24
oversophistication, speculative, of pulse diagnosis      194

pain, corollary of      158
palpation      34
para-orbs      27
paradigm, orbisiconographic      28
paraorbs      28
past      31, 9
past effects      9
pathology      65
pathology of the forms of energy      113
pathology, framework for      66
pathology, of the orbs      66
patterns, cyclical      22
pedal pulse      206
pedal pulses      36, 38
pedal pulse, defining the      234
pedal pulse, depth of      237
penetration      101
penetration of disease      32
penetration, of a heteropathy      130
perception, positive, of function      8
perfective aspect      19
pericardial orb      74
pericardium      27, 59
peripheral E.P.s      80
periphery      39
personality      111, 123, 27
personality of the patient      14
personality, cohesion of      129, 73, 74
personality, integration of      73
personality, projection of      73
perspective, correct      65
perspective, difference of      8
perspective, intellectual, wrong      193
perspective, wrong intellectual, in pulse diagnosis      195
perspiration      181, 37, 38

perspiration, continuous      40
perspiration, smell of      178
pes sites      116
pharmacotherapy      102
pharynx      131
phase sequences      23
phase sequences      23
phases, evolutive      22
phases, evolutive      22
phenomena, present      19
phenomena, psychic      4
phenomena, vital      4
phenomenon, sensory      57
philtrum      167
phlegm      81, 89, 90
phlegm, murky, hems in the pulmonal orb      89
phlegm, residual in the thorax      175
physics, nuclear      5
physiology      198, 26
pigmentation, basic      124
pivot      111, 112, 22
pleasure      57, 61
plexus, ocular      66
poison      10
poisoning      139
poison, infectious      113
polarity      1
pollex, finding the      234
pollicar pulse      206
pollicar pulse, finding the      234
population, crowded      64
pores, stopped-up      181
pores, wideness of      127
positive      19
postulates, general      56
postulates, theoretical      100
postulate, abstract      57
potential structivity      88
potentiality      22
potential, structive      21, 27
potentiation of power      94
power      20
practices, magic      18
precision      1, 12, 121
precision, of pulse diagnosis      196
predisposition, constitutional      46
pregnancy      191, 247
preponderance, extreme, of yin      158
prerequisites, for mastering pulse diagnosis      193
prescriptions, cooling      92
prescriptions, cooling from within      106
prescriptions, diaphoretic      145
prescriptions, hot, have harmed the yin      144
prescriptions, laxative      92
prescriptions, of drugs      49
prescriptions, preventing excessive perspiration      105
prescriptions, purging      145
prescriptions, reductive      96
prescriptions, transforming excess humidity      105
prescriptions, warming from within      105
presence of mind      66
present      31
present phenomena      19
present situation      9
principles      17
probability      3, 8
processes, digestive      108
production of calor      103
production sequence      126, 23
profligacy, alcoholic      97
profligacy, sexual      96, 97
```

prognosis   1, 32, 8
prognosis, detailed   3
prognosis, reassuring   124
prognosis, sure   6
projection, active, of the personality   66
projection, of a heteropathy onto the surface of the tongue   142
projection, of the personality   73
prolongation, of illness   101
prolonged illness   161
proto-science   5
protuberances, on the surface of the tongue   139
prudery   122
psyche   9
pulmonal orb   165, 178, 38
pulse diagnosis   12, 13
pulse diagnosis, complete, time required   200
pulse diagnosis, in Japan   199
pulses of the ear   204
pulses of the foot   **204**
pulses of the hand   **204**
pulses, accelerated   227, 230, **232**, 247
pulses, adherent   227, 230
pulses, agitated   227, 230
pulses, brief   227, 229
pulses, deep   227
pulses, dispersed   230, 230
pulses, evanescent   226, 228, 230
pulses, exhausted   226, 226, 230, **232**, 246
pulses, fixed   227, 229, 247
pulses, flooding   227, 228, 229, 246
pulses, frail   226, 230
pulses, grating   218, 227, 228, 230
pulses, in gynecology and obstetrics   247
pulses, infirm   226, 230, 246
pulses, intermittent   227, 230
pulses, languid   228, 229
pulses long   227, 229

pulses, medium   239, 250
pulses, middle   **209**
pulses, minute   226, 230
pulses, mobile   230
pulses, onion-stalk   226, 230, 247
pulses, palpation of   **193**
pulses, pedal   36
pulses, pedal, requiring greater pressure   209
pulses, racing   230
pulses, radial   **205**
pulses, recondite   230, 247
pulses, replete   227, 230, **232**
pulses, representative, on the head, hand and foot   **204**
pulses, slippery   228, 230, 227
pulses, slowed down   230, **232**
pulses, soft   226, 230
pulses, stringy   218, 227, 229, 247
pulses, submerged   **209**, 216, 227, 229, **232**, 239, 250
pulses, superficial   **209**, 227, 229, **231**, 239, 246, 250
pulses, tense   228, 230
pulses, tympanic   227, 230
pulse, accelerated   **211**, 226
pulse, adherent   **223**
pulse, agitated   **222**
pulse, brief   **214**
pulse, depleted   **212**
pulse, depth of   **209**
pulse, dispersed   **220**
pulse, evanescent   **215**
pulse, exhausted   **212**
pulse, fixed   **219**
pulse, flooding   **214**

pulse, frail   **219**
pulse, grating   **213**
pulse, infirm   **220**
pulse, intermittent   **223**
pulse, languid   217, 225
pulse, large   **215**
pulse, length of   **209**
pulse, long   **213**
pulse, minute   **220**
pulse, mobile   **222**
pulse, onion-stalk   **218**
pulse, pedal, finding the - pulse   234
pulse, racing   **223**
pulse, recondite   **221**, 226
pulse, replete   **212**
pulse, short   218
pulse, site of the   29
pulse, slippery   **212**
pulse, slippery   226
pulse, slowed down   **211**, 225
pulse, small   **221**
pulse, soft   **219**
pulse, specific   29
pulse, stringy   **217**
pulse, submerged   **210**, 226
pulse, superficial   **210**, 226
pulse, tense   **216**, 226
pulse, tympanic   **218**
pulse, vibrating   216
pulse, width of   **209**
purgation   53
purgatives   107
purges, with cold, bitter laxatives   106
purging, excessive   186
qualification, synthetic, of factors   9
qualitative conventions   103
qualitative standards   **17**
qualitative standards   32
qualitative statements   12
quality   17, 28, .31, 32
quality standards, of the triple yang, and tripe yin   100
quality, specific, of a personality   129
quantitative statements   12
questioning, cf. interrogation   179
quiescence   20

race   124
radiation   18
rapport, re-establishing the   78
rational considerations   31
rational integration, stringend   7
re-action   18
receptors, sensory   19
recovery, of the orthopathy   217
red   125
redundancy   254, 49
redundancy, energetic   25, 53
redundancy, of active energy   35
refinement, degree of - , of the active energies   146
reflection   **62**, 30
reflection, exaggerated   190
reflection, excessive   62
regularity, movement of the body   123
regulation, of the energy flow   108
regulation, quantitative distribution of energy   109
relations   13
relationships   13
relations, functional   26
relection, continuity of   123
remedies, aiding diuretic elimination   99

271

remedies, augmenting structive energy 97
remedies, bolstering the active energies 98
remedies, bolstering the structive basis 89
remedies, bolstering the yang 97
remedies, clearing the heat 99
remedies, clearing the passages of energy 89
remedies, cold 44
remedies, cold 49, 90
remedies, completing 76
remedies, completing the active energies 82
remedies, cooling 83, 90
remedies, diuretic 83
remedies, draining the humidity of phlegm 89
remedies, dynamizing 82
remedies, enhancing the structive energies 91
remedies, exteriorizing activity 82
remedies, hot 49
remedies, humectating 76
remedies, laxative 79
remedies, leading back the glare to its source 97
remedies, leading down the active energy 89
remedies, lifting up 82
remedies, moistening the pulmonal orb 89
remedies, nourishing 98
remedies, suppletive 98
remedies, transformative 90
remedies, transforming water 97
remedies, warm 97, 44, 82, 90
remedies, warm and opening 78
renal orb 163, 188, 46, 6
renal orb, affections of 184
renal orb, predominance of the energies of 166
repletion 150, 173, 21, 213, 230, 32, 49, 79, 81, 82, 99, 85
repletion of calor 222
repletion of energy in the large intestine orb 92
repletion of the energies of the orbs 51
repletion of the individually specific structive energy 51
repletion of the surface 181
repletion of xue 178
repletion symptoms 174, 48, 50, 52
repletion, by an exogenous heteropathy 183
repletion, especially of the oo. cardialis et intestinorum 175
repletion, false 54
repletion, spurious, of the yang renale 98
reserves, constitutional, reflected upon the tongue 138
reserves, orthopathic 114
reservoir, constitutional 36
reservoir, regulating 84
resilience 111
resistance 24
resoluteness 68
response, pathological 57
restitution, of the energy flow 77
reticular conduits 103
reticular conduits, affections superficial of 170
return of cold 109
return of yang 151
reversal of direction 53
rhythmic control 108
rhythmic cue 87
rhythmic distribution of energies 160
rhythm, disruption of 87
rhythm, respiratory 174
right (side) 20
ritual, religious 18
rootless yang 182
roots 243

root, of an individual's life 94
rope, twisted 216
saliva, inspection of **171**
salty food, addiction to 175
sapor 28
sapors 188, 21, 21
science, critical 124
science, exact 5
science, rational 56
scientific system 31
scleras 162
season 28
secretions 116
secundovection 126
sedation 69
self observation 12
self-assertion 74
self-confidence 74
sensations, of temperature **179**
senses 121
sensitivity of the fingers, impaired 200
sensitivity of the fingers, in pulse diagnosis 194
separation, of clear and murky energies 82
sequences, phase- 23
sequence, pathological 24
sexpartite conventions 101
sexpartite cycle 100
sexpartite terms 102
sexual excesses 40
sex, differences of - influencing reading the pulse 246
shape of the body of the tongue, in diagnosis 138
shape, of the body 80
shoulders 103
sickroom, odour of 178
side, lower 20
side, upper 20
significance, universal 17
signs, reassuring, of diagnosis 126
signs, somber 126
similarity 15
simplicity 11
sinarteries 113, 114, 66, 73
sinarteriology 100, 102
sinartery 28
sinking down 21
sinuses 131
sites of the eye, correspondences of **162**
situation, pathological 57
situation, present 9
skills, extraordinary 121
skin 113, 162, 169, 175, 178, 27, 39, 48, 90
skin, colour of 124
skin, colour tint of 126
skin, healthy tints of 126
skin, inspection of 171
skull, top of 66, 69
sleekness, of shape and bodily form 127
sleep **190**
small intestine orb, special symptoms related to 78
small intestine 27, 59
small intestine and urinary bladder orbs 111
smallness 20
smell 28
softening, of the energies of the o. hepaticus 71
softness 21
soma 9
somatization 19
sorrow 57, **62**
sour food, addiction to 175
species affection 184

species-symptom   43
species-symptoms   40
speech, auditive diagnosis of   **173**
speech, distinct articulation of   123
spleen   27
spleen orb   62
splendor yang syndrome   211
spring   20, 23, 58
stability of function   15, 4
stages of disease, most dangerous   111
stagnating xue   159
stagnation, breaking up of   77
stamina   111
standards   32
standards, conventional   **17**
standards, qualitative   **17**
standards, qualitative   20, 22, 32
statements, qualitative   13
statements, quantitative   12
stimuli, outward   114, 80
stomach   27
stomach orb   165, 167, 178
stomach orb, radiation of the active energies of the -   142
stomach qi, loss of   126
stomach, entrance of   132
stomach, exit of   132
stomach, middle of   132
storage capacity, for energies   94
storage of fluids   98
strain, constitutional   105
strength of the orthopathy   180
strength, of muscles and sinews   127
stress   255, 40, 46, 63
stress, abnormal   94
stress, emotional   81
stress, extreme   89
stress, nervous   97
stringency   121, 3, 17
stringency, of pulse diagnosis   196
stringency, rational   121
stripping the patient   122
struction   **18**
struction   34
structive aspect   103
structive check   23, 24
structive energies   104, 111, 94
structive energies, deficiency of   159
structive energies, depleted   153
structive energies, exhaustion of   255
structive energies, general deficiency of   140
structive energies, imminent depletion of   154
structive energies, of the renal orb   97
structive energies, state of   130
structive energies, symptoms of primary affections of the   180
structive energies, very powerful   190
structive energy   109, 228, 115
structive energy, depletion of   139
structive energy, individually specific   21, 114, **115**, 61, 66, 67, 69, 70, 73, 75
structive energies, deficiency of   160
structive fluids   168
structive potential   21, 219, 27, 94, 96, 181, 156
structive potential, impaired   213
structive potential, transformation of   70
structive reserves   168
structive restiveness   48
structivity   103, **18**, 22
structivity, actual   23
structivity, extreme   59

structivity, potential   23
structivity, total loss of   37
structure, particular, of the coating of the tongue   130
substratum   17, 27, 9, 2
summer   20, 23
sun   20
surface   20, 39, 42, 58
surface, of the body   103, 114, 27, 57
sustenance, of the body   115
sweets   60
symbols   17, 18
symptoms   101, 31, 32, 56
symptoms, congestive   67
symptoms, critical, of the pulse   252
symptoms, dangerous   61
symptoms, false   46
symptoms, related to the cardial and large intestine orbs   79
symptoms, related to the orbis aulicus   104
symptoms, specific, of the stomach orb   84
symptoms, striking   33
symptoms, thermic   44
symptoms, transitory   43
synthesis of individual factors   15
synthesis, inductive   11, **4**, 5
synthesis, inductive, in medical practice   7
synthetic view   155
systematization   7
system, metric   17

taste quality   28
technical capacities   94
techniques, complicated   121
technology, complex   14
teeth   204, 94
teeth and gums, inspection of   **167**
temperate diseases   65
temperature, sensations of   **179**
temple pulse   **203**
tendency, energetic   31
tension   62, 63
tepid diseases   113
terror syndrome   108
theoretical background, of pulse diagnosis   198
theories, abstract   113
theory, sinarteriological   102
therapeutic agents   10
therapeutic measures, wrong   110
therapy   32
therapy, wrong   107
thermic symptoms   44
three heated spaces   **116**
throath, inner inspection of   **168**
time   28
tongue   13, 34, 73
tongue diagnosis   **129**, 130
tongue, conduits touching the -   129
tongue, diagnostic correspondence of   132
tongue, mobility of   140
total loss of energy   38
total loss of structivity   37
total loss of yang   112, **36**
total loss of yin   **36**
traits, general, common   15
transformation   23
transformation of energy   108
transformation of fluids   98
transformation of food   91
transformation of structive potential   70
transformation, of energy   80
transformation, of sticky mucus   77

transition 23
transportation of food 91
treatment, effective 6
treatment, incorrect 105
treatment, pharmacotherapeutic 100
tricalorium **116**, 27, 59
true energy 36
true symptoms 53
true yang 33
true yin 33
trunk 21
unfoldments, specific 126, 29
unity 22
univocality 13
univocality 17, 7
uplifting 21
upper side 20
urinary bladder 27
urinary bladder orb 98
urination, inspection of **172**
use, excessive, of tonics 222
varied diseases 65
ventus heteropathies 184
ventus heteropathy 189
victory/return situation 109
violation sequence 23, 24
vision **189**
vital resources, withering of 96
vocal manifestation 28
voice, auditive diagnosis of **173**
vomitus, inspection of **171**
warm ariditas 61
warm heteropathy 113
warmth 20
warmth, lack of 89
water 20, 38, 58
water, cold 49
weak function, of the orbes lienalis et stomachi 98
weakness 20, 221
weaknesses, constitutional 9, 81, 53, 74
weakness, of the orthopathy 166
white 125
width, of the pulse **209**
will power 111
wind 56, 57, 58, 90
wind heteropathy in the hepatic orb 167
wind, cold-induced 173
winter 160, 20, 23
winter 23, 58
wood 58
wounds 223
wrath 191, 57, **61**
wrath, irascibility 56
wrath, suppressed 68
wrists, appearance of 169

yang 103, **18**, 32, **33**
yang, collapsing 35
yang fluids, deficiency of 136
yang, vigorous 109, 35
yang symptoms 48
yang, triple 100
yang, uncontrolled, smashes into the species 215
yellow 125
yielding yin 100, 109
yin 103, 32, **33**
yin enfeebled 35
yin flectens diseases **109**, 110
yin fluids 139
yin reduced 35
yin, vigorous 35, 109

yin2 **18, 18**
yin, triple 100
zero 22

INDEX OF SYMPTONS

abdomen hard 115
abdomen swollen 36
abdomen, bloated 50, 51
abdomen, congested 52
abdomen, distended 175, 55, 71
abdomen, distended 97, 103
abdomen, hard 105, 175, 52
abdomen, hard and tender 151
abdomen, painful 106
abdomen, painful 153, 191
abdomen, pains in the 165
abdomen, swollen 55
abdomen, tender 115, 103
abdomen, tense 105, 106, 115, 153, 51, 52
abdomen, tumescent 82
abdomen, turgescent 62
abdominal pains 185
abdominal pains, after birth 184
abhorrence of cold 47, 48
abhorrence of heat 180, 47
absence, of menstruation 191
absentmindedness 124
accumulation, of pituita (phlegm) 110
actions, contradictory 63
acuity of vision, reduced 189
aggravation by cold 37, 41
aggravation by heat 37
aggravation of symptoms at night 180
aggravation of symptoms during the day 180
aggravation of symptoms, at dusk 117
agitation 128
alopecia 156
alternation of cold and fever 110
alternation, between constipation and diarrhea 63
alternation, between fever and cold 42
alternation, between heat and cold 180
alternation, of heat and shivering 107
anguish 222
anorexia 42, 54
anus, inflamed 92
anus, swollen 92
anxiety 115, 126
aphasia 140
aphthae 75, 78
apoplectic stroke 103
apoplexy 140, 141, 162
appearance, swollen 97
appearance, turgid 97
appearance, wasted 33
appetite **186**
appetite, complete loss of 83
appetite, increased 85
appetite, lack of 107
appetite, loss of 68, 43, 50, 60
appetite, poor 71
appetite, reduced 52, 62, 77, 82, 98
apprehension 115, 126
arthritic swellings 169
ascites 81, 95, 98
ascites, especially in the legs 97
asthma 174, 50, 75, 95
asthmatic states 75
asthma, aggravated by movement 75
atrophies 68
atrophy 169
atrophy of the genitals 36
atrophy, of the penis 63

back, inability to bend the 128
back, painful 97
back, stiff 51
back, weak 71
bad breath **178**
bad smell from the mouth 85
behaviour, erratic 63
behaviour, noisy 34
being cold 179
bent up in bed, patient 128
bitter taste 115
bland taste of food 36
bleeding gums 168
bloody secretions, from the nose 90
blindness at night 190
bloating, of the midriff region 51
block of digestion 108, 71
bloody faeces 92
blood, admixtures, in the sputum, nasal discharge, urine, faeces 116
blood, coughing up of 72
body bloated 53
body of the tongue, deeply red 36
" ,dry 36
" ,pale 35, 36
" ,red, slightly moist 35
" ,black **137**
" ,black 48
" ,blood-cloured **136**
" ,blue **137**
" ,blue in the centre only 137
" ,blue red stripes on the 77
" ,bright red 42
" ,covered by sticky mucus 145
" ,dard red 51, 53
" ,dark 52
" ,deep crimson **135**
" ,deep red 72
" ,drastically shrunken 154
" ,dry 37, 51, 70
" ,elastic 140
" ,hard 45, 140
" ,intensely red 111, 114, 115, 116, 140, 150, 34, 72, 76, 77, 78, 78, 88, 90, 91, 97, 97
" , pale **135**, 34, 41, 45, 59, 77, 78, 82, 89, 92, 95, 96, 98
" ,pale red 84
" ,paretic **141**
" ,pink 45
" ,puffed **139**
" ,purple 116, **137**, 142, 51, 52
" ,quivering **141**
" ,red 37, 38, 38, 59, 61, 69
" ,scarlet 115, 117, **136**, 34, 53, 76, 85, 136
" ,shrunken **140**, 45
body of the tongue, shrunken, parched 131
body of the tongue, soft 34
body of the tongue, stiff 140
body of the tongue, swollen 34
body of the tongue, swollen 43
body of the tongue, whitish 97
body of the tongue, with cinnabar coloured dots and streaks 145
body of the tongue, with purple spots on its margin 51
body, cold 148
body, decrepit 124
body, emaciated 52

275

body, hot   53
body, limp   124
borders of the eyelids, red   117
breath loud   34
breathing audible   54
breathing heavy   36
breathing irregular   63
breathing though mouth   50
breathing, accelerated   63, 174
breathing, difficult, through the mouth   174
breathing, feeble   34
breathing, heavy   34, 115, 37, 59
breathing, impeded   139, 50, 90
breathing, inaudible   37
breathing, irregular   190, 50
breathing, laboured   150, 164, 35, 54, 75, 77, 82, 84, 96
breathing, loud   104
breathing, rapid   59
breathing, shallow   51
breath, accelerated   124
breath, exhaled, feels hot   90
breath, fetid   41
breath, gasping for   51
breath, irregular   124
breath, panting   106
breath, panting, after slight movement   97
breath, rattling   34
breath, shallow   106, 62
breath, shortness of   71, 87, 96, 50, 51, 63
bronchitis   87
bronchopyelitis   87
buzz, of respiration   174

calor above, algor below   110
calves, aching   117
canthi, pale   163
cheeks red   35
cheeks, faintly pink   71
cheeks, intensely red   97
cheeks, red   36
cheeks, red spots on   50, 70
cheeks, red, in the afternoon   88
chest, pressure on   84
chilliness   180
chills   189
cholera   60, 81
chordapsus   68
clearing of throat, frequent   175
coating of the tongue black   34
coating of the tongue cracked   34
coating of the tongue dry   34, 35, 61, 76
coating of the tongue entirely lacking   154
coating of the tongue excessively thick   145
coating of the tongue missing   137
coating of the tongue moist   35, 37
coating of the tongue of loamy colour   34
coating of the tongue sleek   34
coating of the tongue slippery   34
" ,slippery or sticky on a blue body   137
" ,thin   40
" ,thin, whitish   145
" ,with protuberances   34
" ,with white and yellow patches   152
" ,yellow   34, 35
" ,absence of   **144**
" ,ash-coloured   **150**
" ,black   115, **150**
" black, limited to the tip   151
" ,black, with pointed protuberances   117
" ,colourless   75
" ,colourless   98
" ,cracked   76
" ,different colours showing simultaneously   **152**
" ,dry   106, 116, 185, 53, 61, 69, 92
" ,fast   **143**
" ,glistening   70
" ,glistening   98
" ,grey   40
" ,increased in thickness   114
" ,increased in thickness   44
" ,lacking   44
" ,leathery and yellow   117
" ,little   97
" ,loose   **143**, 143
" ,lustrous   145
" ,missing   35
" ,missing   78
" ,missing, on a pale body of the tongue   135
" ,moist   142
" ,moist   **146**, 34, 43, 45
" ,murky-coloured   43
" ,no   72
" ,not extending to the tip   41
" ,parched   115
" ,parched and black   151
" ,partial or complete   **144**
" ,putrid, slimy   **146**
" ,reduced   70, 76, 77, 88, 91, 97
" ,reduced in thickness   72
" ,rough   53
" ,slightly sticky   115
" ,slippery   182, 41, 44, 70, 85, 90, 92
" ,sticky   117, 142, **146**, 53, 69, 71, 83, 83, 84, 89
coating of the tongue, thick   **146**
" ,thin   98, 114, **146**, 41, 58, 59, 68, 71, 90, 90, 92, 95, 96, 98
" ,thin white   41, 83, 84
" ,thin, yellow   71
" ,true   143
" ,wet   98
" ,white   114, 142, **147**, 176, 185, 41, 44, 58, 59, 70, 71, 71, 77, 79, 82, 82, 83, 84, 85, 90, 91, 92
" ,white and sticky   77
" ,white and thin   78
" ,white to yellow   151
" ,whitish   114, 61, 90, 95, 40, 75, 96
coating of the tongue, whitish, moist   59
" ,whitish, thin   89
" ,with pointed protuberances   115
" ,with pointed protuberances   61
" ,yellow   106, 115, 117, 139, 182, 185, 40, 42, 43, 59, 61, 69, 69, 78, 83, 85, 89, 92, 99
" ,yellow and dry   115, 90
" ,yellow and sticky   92
" ,yellow to black   44
" ,yellowish   53
" ,yellow, heavy   149
" ,to grey   116
cold   42
cold beverages, desire for   48
cold extremities   75
cold within   34
cold without   34
coldness of the body   34
collapse, sudden   141
coloration, diffuse   161
coma   116
complexion, bluish-green   126
" ,dark   46

"   ,dark, blackish   **160**
"   ,dull   161
complexion, greenish   44, 53
"   ,greenish white   33
"   ,green, blue-green   **158**
"   ,intensely red   33
"   ,intermittently red   33
"   ,looking dirty   **158**
"   ,lustreless   161
"   ,pale   117, 36, 38, 44, 51, 82, 96
complexion, red   126, **158**, 44
"   ,sallow   159, 33, 59, 77
"   ,scarlet   **158**
"   ,shiny   163
"   ,shiny, white   148
"   ,waxy   89
"   ,white   126, **160**, 89
"   ,yellow   **159**, 83
"   ,yellowish   117, 53, 60
confusion, mental   164
congestion   170, 69, 169, 68
congestions, blocks of energy   74
congestion, in the chest   98
consciousness, impaired   117, 61
constipation   105, 106, 107, 115, 117, 117, 149, 184, 185, 187, 35, 43, 45, 46, 48, 52, 53, 54, 63, 68, 85, 91, 92, 97
contraction, of the scrotum   70
contravection   110
contravections   109
contravective energy   52
convulsion   59, 116, 126, 50, 51, 51, 60
coordination disturbed, of the muscles of the eyes, mouth, face   141
cough   114, 116, **176**, 35, 43, 44, 61, 63, 72, 84, 87, 88, 89, 97, 98
cough, accompanied by perspiration and enuresis   96
"   ,blaring   90
"   ,chronic   128
"   ,chronic   88
"   ,producing thin phlegm   90
"   ,with copious expectoration   91
"   ,worse during the night   91
covered up tightly, patient in bed   128
crying   34
crying   46
crying and laughing, without reason   76
curling up in bed   44
curling up in bed, patient   111
cyanosis, of lips and nails   98
daze   58
dazedness   115, 117, 221, 40, 59, 59, 60, 83, 91, 96, **188**, 68, 69
deafness   70
deafness, temporary   50
defecation, brings no relief   92
defecation, frequent   82
defecation, inanbility of   51
demanding hot beverages   34
demeanour, erratic   61
dementia   75
desire for cold beverages   37
desire for cold drinks   76, 85
desire for cold food   45
desire for hot beverages   187
desire for small quantities of hot beverages   111
desire for warm beverages   37
desire for warm drinks   82
desire for warm food   45
desire to shut oneself off   63
despondency   51, 63

diabetes   110, 117, 95
diaphoresis brings relief   106
diarrhea, morning-   51
diarrhea   71, 108, 112, 117, 148, 150, 35, 40, 41, 41, 43, 45, 46, 50, 54, 59, 59, 60, 60, 62, 63, 78, 81, 82, 82, 83, 84, 91, 92
diarrhea, brings no relief   68
diarrhea, containing undigested food   98
diarrhea, continuous   110
diarrhea, general   36
diarrhea, in the morning   36
diarrhea, including undigested food   84
diarrhea, liquid   48
diarrhea, persistent   92
diarrhea, severe   215
diarrhea, thin   48
diarrhea, very intense   110
diarrhea, with shivering   110
digestion, depressed   51
digestion, sluggish   60, 85
digestion, weak   82, 83, 82
diphtheria   168
distension, abdominal   78
distrust   76
dizziness   107, 126, 128, **183**, 36, 36, 50, 50, 51, 51, 54, 58, 71, 78, 97
dreams, numerous   70
dropsy   163
dumbness   58
dysentery   60, 92
emaciation   160, 62
"   ,general   82
emphysema   128
enfeeblement   63
enuresis   51, 95, 98
epilepsy   127, 68, 68
epistaxis   75, 76, 87
eructation   104, **177**, 68, 81, 83
"   ,foul   50, 63
eructations, malodorous   71
eructations, of clear fluids   85
eructations, sour   50, 63, 71
eructation, sounds of   **176**
exhaustion   71
evacuations, murky   60
evening meal, undigested   177
exanthema   115, 44, 47, 116
exanthema, pustule-   58
exanthema, spurious   53
excitability   68
excitation   76
excretion of urine, copious   175
exhaustion   108, 51
exhaustion, mental   51
exophthalmus   164
expecoration of malodorous pus   90
"   ,bloodstreaked   61
"   ,clear to whitish   45
"   ,containing bloody streaks   88
"   ,copious   45
"   ,copious   91
"   ,frequent   171
"   ,lacking in spite of cough   176
"   ,much   62
"   ,of great quantities of thin phlegm   97
"   ,of opaque phlegm   175
"   ,of thick, sticky phlegm   89
"   ,of thick, yellow phlegm   90
"   ,thick   176
"   ,thin   45
"   ,thin, clear   89

```
"       ,yellow           176
"       ,yellow and thick      45
extremities warm       37
extremities, cold         110, 150, 176, 185, 41, 43, 47, 58,
82, 92, 98
extremities, contracted       69
"       ,painful       110
"       ,paretic       51
"       ,swollen       53
"       ,twitching       50
"       ,warm       45
"       ,weak       91
"       ,cold       68
eyelids, dark coloured       163
"       ,painful       69
"       ,paralysis of       58
"       ,red-borderd       69
"       ,red-bordered       72
"       ,shining       163
"       ,sore, inflamed       163
"       ,twitching       50
eyes, clear       44
eyes, tearing       44
eyes, tearing       58
eyes, white open       44
eye, entire, red and swollen       163

face sunken       54
face, fallen       62
face, flushed       117
face, haggard       52, 53
face, hot       70
"       ,hot, red       69
face, pale       62, 95
face, red       111, 117, 42, 46, 53, 54, 61, 62, 70, 76
face, sallow       95
face, tumescence of       91
face, white, diaphanous       96
facing away, patient - from the room       128
faeces, containing dry clots       48
faeces, bloody       92
faeces, difficult to expell       34
faeces, dried up       90
faeces, extremely malodorous       48
faeces, hard       34
faeces, liquid       45
faeces, malodorous       34
faeces, purulent       92
faeces, red and white       60
faeces, smelling of fish or meat       34
faeces, soft       83, 84
faeces, solid       90
faltering menstruation       191
fatigue       117, 148, 62, 83
fatigue, extreme       83
"       ,extreme       91
"       ,great       90
"       ,intense       77
fear       75
feeling of a lump in the stomach       85
feeling, oppressive, in the region of the heart       190
feet, weakness of       36
fever       104, 105, 107, 114, 116, 117, 180, 221, 34, 42,
44, 58, 61, 83, 90, 90, 92
fevers, adynamic       115
"       ,intermittent       51
"       ,malarialike       115
"       ,periodic       115
"       ,periodic       88, 78
fever,       40
"       ,accompanied by perspiration       61
```

```
"       ,after extreme loss of body fluids       36
"       ,high       115, 47
"       ,high during the night       115
"       ,high, during the hours of the night       116
"       ,light       148
"       ,no       111
"       ,nocturnal       51
"       ,periodic       185, 35
fever, rising and falling periodically       115
"       ,rising highest during the night       117
"       ,slight       35
"       ,with restlessness       35
"       ,with shuddering       41
"       ,with shuddering       90
"       ,without perspiration       43
"       ,without perspiration       59
"       ,tips cold       256
fingers and toes, cold       150
flanks, painful       68
flare, of the ministerial fire of the pericardial orb
109
flexus       109
flexus spasms       117
fluid stools       50
fluids (juices), deficiency of       51
fluor albus       191
flutter of the heart       117
fontanels, depressed       155
fontanels, protruding       155
food, undigested, blocking the intestines       110
food, vomited immediately after ingestion       110
forehead, temperature higher than palms       256
forgetfulness       51, 62, 75, 75, 77, 97
fright       222
fullness       42
functions, sexual       94

gasping       175
gasping for air       167
gasping for breath, patient       128
gaze, tired       124
gaze, unsteady       124
glimmer, unusual of the eyes       163
gnashing the teeth       168
gooseflesh       59
gums, bleeding       85
gums, painful       85
gums, swollen       168, 85
gums, ulcerated       85
gums, white as the teeth       168
hair brittle       156
hair, dry       156
hair, stiff       156
hands and feet, clammy       63
hands and feet, cold       111, 84
hands and feet, remarkably warm       108
hands and feet, tumescence of       91
hands, groping aimlessly       106
hands, restlessly groping       128
hardness of hearing       117, 162, 189
headache       104, 114, 116, 149, **183**, 189, 40, 41, 42, 43,
51, 58, 59, 59, 68, 69, 90, 148, 40, 104, 61
headache, piercing       69
head, hot       69
hearing, hardness of       78
hearing, reduced acuity of       95
heart ache       75
heart attacks       110, 75
heat       35
heat congestion       106
heat on top, cold in the extremities       109
```

heat sensations 51
heat within 34
heat without 34
heat, inner 44, 52, 63
heat, oppressive 106, 117, 180, 41, 42, 72, 40
hematomas 169, 51, 68
hematuria 75, 76, 95, 140
hemoptea 176, 75, 76, 81, 87, 68
hemorrhage, profuse, from the nose and mouth 69
" ,sudden 69
hemorrhoids 167
hernias 68
hiccup 177, 83, 85
hiccup, sounds of **176**
high temparature 61
hight fever, yet no shuddering 106
hips, aching 117
hoarseness 88
horizontal position, unbearabe 50, 174, 175
hot flushes 105, 111, 180, 97
hot palms 255
hunger pangs 75
hunger, despite the absence of appetite 110
hunger, yet no appetite 188
icterus 169, 60, 81
ideas, whimsical 51
imagianation, lack of 51
impotency 36, 95, 96
inability of defecation 51
indurations 68
indurations, below the skin 58
indurations, in the abdomen 68
infiltrations, liquid, throughout the body 97
influenza type affections 87
initiative, lack of 51
insanity 117
insomnia 111, 115, 117, 117, **190**, 43, 51, 68, 71, 75, 78, 88, 97
irascibility 61, 72
iris, outcurving 163
irresolution 63
ischiatic pains 184
joints, painful 107, 175, 60
joints, tense 107
knees, weak and painful 71
lassitude 111, 174, 184, 59, 98
lassitude, fatigue 182
" ,great 115
laughter, convulsive 51
leaning back, when sitting 128
leaning forward, patient, when sitting 128
legs swollen 36
legs, stretched out, patient in bed with - 128
legs, weak 97, 78, 96
lethargy 91
limbs, heavy 184, 190
limpness, numbness, of hands and feet 50
lips, as if painted with cinnabar 36
lips intensely red 35
lips, as if covered by a black veil 167
lips, bluish 44
lips, cracked 117, 33, 44, 47, 51, 92
lips, deep red 42
lips, dry 33, 44
lips, green, blue-green **167**
lips, incessantly licked 142
lips, pale **167**, 36, 44, 51
lips, scarlet 97
lips, swollen 44
lips, violet 44

lip, upper, white spots inside 167
listlessness 117, 148, 62
loins, aching 96, 97
loins, painful and weak 91
loins, weak 78
loquaciousness 34
loss of appetite 117, 41, 43, 60, 83
loss of hair 156
loss of semen 51, 75, 75, 91, 95, 97
loss of semen during sleep 36, 97, 63, 78
loss of sensitivity 68
loss of voice 88
lower extremities, painful and weak 91
lower eyelid, swollen 164
lump in the stomach, feeling of 83, 85, 115, 71
lump, in the plexus region 77
madness, raving 105, 116
malaria 127, 60, 60
measles 166
membrane on the fauces 168
menses, irregular 77
menstruation, advanced 190
menstruation, faltering 191
mental disease 75
micturition impaired 117
micturition, difficult 190
micturition, disturbed 76
micturition, frequent 105, 46
micturition, impeded 36
micturition, irregularities 103
middle finger cold 256
middle finger hot 256
mind, disturbed 76
miscarriage 81
mouches volantes 36
mouth and tongue, dry 117
mouth, breathing through the 174
mouth, dry 190, 36, 41, 42, 46, 69, 70, 88, 97, 92
mouth, open 167
mouth, surroundings of, bluish tinge 167
movements, erratic 61
movements, uncoordinated of the eyes 164
muscles, painful 51
muscles, tense 51
muttering 174
mutter, repetitive 174
napping, with half open eyelids 164
natural warmth, lack of 89
nausea 104, 115, 117, 149, 41, 42, 43, 45, 60, 75, 77
neck, stiff 107, 41, 69
neoplasias 68
nervousness 111, 77, 78
night blindness 70
nightmares 36, 71, 75, 76
noise, rumbling, in the intestines 78
nose, dry 61, 90
nose, hot 176
nose, stopped up 40, 60
nose, stuffed-up 58, 61
nose, swollen 60
nostrils, runny, cold 166
numbness 58
oppressive heat 34
orbit, swelling of 163
pain 170, 230
pain, improved by pressure 78
pain in the neck, intense 104
pains **182**
pains around the navel 51
pains around the small ribs 51
pains in the abdomen 51

279

```
pains in the body            90
pains in the centre of the abdomen       51
pains in the chest           51
pains in the joints          104, 41
pains in the loins           59, 36
pains througout the body     41
pains, abdominal             150, 35, 40, 41, 59, 59, 60, 68, 79
pains, abdominal, improved by pressure     34, 50
pains, abdominal, increased by pressure    34
pains, abdominal, sudden     43
pains, abdominal, with diarrhea          41
pains, abdominal, aggravated by pressure   43
pains, acute                 128
pains, acute of the heart    75
pains, around the small ribs            115
pains, below the small ribs             69
pains, burning               75
pains, diffeuse              40
pains, diffuse throughout the body       104, 184, 43, 59
pains, improved by pressure              54
pains, in the abdomen        165
pains, in the back           184, 59, 79
pains, in the body           148
pains, in the chest          61, 89, 90
pains, in the extremities    51
pains, in the eyes           189, 71
pains, in the flanks         51
pains, in the head and neck             104
pains, in the joints         184
pains, in the loins          95
pains, in the neck           59
pains, in the penis          78
pains, in the stomach        63
pains, ischiatic             41
pains, lancinating, around de navel     51
pains, of hands and feet     169
pains, piercing, in the chest           87
pains, radiating into the loins         79
pains, radiating into the shoulders     184
pains, radiating into the testicles     79
pains, sharp, in the chest              72
pains, stabbing              77
pains, stabbing, in the abdomen         105
pains, stabbing, in the heart           76
pains, throughout the body              43
pains, wandering, in all joints         58
pain, abdominal              55
pain, improved by the application of pressure      85
pain, in the abdomen         70
pain, in the lower abdomen, dull        78
pain, in the region of the heart        110
pain, in the stomach         71
pain, in the stomach region, improved by warm applications  85
pain, intense, during an advanced stage of phthisis     184
pain, persistent, in the stomach region          84
pain, prolonged              216
palms hot                    36
palpitations                 108, 111, 115, 126, 190, 36, 50, 62, 75, 76, 77, 78, 89
palms cold                   256
palms, temperature higher than forehead          256
panting           104, 115, 124, 164, 174, 182, 190, 34, 35, 46, 52, 89
panting, loud                90
paralysis                    95
paralysis, of the eyelids               58
paralysis, of the facial muscles        58
paralysis, of the feet                  36
paralysis, unilateral                   69
pareses                      58, 69, 70, 95
pareses, spastic             127, 68
pareses, unilateral          69
paresthesias, of the extremities         70
parotitis                    162
patient enfeebled            33
patient in bed, with legs extended       44
patient reclining            33
patient, reluctant to move              33
periodic fevers              180
persecution mania            63
perspiration                 110, 115, 116, 166, 181, 44, 59, 60
perspiration,                41
perspiration, absolute                  182
perspiration, cold           37
perspiration, constant       41
perspiration, constant       59
perspiration, during sleep              181, 35, 36, 51, 62, 63, 76, 78, 88, 91, 97
perspiration, excessive      105
    ",fitful                 41
    ",flush of, brings relief            60
    ",great propensity for               84
    ",heavy                  36, 51, 59
perspiration, hot            37
    ",lack of                48
    ",limited to the forehead            182
    ",limited to the head                182
perspiration, no             104, 149, 34, 41, 43, 61, 90, 114
perspiration, of salty taste            37
perspiration, profuse        105, 106, 141, 59
perspiration, reduced        114
perspiration, spontaneous               104, 180, 181, 36, 43, 63, 75, 89, 50
perspiration, sticky         37
perspiration, trepidation-              182
phlegm, flowing from the mouth          69
phlegm, rattle of            89
phlegm, rattle of            96
phlegm, sticky               88
phlegm, thin                 90
phthisic disease             218
phthisis                     215, 87
physiognomy, exhausted looking           71
physiognomy, waxen           75
plethora, abdominal          148
pollicar pulses, weak        38
polyuria, during the night              78
pores, wide open             181
pressure, on the chest       42
pressure, on the chest       44
prickling, in the fingers and toes       117
pricks and fissures, on the body of the tongue     138
prolapsus ani                82, 92
prostration                  117, 46
prostration, extreme         63, 92
prostration, great           44, 44, 60, 89
prostration, nervous         174
protuberances, on the body of the tongue          150
puffing                      175
pulsations                   69
pulses, accelerated          105, 114, 115, 116, 177, 182, 190, 34, 35, 36, 37, 40, 42, 45, 46, 47, 53, 61, 69, 70, 72, 75, 76, 78, 79, 83, 85, 88, 90, 91, 92, 97, 98, 99
pulses, agitated             117
pulses, dispersed            75
pulses, evanescent           111, 111, 150, 34, 37, 38, 59, 92, 117
pulses, exhausted            148, 177, 36, 37, 38, 59, 75, 78, 89, 96, 98
pulses, feeble               54
```

pulses, fixed   51
pulses, flooding   105, 115, 116, 117, 34, 35, 36, 37, 38, 45, 47, 61
pulses, frail   108, 115, 117, 53, 77, 82, 83, 83, 85, 91
pulses, full   117
pulses, grating   34, 51, 53, 77
pulses, hard, narrow, weak   182
pulses, infirm   34, 37, 43, 47, 75, 77, 82, 89, 91, 95, 96
pulses, languid   104, 108, 115, 116, 190, 41, 45, 53, 58, 71, 78, 92
pulses, large   34, 75
pulses, minute   107, 111, 117, 117, 150, 190, 34, 35, 37, 38, 45, 47, 53, 70, 71, 72, 75, 77, 78, 82, 83, 83, 84, 88, 91, 92, 95, 97, 98
pulses, mobile   116
pulses, onionstalk   37
pulses, powerful   54
pulses, racing   37, 38, 45, 75
pulses, replete   105, 106, 115, 174, 177, 34, 37, 38, 41, 48, 92
pulses, slippery   177, 34, 48, 76, 77, 79, 84, 85, 89, 92, 97
pulses, slowed down   177, 185, 191, 34, 35, 41, 45, 47, 54, 59, 70, 85, 98
pulses, stringy   107, 115, 117, 126, 42, 54, 68, 69, 70, 70, 71, 72, 79
pulses, strong   34, 45, 48
pulses, submerged   105, 106, 115, 150, 175, 182, 185, 34, 35, 41, 45, 47, 48, 53, 54, 59, 70, 77, 79, 84, 92, 96, 97, 98
pulses, superficial   104, 105, 114, 148, 182, 34, 37, 40, 41, 43, 47, 58, 59, 61, 90
pulses, tense   104, 110, 116, 40, 41, 43, 46, 59, 77, 90
pulses, weak   34, 35, 36, 45, 53, 185
pupils, contracted   50
pupils, dilated   50,
pupils, widely dilated   164

redness, of the canthi   163
redness, of the eyes and eyelids   189, 117
refusing food   34
relief after diaphoresis   106
reluctance to eat   85
reluctance to speak   174, 42, 46, 82, 89
repletive symptoms   53
respiration unstable   175
respiration, accelerated by slight movement   91
respiration, audible   117, 174
"   ,difficult   175
"   ,loud   174
"   ,nervous   175
"   ,noisy   174
"   ,slow   175
restiveness   107, 111, 40, 42, 43, 44, 46, 51, 61, 63, 71, 98
restless patient   33
restlessness   115, 117, 35, 46, 48, 63, 88
retching   104, 107
retching, sounds of   **176**
retention, complete, of urine   186
ringing of the ears   189
rise in temperature, slight   63
rise of temperature in the afternoon   116
rise of temperature in the afternoon   117
rise of temperature in the afternoon   180
rumble, noisy in the intestines   77
rumbling noise, in the intestines   82, 92, 59, 71
sadness   51
saliva, bubbly   171
saliva, continuous secretion of   171

saliva, foamy   171
saliva, much   45
satiety   84
scleras, red   42, 61, 44
scleras, white, strikingly limpid   163
scleras, yellow   163
scleras, yellow   83
sclerosis, multiple   138
scrotum, shrunken   51
secretion of saliva, reduced   85
secretions, bloody or pussy, from the nose   90
sensations, pricking, in the hands and feet   69
senses, dulled   174
sensitivity, excessive, to light   189
sensitivity, great to draft   104
sensitivity, loss of   69
septicemia   128
shivering   148, 169, 179, 34, 98
shivering, slight   116
shock   117, 140
shortness of breath   98, 175, 221, 34, 46, 52, 62, 63, 77, 84, 89
shortness of breath, when in a horizontal position   89
shoulders, pulling up the - when breathing   174
shuddering   104, 114, 128, 148, 149, 179, 180, 40, 41, 48, 58, 59, 59, 61, 77, 90
"   ,but no fever   111
"   ,moderate   107
"   ,without perspiration   43
sighing, frequent   174
sight, murky   42
sitting in water, sensation of   184
skin, cold   36, 37, 75, 96
skin, cool   38
skin, dry   51, 52
skin, hot   90
skin, itching   83
skin, purple   59
skin, warm   37
sleepiness   111
sleeplessness   41
sleep, disturbed   97, 77
sleep, fleeting   75
sleep, little   70
sleep, shallow   75
smallpox   166
smell of food, abhorrence of   83
smell of fresh meat   178
soles and palms, warmer than the back of feet and hands   117
soles hot, calves cold   256
somnolence   111, 190
spasms   59
spasms, abdominal   40
spasms, in the plexus region   107
spasms, infantile   127
spasms, with stiff neck   69
speech confused   115
speech confused, raving   174
speech, blurred   69
speech, confused   106, 117
speech, faltering   34, 82
speech, frequently interrupted   174
speech, halting   34, 82
speech, incoherent   110, 124, 174, 61
speech, raving   187, 34, 35, 76, 63
speech, reluctant   34, 84
speech, slow   50
spontaneous perspiration,   36
sputum sticky   84
sputum, bloody   63

sputum, clear   84
sputum, great qunantities of   50
sputum, with admixtures of blood   116
squinting   164
stare   106
stare, fixed   128, 164
stases   254
stiff neck   104
stomach ache   81, 92
stomach ache, aggravated by pressure   92
stomach region, turgescence in   83
stomach, feeling of coldness in   82
stomach, feeling of splashing fluid in   82
stomach, pains in the   63
stomach, rumbling in   50
stools, black   105, 51
stools, diarrheic   51
stools, dry   51
stools, easily avacuated   116
stools, fluid   81
stools, liquid   153
stools, loose   85
stools, malodorous   153, 92
stools, of black colour   116
stools, of white colour   51
stools, sticky   105
stools,hard   51
stroke   62
stroke   68
surfeit   108, 85
swearing   34, 46
sweetish taste   83
swellings, painful   222
swelling, of the eyelids   164
symptoms, congestive   67
symptoms, contravective   110
syncopes   68
syncope, sudden, with cold extremities   69

tachycardia   63
taste, bitter   107, 126, 188, 42, 43, 69, 71, 72, 83
taste, pungent   188
taste, salty   188
taste, sour   188
taste, stale   177
taste, stale   185, 188
taste, sweetish   188
teeth black   117
teeth, decayed   160
teeth, gnashing the   168
teeth, lookin like dried bones   168
teeth, looking like dry or polished stones   168
temperature difference, between abdominal side and back   180
temperature difference, between palms and back of hands   180
temperature falling immediately after a fit of perspiration   182
temperature subnormal after perspiration   182
temperature, elevated   46
temperature, high   40
temperature, rising and falling periodically   106
temperature, rising periodically at dusk   107
tenderness of the tongue   138
tensions, spastic   68
tension, abdominal, improved after defecation   78
tension, in the abdomen   70
tension, in the chest   107
tension, in the stomach region   84
tetanus   127, 128, 58

thirst   105, 112, 114, 185, 34, 35, 41, 41, 42, 45, 46, 48, 59, 61, 76, 83, 85
thirst, absence of   148, 152
thirst, after vomiting   187
thirst, desire for cold beverages   48
thirst, increasing in the afternoon   60
thirst, intense   104, 106, 90
thirst, lack of   37
thirst, massive   187
thirst, moderate   115
thirst, no   108, 150, 41, 45, 71
thirst, persistent   182, 182
thorax, congested   117
thorax, tense   50, 51
throat, dry   88, 107, 36, 42, 70, 72, 78
throat, irritated   52
throat, painful   168, 46, 72, 90
throat, sore   175, 97, 111, 117, 162, 176, 50, 58, 61, 61, 78
throat, swollen   46, 90
throwing off blankets, patient   128
tic convulsif   51
timidity   51
tinnitus   189, 50, 68, 69, 70, 78, 96, 97
tip of the nose, yellow   159
tired looking patient   33
tongue retracted   **142**
tongue, dry   42
tongue, margins of, intensely coloured   69
tongue, oscillating   69
tongue, oscillating between the lips   **142**
tongue, protruding   **141**
tongue, sticky   83
tongue, surface of - slippery   137
tongue, tip of, intensely coloured   69
tongue, ulcers on   75
tongue, white   37
toothache   85
treeth, decayed   178
trembling, intense   127
tremors   68
turgescence   68
turgidness   63
twitching of muscles   51
twitching of the head, uncontrolled   155
twitching of the mouth   127
twitching of the muscles   70
twitching, of the eyelids   127
twitching, of the fingers   127
twitching, of the muscles   69
tympanites   53, 54, 68, 81

ulcers, internal   171
ulcers, of the lungs   87
unconsciousness   62, 58
unconsciousness, sudden   59
urge to defecate, uncontrollable   98
urge, continuous to urinate   96
urge, frequent, to clear one's throat   88
urinary sediments   99
urination, accompanied by heat and pain in the penis   99
"   ,copious, limpid   172
"   ,difficult   69
"   ,infrequent   99
"   ,light coloured   172
"   ,little or faltering   117
"   ,reduced   184
urine of reddish colour   34
urine reduced in quantity   34
urine, clear   45, 92, 34, 95
urine, copious   34, 105, 111, 45

urine, copious, clear   43
urine, dark coloured   184
urine, dark yellow   45
urine, diminished quantity of   99
urine, excretion increased   185
urine, excretion of great quantities   151
urine, incontinence of   95
urine, light   82
urine, light coloured   111
urine, limpid, frequent excretion of   186
urine, little   105, 105, 115, 45, 97
urine, murky   99
urine, of red colour   48
urine, plentiful   82
urine, quantity of   **186**
urine, red   90
urine, reddish   115, 45, 46, 59, 69, 76, 78, 92, 99, 40
urine, reddish, reduced in quantity   46
urine, reduced excretion of   148
urine, reduced in quantity   40, 83, 59
urine, retained   90, 43, 95, 149, 51, 99
urine, scanty   95
urine, small quantities of   46, 78
urine, sparing   48, 90, 92, 172
urine, yellow   115, 117, 46
urine, yellow   69, 97, 99
vertigo   189, 68, 69, 69, 72, 77
vigour of heat   117
vision, blurred   164, 54
vision, impaired   71
voice clear yet feeble   173
voice loud   34
voice low   34
voice piercing   34
voice powerful   34
voice sonorous   150
voice weak   34
voice, low, weak   174
voice, feeble   174
voice, high pitched   173
voice, hoarse   173
voice, hoarse   58
voice, jangling   173
voice, loss of   87
voice, loud   117, 54
voice, loud, jangling   174
voice, low   42
voice, piping   173
voice, raucous   117, 173, 50
voice, strong   47
voice, weak   42, 50, 54
voice, whispering   89
volubility   174
voluptuous dreams   97
vomiting   108, 111, 149, 150, 41, 43, 50, 59, 59, 60, 69, 77, 81, 83, 92
vomiting of worms   110
" ,immediately after ingesting food   85
" ,noisy   85
" ,of bile   68
" ,of mucus and saliva   77
" ,of undigested food   63
" ,sounds of   176
warmness of the body and the extremities   34
weakness, general   175, 97
weakness, in the hips and loins   63
weakness, of the limbs   98
weakness, of the loins   184, 36
wrath, fits of   69
yang cap syndrome   111, 159

INDEX OF LATIN TERMS

accipiens hominum   **204, 205**
aestus   159, 57, **59**, 60, 61
aestus structivus   59
aestus subreptus   60
aestus venti   58
algor   32, 41, **44**, 57, 87, 104, 106, 108, 109, 110, 111, 113, 128, 130, 135, 137, 138, 142, 147, 158, 158, 160, 163, 166, 167, 169, 171, 172, 174, 176, 178, 184, 185, 187, 191, 219, 224, 228, 230, 256, 45, **58**, 59, 78
algor externus   147, 67
algor falsus   44, **46**, 47, 48, 49
algor inanitatis   110, 138, 187, 191, 211
algor inanitatis calorii inferius   186
algor inanitatis intestini tenuis   78
algor inanitatis orbis vesicalis   98
algor inanitatis orbium lienalis et stomachi   110
algor internus   173
algor intestini crassi   92
algor intimae   185, 46
algor intimae et speciei   **42**
algor laedens   **100**, 101, 102, 103, 104, 113, 152, 188, 211, 224, 39, 43, 46, 47, 53, 65
algor merus et falsus   47
algor repletionis   211
algor sinarteriae yin flectentis pedis   70
algor speciei   217, **41**
algor speciei et algor intimae   **43**
algor stomachi   84
algor venti   107, 147, 152, 166, 173, 175, 184, 256, 58, 90
algore percussio   191
anhelitus   174
animatio xue   77
aqua   160
aqua mera yin maioris   151
aqua renalis   109, 70, 98, 91
ardor   107, 127, 136, 139, 149, 151, 152, 154, 163, 167, 175, 176, 183, 184, 47, 58, **61**, 74, 76, 97, 138
ardor calorii superius   182
ardor inanitatis   168, 36
ardor inanitatis yin   136
ardor orbis hepatici   158, 67, 69, 72
ardor o. cardialis   38
ardor structivus   159, 38
ardor vigens orbis stomachi   168
ariditas   142, 160, 58, **60**
ariditas frigidula   61
ariditas pulmonalis   88
ariditas temperata   61
ariditas venti   58
arteria dorsalis pedis   205
arteria radialis   204
ascaris lumbricoides   165
asperatio profluvii   92
augmentatio qi   84, 85
calor   149, 159, 41, 103, 109, 110, 111, 130, 135, 136, 137, 138, 141, 146, 147, 150, 152, 158, 163, 166, 167, 168, 169, 170, 171, 172, 173, 174, 177, 178, 185, 211, 213, 222, 224, 228, 230, 255, 256, **44**, 45, 78
calor falsus   151, 44, **46**, 46, 49
calor heteropathicus   117
calor humidus   106, 110, 136, 136, 137, 139, 148, 149, 153, 165, 182, 186, 187, 189, 191, 255, 83
calor inanitatis   117, 159, 256, 88
calor internus   147
calor intestini crassi   92
calor intimae   214, 186, 48

calor intimae et speciei   **42**
calor merus   46, 47
calor orbium cardialis et lienalis   142
calor orbis hepatici   188
calor orbis pulmonalis   148, 176, 188
calor pituitae orbis cardialis   141
calor repletionis   110, 159, 187
calor repletionis intestini tenuis   78
calor repletionis intimae   112
calor repletionis orbis vesicalis   99
calor speciei   181, 256, **43**, 41
calor stomachi   85
calor venti   163, 166, 189, 58
calor vigens   128, 139, 140, 214
calor xue   156
caloria   114
calorium inferius   116, 117, 151
calorium medium   116, 117, 137, 149
calorium superius   116
calor inanitatis yin   215
cardinales pulmonalis et pericardialis   116
cardinales renalis et hepatica   116
cardinales splendoris yang pedis et manus   167
cardinales yang maioris   103
cardinales yin maioris manus   116
cardinalis fellea   183
cardinalis pulmonalis yin maioris manus   116
cardinalis yang maioris   104
cardo   111
caro   80
causae   31
cella ampla   **204**
ch'i = qi
ching = jing
clusa fortunae   169, 170
clusa qi   169, 170
clusa superior   183, **203**
clusa venti   169, 170
cl(a)usa   **206**
cogitatio   190, 221, 57, **62**, 81
compositio   108, 71, 84
concha Ostreae   38
concretiones   219, 230, 68
concretiones et congelationes   223
congelationes   68
contravectio qi   128
conventus 12 cardinalium   205
conventus omnium yang   155
corpus linguae   130
cutis pedalis   **254**
demissio aquae   98
emissio ardoris   76, 97
demissio yang   71, 89
demittentia   38
deversari   125
dispulsio   49, 68, 71, 85
dispulsio algoris   85, 92
dispulsio algoris venti   90
dispulsio ardoris   85
dispulsio caloris   90
dispulsio oo. hepatici et felleus   69
dispulsio orbis pulmonalis   72
dispulsio repletionis orbis pulmonalis   89
distensio orbis pulmonalis   164
dolor   158, 160, 168, 222
dominari   125
ejaculatio praecox   95

```
elevatio yang       82
emotio      29
exstillatio humoris      83
exstillatio pituitae     89
exstillation humoris     76
flexus       109, 109, 110, 117, 221, 48, 58, 98
flexus algoris      59
flexus occaecans    68, 69
flexus pavoris      256
flos        127, 29
foramina    29
foramina originalis      257
hsüeh = xue
humor 134, 146, 148, 153, 159, 171, 172, 176, 178, 183, 184,
185, 217, 218, 219, 221, 225, 230, 57, 60, 60, 81
humor algidus       108, 152, 159
humor externus      60
humor inferior      60
humor internus      147, 60
humor lienalis      84
humor orbis stomachi     188
humor superior      60
humor vigens        187
humus       98

ignis cardialis     111
ignis ministri orbis pericardialis     109
impedimentale laetitiae     204
impedimentale maius         204
inanitas    106, 108, 111, 128, 135, 147, 160, 161, 167,
170, 173, 174, 177, 185, 187, 205, 21, 21, 210, 211, 212,
219, 220, 221, 224, 228, 230, 254, 255, 32, 49, 183
inanitas algoris    222
inanitas falsa      53, 54
inanitas intestini crassi      92
inanitas intimae    148, 215, 42
inanitas intimae oo. cardialis et intestinorum      175
inanitas jing       156
inanitas lienalis   91
inanitas orbis cardialis       188, 51, 77
inanitas orbis cardialis et orbis lienalis     77
inanitas orbis hepatici        190, 51
inanitas orbis lienalis        149, 159, 164, 51
inanitas orbis pulmonalis      128, 138, 51
inanitas orbis renalis         163, 186, 51
inanitas orbis stomachi        188
inanitas orbium     51
inanitas qi      50
inanitas qi lienalis et stomachi       50
inanitas qi medii       50
inanitas qi primi       50
inanitas qi pulmonalis        50
inanitas qi renalis       50
inanitas renalis    96
inanitas renalis cum humo dilabente     98
inanitas speciei    181, 210, 230
inanitas speciei et intimae      43
inanitas speciei et repletio intimae      43
inanitas stomachi   85
inanitas xue        169, 184, 189, 191, 51
inanitas yang       150, 180, 181, 182, 255, 34
inanitas yang cardialis        75, 75
inanitas yang orbium lienalis et renalis       84
inanitas yang renalis      184, 189, 95
inanitas yin        136, 180, 181, 19, 34, 35, 88
inanitas yin orbis renalis     175
inanitas yin renalis       184, 189, 97
inductoria dorsalia      256
inspectio       123
inspectio indicis infantum      169
intima       101, 107, 114, 130, 144, 146, 148, 152, 153,

161, 163, 175, 20, 210, 223, 28, 32, 39, 41, 45, 58, 89, 90
ira         191, 56, 57, 61
lacus pedalis       206, 254
lacus ulnaris       206, 254
linea piscis        205
madefactio orbis pulmonalis       89
maeror      57, 62
mare        84
medicamenta adiuvantia        49
medicamenta adjuvantia yang       112
medicamenta demittentia       96
medicamenta exstillantia humoris       106
medicamenta liberantia speciei         112, 145, 149, 105, 108,
109, 181
medicamenta purgativa         110, 112
medicamenta refrigerantia     110, 149, 81
medicamenta refrigerantia ardoris      48
medicamenta refrigerantia caloris      106
medicamenta refrigerantia et laxantia      92
medicamenta refrigerantia intimae      106, 108
medicamenta regulatoria       107, 108, 109, 112
medicamenta regulatoria et asperantia cutis        105
medicamenta rigantia      49
medicamenta rigantia yin       112
medicamenta sive rigantia yin      48
medicamenta supplentia        110, 49
medicamenta supplentia qi       112
medicamenta sustinentia xue       112
medicamenta tepafacientia     108, 105, 110, 112
medicamenta transformatoria      105
medicamenta transformatoria humoris       106
merum       36
m. demittentia      38
morbi temperati     113, 113, 114, 116, 188, 224, 65, 73
morbi varii     101, 102, 140, 39, 46, 48, 65, 66
morbus temperatum       42, 144, 162, 49
humus aridus        84
nervocardinales     141, 142
nervus      127, 128, 163, 184, 66
orbes aulici        103, 113, 158, 21, 52
orbes cardialis et intestini tenuis     73
orbes cardialis et lienalis       140
orbes cardialis et renalis        103, 78
orbes et cardinales lienalis et cardialis       139
orbes felleus et tricalorii       109
orbes hepaticus et felleus     66
orbes hepaticus et pericardialis       106, 109
orbes horreales     27
orbes intestini crassi et stomachi       108
orbes intestini crassi et vesicalis     78
orbes intestini tenuis et vesicalis       103, 111
orbes intestinorum     115, 133, 144, 151, 153, 156, 185,
54, 60
orbes lienalis et pulmonalis     165
orbes lienalis et stomachi       159, 186, 187, 239, 80, 98
orbes pulmonalis et intestini crassi      60
orbes pulmonalis et lienalis     108
orbes renalis et cardialis       112
orbis       26
orbis aulicus       104, 39, 78
orbis cardialis     110, 113, 126, 129, 136, 162, 229, 239,
27, 38, 59, 61, 74, 75, 76, 77, 78, 98
orbis cardialis et intestini tenuis       75
orbis cardialis et renalis       111, 62
orbis felleus       133, 158, 188, 239, 27, 83
orbis felleus et tricalorii       106
orbis hepaticus     126, 154, 158, 218, 229, 230, 27, 61,
62, 67, 68, 71
orbis hepaticus et felleus       58, 62, 68, 69, 71
orbis horrealis       39
```

orbis intestini crassi   152, 168, 27, 87, 89, 90, 91, 27
orbis intestini tenuis   59, 79
orbis intestini tenuis, special symptoms of   78
orbis lienalis   108, 129, 134, 149, 158, 159, 167, 188, 217, 229, 230, 27, 60, 62, 75, 82, 84, 91, 83
orbis lienalis et cardialis   75
orbis lienalis et pulmonalis   105
orbis lienalis et stomachi   43, 60, 89
orbis pericardialis   113, 133, 140, 174, 27, 59, 73, 76
orbis pulmonalis   108, 113, 115, 133, 148, 160, 165, 166, 175, 229, 230, 239, 27, 72, 84, 87, 89, 90, 91
orbis renalis   109, 111, 133, 136, 138, 139, 149, 151, 155, 166, 167, 229, 230, 239, 244, 27, 35, 36, 38, 58, 6, 61, 62, 67, 70, 78, 84, 94, 95, 96, 98
orbis stomachi   129, 133, 134, 135, 149, 152, 153, 167, 168, 177, 27, 54, 82, 83, 84
orbis stomachi et intestini crassi   105
orbis tricalorii   27, 59, 73
orbis vesicalis   133, 151, 186, 27, 58, 94, 98
organum   29
ostium pollicare   131, 198, **204**, 205, **205**, 206, 239
o. pulmonalis   38
pacatio orbis hepatici   69
pacatio shen   76
pacatio venti hepatici   69
palpatio   **193**
para-orbis cerebri et medullae   28
para-orbis felleus   28
para-orbis uteri   28
paraorbes   27
paraorbes cerebri et medullae   155
paraorbes ossum et meduallae   39
pars kardiaca   132
pars pylorica   132
patefactio   89
pavor   108, 222, 57
pel pedalis   116
percussio aestus   59
percussio algoris mensum aestus   59
perfectio   127, 29, 73, 83, 87
pes   **206**
pituita   110, 127, 136, 137, 139, 141, 144, 146, 147, 148, 149, 152, 163, 171, 174, 175, 176, 183, 187, 212, 213, 222, 223, 230, 54, 76, 81, 87, 89
pituita algida   90
pituita algoris   90
pituita flexus   110
pituita humida   142
pituita humoris algidi   152
pituita subrepta   150, 174
plenus   27, 28
plexus ocularis   131
pollex   205, **206**
porta auris   **204**
porta sagittarii   **204**
processus styloides radii   198, 204
pulsus agitatus   **222**, 227
pulsus asper   **213**, 228
pulsus asperi   51, 53, 77
pulsus brevis   **214**, 227
pulsus celer   **211**, 35
pulsus celeri   105, 114, 115, 37, 46, 47, 69, 70, 72, 75, 78, 79, 83, 85, 88, 90, 97, 99
pulsus celeri et inanes   36
pulsus cepacaulici   226, 37, **218**
pulsus chordales   107, 115, 117, 53, 54, 68, 69, 70, 71, 72, 79
pulsus chordales atque lubrici   79
pulsus chordales et tardi   70
pulsus chordalis   126, **217**

pulsus concitati   37, 75
pulsus concitatus   **223**, 38
pulsus diffundens   **220**
pulsus diffundentes   75
pulsus evanescens   **215**
pulsus evanescentes   92
pulsus exundans   **214**, 227, 228, 35
pulsus exundantes   105, 106, 115, 37, 47
pulsus exundantes et inanes   117, 36
pulsus firmus   214
pulsus fixi   51
pulsus fixus   **219**
pulsus haesitans   **223**, 227
pulsus inanes   148, 177, 226, 37, 59, 75, 78, 89, 96, 98, **212**, 38
pulsus intenti   104, 110, 43, 46, 59, 77, 90
pulsus intentus   **216**
pulsus intermittens   **223**, 227
pulsus invalidi   226, 37, 43, 47, 75, 77, 89, 91, 96, 82
pulsus invalidus   **220**
pulsus languidi   104, 108, 115, 190, 53, 71, 78, 82, 92
pulsus languidus   **217**
pulsus lenes   108, 115, 117, 226, 53, 77, 82, 83, 85, 91
pulsus lenis   **219**
pulsus longus   **213**
pulsus lubrici   77, 177, 48, 79, 84, 85, 89, 97
pulsus lubrici aut repleti   48
pulsus lubrici et celeri   76, 92
pulsus lubricus   **212**, 228
pulsus magni   75
pulsus magnus   **215**
pulsus mediani   **209**
pulsus mersi   105, 106, 115, 150, **209**, 47, 48, 53, 54, 77, 79, 84, 92, 96, 97, 98
pulsus mersi aut chordales et tardi   70
pulsus mersi et intenti   59
pulsus mersi et tardi   59

pulsus mersus   **210**, 35
pulsus mersus inanis   211
pulsus minuti   107, 117, 150, 37, 47, 53, 70, 71, 75, 77, 78, 82, 84, 88, 92, 95, 97, 98, 83
pulsus minuti et lenes   117
pulsus minuti sive agitati   117
pulsus minutus   **220**, 35
pulsus mobilis   **222**
pulsus molles   226
pulsus mollis   **219**
pulsus movens   214
pulsus parvus   **221**
pulsus rapidus   214
pulsus redundans   214, 214
pulsus repleti   105, 106, 115, 177, 37, 92
pulsus repletus   **212**
pulsus splendoris yang manus   204
pulsus subreptus   **221**
pulsus subtilis   214
pulsus superficiales   104, 105, 114, 148, **209**, 37, 43, 47, 59, 90
pulsus superficiales sive exundantes   61
pulsus superficialis   **210**
pulsus tardi   185, 47, 54, 85, 98
pulsus tardus   **211**
pulsus tardus   35
pulsus turbulentus   214
pulsus tympanicus   **218**
pulsus yin flectentis pedis   204
pulsus yin maioris manus   204
pulsus yin maioris pedis   204
pulsus yin minoris manus   204
pulsus yin minoris pedis   204

purgatio 177
qi aquaticum 188
qi ascitum 205
qi constructivum 103, 113, 115, 136
qi defensivum 103, **114**, 87
qi frumentarium 145, 148
qi heteropathicum 142, 143, 145
qi medium 213
qi merum orbis renalis 221
qi nativum 166, 205, 220, 244, 47
qi orbis hepatici 68
qi orthopathicum 127, 139, 145, 148
qi primum 183, 186, 220, 224, 230, 47, 89, 96
qi renale 95, 96
qi renale dilabens 156
qi stomachi 130, 142, 143, 144, 145, 154, 187, 204, 205, 218, 224, **243**
qi subreptum 64
refrigeratio 71
refrigeratio ardoris 72
refrigeratio caloris 69, 83, 92
refrigeratio caloris et exstillatio humoris 99
refrigeratio et laxatio caloris repletionis 79
refrigeratio orbis cardialis 76
refrigeratio orbis hepatici 72
refrigeratio orbis pulmonalis 90
refrigeratio orbis stomachi 85
rententio xue 105
repletio 127, 135, 147, 161, 21, 21 224, 32, **49**
repletio falsa 53
repletio intestini crassi 92
repletio intimae **42**
repletio orbis cardialis 51
repletio orbis hepatici 51
repletio orbis lienalis 52
repletio orbis pulmonalis 52
repletio orbis renalis 52
repletio orbium 51
repletio qi hepatici 51
repletio qi intestinorum 50
repletio qi pulmonalis 50
repletio qi stomachi 50
repletio speciei 104, 181
repletio speciei et inanitas intimae **43**
repletio speciei et intimae **43**
repletio stomachi 85
repletio xue 51
repletio yang 189
repletio yin 19
repletus 27
respiratio minor 175
retentio aquae 104
rigantia yin 96
rigatio 71
rigatio et sustentatio yin renalis 97
rigatio yin 72, 76, 89, 91
rivulus maior **204**, 205, 222
rubella 58
rubor 168
sequentia cohibens 24
sequentia efficiens 23
sequentia vincens 24
sequentia violationis 24
sinarteria cardinalis 29
sinarteria yin flectentis 158
sinarteriae 100, 115, 39
sinarteriae yin flectentis 183
sinus maxillaris 131
sitis diffundens 110, 117, 186

sitis diffundens, variatio inferior 95
sollicitudo 221, 57, **62**
species 104, 20, 20, 28, 32, **39**, 41, 90, 101, 103, 105, 107, 112, 114, 130, 144, 148, 151, 152, 161, 181, 210, 255, 45, 58, 59
splendor yang 100, **105**, 106, 107, 108, 115, 149, 152, 153, 160, 166, 167, 168
stirps 243
struere 19
sudatio 177
suppletio qi cardialis 75
supplentia yin 96
suppletio et augmentatio orbium cardialis et lienalis 77
suppletio et sustentatio 47
suppletio ignis 98
suppletio orbis lienalis 84
suppletio qi 82
suppletio qui medii 85
suppletio transvectus humi 91
suppletio xue 76
suppletio yang renalis 96
suppletio yin 112
sustentatio orbis pulmonalis 91
sustentatio yin 71
tegmen linguae 130
tepefactio et animatio yang medii 82
tepefactio et patefactio orbis intestini tenuis 78
tepefactio et transformatio pituitae algidae 90
tepefactio orbis et cardinalium hepatici 70
tepefactio orbis renalis 84
tepefactio orbis stomachi 85
tepefactio yang 97
tepefactio yang cardialis 75
tepefactio yang renalis 96
timor 57, **62**
tinnitus 36
transformatio et exstillatio pituitae 77
transformatio humoris 83, 97
transformatio pituitae 84
tricalorium **116**
turgor 168
tussis 175
urina puerum 38
valles coniunctae **204**
vento percussio 103, 104, 141, 162, 162, 68
ventus 104, 126, 147, 149, 158, 170, 171, 172, 178, 184, 218, 223, 228, 230, 254, 43, 56, 57, 58, 90
ventus hepaticus 141, 164, 167, 69, 158, 127, 140, 155, 58, 67, 127, 141
ventus pavoris 158
vertigo oculorum 68, 70
vicus quintus pedis **204**
vigor caloris 117, 139
vigor caloris humidi 163
vigor caloris qi constructivi 136
vigor heteropathiae 215
vigor yang 35
voluptas 57, **61**
vorago maior 205
xue cardiale 77
xue orbis cardialis 190
yang.....17, **18**
yang dilabens 215
yang hepaticum 214, 67, 70
yang impedimentalis **204**, 205, **205**, 222
yang lienale inanis et dilabens 81
yang maior 100, 103, 104, 105, 106, 107
yang merum 33, 35, 38, 47, 94
yang minor 100, 106, **106**, 107, 183

yang vigens   211, 222
yin deficiens   117
yin flectens   100, **109**, 116
yin hepaticum   154, 183, 70
yin maior   100, **108**, 109, 116, 150, 153, 159, 160
yin merum   224, 33, 35, 36, 94, 97
yin minor   100, 108, **110**, 111, 112, 116, 160
yin orbis hepatici   67
yin renale   154, 168, 97
yin2   17, **18**

INDEX OF TRANSCRIBED CHINESE TERMS AND NAMES

Bencaogangmu   197
Binhu moxue   **197**
Chen Wuze   57
Cheng Zhongling   37, 40
Gushi yijing   54
Huangdi Neijing Suwen   100, 197, 34, 39, 49, 66
Huangfu Mi   100, 101
Jingyue quanshu   41, 47, 48, 54
Jinkuei yaolue   57
Li Shizhen   197
Mojing   **197**, 208
Nanjing   205
Neijing cf. Huangdi Neijing as well as Huangdi Neijing Suwen and Lingshu
Relun   100
Sanyin ji yibin yuanlun   57
Shanghan zabinglun   66
Shanghanlun   **100**, 205, 34, 39, 45, 57
Sung   57
Wang Shuhe   197
Xu Lingtai   38
Ye Tianshi   113
Yixue xinwu   37
Yu Genchu   52
Zhang Jiebin   41, 46
Zhang Jingyue   52
Zhang Zhongjing   **100**, 101, 57, 66
Zhongyi zhenduanxue jiangyi   52, 54
aiqi   176
anzhen   **193**
ba gang   31, **32**
beishu   256
ben   243, 29
bi   184
biao   28, 39
bingyin   **56**
bu   49
ch'i = qi
changmo   **213**
chaore   180
chenmo   **210**
chi   **206**
chifu   **254**
chimo   **211**
ching = jing 1
chuan   174
chung   127, 29
cumo   **222**
cun   **205**
cunkou   **205**
daimo   **223**
daiyang   111
damo   **215**
daohan   **181**
dongbi   184
dongmo   **222**
duanmo   **214**
duanqui   175
ehan   48
eni   176
fare   180
feng   **58**
fengguan   170
fengzhen   58
fu 1   21, 21, 27, 39
fumo 1   **210**

fumo 2   **221**
fushu   60
ganou   176
gemo   **218**
guan   129
guan   **206**
guan   29
hai   84
han   **58**
houmo   **218**
hsüeh = xue
hua   127, 29
huamo   **212**
huanmo   **217**
hun   21
hungmo   **214**
huo   **61**
jiangyao   38
jiemo   **223**
jimo   **223**
jin   146, 21
jing 1   100, 156, 164, 188, 21, 213, 218, 219, 67, 70, 75, 94
jing 2   **63**
jing 3   103
jingluoxue   101
jinmo   **216**
juanmo   **219**
juehan   182
jueyin   **109**
jumo   **219**
juomo   **220**
kai qiao   29
kung   **62**
laomo   **219**
li   28, 39
liuyin   57
liuyin   **58**
luo   103
man   27, 28
mingguan   170

neike   66
neishang   74
neiyin   57
ni   52
nu   **61**
ou   176
pi   54
po   21
qi   104, 109, 113, **114**, 125, 136, 146, 168, 210, 214, 228, 50
qie   122
qiemo   **193**
qiezhen   **193**
qifen   104
qiguan   170
qiheng zhi fu   27, 28
qing   29, 38
qiqing   **61**
rou   71
rung   127
san   49
sanjiao   114, **116**
sanmo   **220**
semo   213

```
shang        74
shangguan        132
shanghan     101, 104, 113, 65
shangqi      175
shaoqi       175
shaoyang     106
shaoyin      110
shen         123, 129, 21, 217, 243, 244, 47, 71, 73, 74, 76
shetai       130
shezhi       130
shi 1        21, 27, 49, 60
shi 2        213
shimo        212
shiqibing        64
shu     59
shu2         111
shumo        211
shuyue zhongshan     59
si      62
sizhen       122
tai     123
taiyang      103, 20
taiyin       108
tan     76
tu      176, 98
waiwei       74
waiyin       57
wang         122
wangzhen     123
wei 1        114, 21, 210, 211
wei 2        103, 168
weimo        215
weiqi        243
weiqi        87
wên          122, 173
wên          122, 179
wenbing      113, 65
wenxie       113
wufeng       179, 41
wuhan        179, 47, 48
wure         180, 47
wuxing       17, 17, 22
xi      61
xiaguan      132
xiangkexu        24
xiangkexu        24
xiangshengxu     23
xiangshêngxu     24
xiangwuxu        24
xianmo       217
xiao         49
xiao 2       174
xiaomo       221
xie          49, 56
ximo         220
xing         143
xingbi       184
xinxia       54
xu 1         21, 49
xu 2         23
xue          100, 104, 105, 109, 113, 114, 115, 116, 127, 136,
137, 139, 146, 155, 159, 168, 178, 191, 21, 213, 214, 218,
219, 228, 37, 50, 52, 54, 61, 66, 67, 70, 73, 75, 77, 104,
73
212
yang         17, 18, 19, 33
yangming     105
yangqi       59
ye      21
yin 1        31, 33, 56, 8

yin 2        17, 18, 56
yin 3        57
ying         103, 113, 114, 115, 21, 228, 75, 80
yinshu       59
you     62
yuanxue      257
yuji         205
zabing       39, 65, 66, 21
zang         21, 26, 27, 39
zangxiang        26
zao     60
zhanhan      182
zhen         76
zhi          29
zhongfeng        103
zhongguan        132
zhuo         43
zihan        181
```